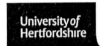

University of Hertfordshire U H

College Lane, Hatfield, Herts. AL10 9AB
Information Hertfordshire
Services and Solutions for the University

For renewal of Standard and One Week Loans,
please visit the web site http://www.voyager.herts.ac.uk

This item must be returned or the loan renewed by the due date.
A fine will be charged for the late return of items.

Commissioning Editor: *Rita Demetriou-Swanwick*
Development Editor: *Veronika Watkins*
Project Manager: *Jagannathan Varadarajan*
Designer: *Stewart Larking*
Illustration Manager: *Merlyn Harvey*
Illustrator: *Antbits*

Acupuncture in Manual Therapy

Edited by

Jennie Longbottom MSc MMEd BSc FCSP MBAcC

Director Parks Therapy Centre, St Neots
Director Alied Acupuncture Training Limited

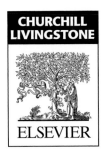

CHURCHILL LIVINGSTONE

ELSEVIER

Edinburgh London New York Oxford Philadelphia St Louis Sydney Toronto 2010

CHURCHILL LIVINGSTONE
ELSEVIER

ISBN 978-0-443-06782-2

British Library Cataloguing in Publication Data
A catalogue record for this book is available from the British Library

Library of Congress Cataloguing in Publication Data
A catalogue record for this book is available from the Library of Congress

Notice
Neither the Publisher nor the Editor and Authors assume any responsibility for any loss or injury and/or damage to persons or property arising out of or related to any use of the material contained in this book. It is the responsibility of the treating practitioner, relying on independent expertise and knowledge of the patient, to determine the best treatment and method of application for the patient.

The Publisher

ELSEVIER your source for books, journals and multimedia in the health sciences

www.elsevierhealth.com

Working together to grow
libraries in developing countries

www.elsevier.com | www.bookaid.org | www.sabre.org

ELSEVIER   BOOK AID International   Sabre Foundation

The Publisher's policy is to use **paper manufactured from sustainable forests**

Printed in Europe

Contents

Contributors

Jo Gibson, Grad Dip Phys
Clinical Physiotherapy Specialist, Department of
Physiotherapy, Royal Liverpool University Hospital,
Liverpool

Lee Herrington, PhD MCSP
Senior Lecturer in Sports Rehabilitation, School of Health,
Sport and Rehabilitation Sciences, Directorate of Sport,
University of Salford, Salford

Mark I Johnson, PhD BSc
Professor of Pain and Analgesia
Faculty of Health, Leeds Metropolitan University, Leeds

Jennie Longbottom, MSc MMEd BSc FCSP MBAcC
Director Parks Therapy Centre, St Neots
Director Alied Acupuncture Training Limited

Alison Middleditch, MCSP MMACP
Director Surrey Physiotherapy, Post Graduate research
post University College, London

Lynley Bradnam-Roberts, PhD Candidate
Movement Neuroscience Laboratory, Department
of Sport and Exercise Science, Faculty of Science,
University of Auckland

Dr. Cherye Roche, DC FCC (UK) FEAC (Ortho)
Private Practitioner and Senior Lecturer/Supervisor
New Zealand College of Chiropractic

Claire Small, MPhty St. MMACP
Clinical Director, Pure Sports Medicine, London

Neil Tucker, MHSc (Hons) BHSc (Pthy) PGDip
(musculoskeletal Physiotherapy), PGCert (acupuncture)
Physiotherapist, Munster Rugby, University of Limerick,
Limerick

Howard M Turner, BSc BAppSc (Pthy) MCSP
Private Practitioner and Lecturer Wilmslow Physiotherapy
Wilmslow, Cheshire

Case study contributors

Siobhan Byrne, BSc (Hons) (Pthy)
Senior Physiotherapist, Chelsea and Westminster
Hospital

Kenny Cross, BSc MMTC MCSP
Private Practitioner, Falkirk

Hannah Edwards, BSc (Hons) MCSP
Senior Physiotherapist in Rheumatology

Dan Franklin, MSc MAAP
Director Morpheus Wellness Solutions, London

Sharon Helsby, MCSP
Clinical Specialist

Kevin Hunt, MSc MCSP
Director Spinal physiotherapy & sports medicine clinic ltd,
Cambridge

Melissa Johnson, MCSP

Daniel Christopher Martin, BSc MCSP MACP
Private practice, Head Physiotherapist, Newport Gwent
Dragons

Lawrence Mayhew, MCSP
Musculoskeletal Physiotherapist, North Tees and
Hartlepool NHS Foundation Trust

Cathie Morrow, MCSP
Extended Scope Practitioner

Brigit Murray, BHS (Pthy)
Associate Physiotherapist, Private Practice, New Zealand

Eghon Murray, MSc BSc
Specialist Musculoskeletal Physiotherapist

Charlie Plummer, MSc MCSP
Director, Boughton Physiotherapy Practice and Sports
Injury Clinic, Maidstone

Andy Reynolds, MSc MMACP MCSP
Senior Physiotherapist

Efterpi Rompoti, BSc (Pthy) MCSP MAACP
Musculoskeletal Physiotherapist, The Sloane Hospital

Sarah Rouse, MSc MCSP

Helen Sankey, MCSP

Rose Sutcliffe, MSc MCSP
Superintendent Physiotherapist, St Luke's Hospital,
Bradford

James Thomson, MCSP

Matthew Walmsley, MCSP
Musculoskeletal Physiotherapist, St Luke's Hospital,
Bradford

Katy Williams, MCSP

This book is dedicated to John … I need never say more.

'For those of you reading this text, I fervently hope that you will not become trapped in the surface of acupuncture therapy, striving only to learn experiential points from teachers and colleagues. Bring the medicine to life.'

—Wang Ju-Yi (2008)

Acknowledgements

I thank all those who have contributed to the development of this book. Each person has offered a wealth of specialized knowledge within manual therapy and acupuncture. As a result, I have learnt from their knowledge, as I hope you will. I would also like to thank those inspirational teachers who brought acupuncture into my clinical management; how did I ever survive without it?

I particularly thank those who have made an incredible impact on my clinical skills during my professional journey: Ann Green, Dr Jeremy Lewis, Alison Middleditch, Mark Johnson to name but a few. I will particularly remember Gill Hughes, whose initial guidance and support to me as a junior physiotherapist made me the clinician I am today. To Andrew Wilson for his professional editing services and who has taught me to proof-read. My sincere thanks to Mark Charboneau, Graphic Designer, St Neots, who provided the art work and inspiration for the cover.

I thank all those students who contributed through their hard work with case studies, and who teach me something new on each course I provide. For Hayley, Myrtle, and John who have listened to my constant doubts and supported me throughout.

This book is primarily written for physiotherapists who use manual skills and acupuncture as an integrated approach to pain management and the facilitation of rehabilitation in musculoskeletal dysfunction. This book has brought together a number of manual therapy experts who have provided the reader with current evidence, and best available practice, for the management of a variety of musculoskeletal conditions affecting various joints of the body.

Physiotherapists working extensively in these areas and students undertaking the Acupuncture Association of Chartered Physiotherapists (AACP) Foundation training course have supplied the acupuncture text. This text has not involved an in depth account of traditional Chinese medical theory, not because of preference or neglect, but because this has been more than adequately covered by a number of excellent well-informed texts previously published. The book emphasizes clinical reasoning, which is a fundamental necessity in all physiotherapy care and in the philosophy of Chinese medicine. Without it we offer nothing more than a point-specific protocol, which will serve to reduce the efficacy, accuracy, and effectiveness of acupuncture intervention.

The addition of acupuncture within my treatment toolbox has not only enhanced my manual skills, but has facilitated a holistic approach to patient management. It has challenged my training and beliefs, informed, complimented, and at times, confused my physiotherapy reasoning, but at all times it has fascinated and enhanced my clinical knowledge … and continues to do so.

Clinical reasoning in Western acupuncture

1

Lynley Bradnam-Roberts

Background

Using acupuncture to treat musculoskeletal disorders should follow a clinical reasoning process (CRP), the thinking behind practice, as identified by physiotherapists for manual therapy interventions (Jones & Rivett 2004), the norm being to identify predominant tissue and pain mechanisms presented by the patient as a means of identifying effective intervention. The layering method is a clinical reasoning model (CRM) developed specifically for clinicians to treat musculoskeletal conditions with acupuncture, using a mechanism-based approach (Bradnam 2007). It aims progressively to target different physiological processes within the central nervous system (CNS) in order to provide the best effect for each individual. The layering method is a Western approach to acupuncture, but does allow a clinician to integrate traditional Chinese acupuncture (TCA) point selection into clinical reasoning.

An orthodox physiotherapy assessment and diagnosis is made with identification of likely contributors to the patients' disability in terms of:

- Associated anatomical structures;
- Tissue sources;
- Tissue healing; and
- Pain mechanisms. (Jones & Rivett 2004)

An acupuncture treatment plan will be formulated to target structures identified as sources of the physical impairment. Applying acupuncture mechanisms in this manner will also allow progression of treatment if the initial approach does not achieve the desired effect; if pain mechanisms change, or if the condition resolves or becomes chronic.

Theoretical knowledge underpinning the model

The following knowledge must underpin the model:

- An understanding of how acupuncture affects the CNS;

DOI: 10.1016/B978-0-443-06782-2.00001-3

- The clinical presentation of pain mechanisms; and
- The tissue healing process and time frames for these processes to be achieved.

The practical implementation of the model relies on:

- A knowledge of acupuncture points;
- A good knowledge of anatomy;
- A knowledge of segmental and peripheral nerve innervation of muscles and skin; and
- A full understanding of the neuroanatomy of the autonomic nervous system (ANS).

Acupuncture mechanisms

Nociception

Three categories of acupuncture mechanisms have been described; peripheral, spinal, and supraspinal (Lundeberg 1998). Firstly, on needling, nociceptive afferents are stimulated and release vasodilatory neuropeptides into the muscle and skin they innervate, forming the basis of the local or peripheral effects of acupuncture (Sato et al 2000). This phenomenon, an axon reflex, releases neuropeptides into human skin such as calcitonin gene-related peptide (CGRP) and substance P (Weidner et al 2000). Sensory neuropeptides modulate immune responses and hence will assist in tissue healing (Brain 1997). Secondly, acupuncture will act within the spinal cord, known as spinal effects or segmental effects. To initiate spinal effects, the sensory stimulus must be applied to tissues that share an innervation with the appropriate spinal cord level (Fig. 1.1). Dorsal horn neurons activated by painful inputs may be inhibited by acupuncture via a gate control mechanism, producing a spinally mediated analgesic response. Neurons of the ANS efferent fibres can be influenced and both sympathetic and parasympathetic activity may be affected, depending on the position of the needles.

- High-intensity (HI) needling may immediately increase sympathetic outflow to tissues supplied by the segment, which is then followed by a decrease in outflow.
- Low-intensity (LI) or non-painful input could reduce sympathetic outflow in the segment (Sato et al 1997).

Lastly, acupuncture may influence alpha-motoneurons housed in the ventral horn of the spinal cord to alter reflex activity in muscles supplied by the segment (Fig. 1.1). At present the effect on motoneurons is still unclear: an immediate change in excitability has not been demonstrated in contrast to clinical observations (Chan et al 2004).

Supraspinal effects

Acupuncture can influence neuronal structures within the brain (Stener-Victorin et al 2002) and these are known as supraspinal effects. Analgesic pathways such as diffuse noxious inhibitory controls (DNIC) and beta-endorphin mediated descending pain inhibitory pathways from the hypothalamus will be activated with appropriate needling (Stener-Victorin et al 2002). Autonomic outflow is also under central control via the medullary vasomotor centre and can be influenced by the acupuncture stimulus.

Neurohormonal responses

Responses affecting the immune, endocrine, and reproductive systems of the body can be affected by acupuncture (Carlsson 2002, Stener-Victorin et al 2002; White 1999). Recent advances in brain imaging technologies such as functional magnetic imaging (fMRI) and positron emission tomography

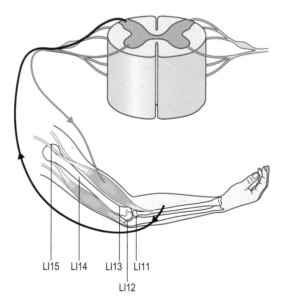

Figure 1.1 • Dermatome and myotome innervation from C5 nerve root.

LI15   LI14   LI13 LI11

LI12

(PET) have allowed investigations of the brain and have elucidated the effect of acupuncture on the CNS. Several analgesic points in the extremities will stimulate blood flow to cortical and subcortical brain regions (Lundeberg 1998). Activation is relatively non-specific and closely related to areas activated by painful stimuli, through what is known as the pain matrix (Lewith et al 2005). Studies show an increase in blood flow in the hypothalamus (Table 1.1) and a decrease in the limbic system (Table 1.2), a brain region where affective and emotional responses to pain are integrated with sensory experience. However, most of the brain regions activated by acupuncture are closely related to those areas mediating placebo analgesia and expectation (Lewith et al 2005), and it is unclear how much of the change is due to the acupuncture stimulus and how much is due to non-specific effects. Recently studies using transcranial magnetic stimulation (TMS) have shown that acupuncture modulates motor cortical excitability and that the effect (excitation or inhibition) is specific to the investigated muscle and the site of needle placement (Lo et al 2005; Maioli et al 2006). Maioli et al (2006) showed that changes lasted for fifteen minutes following the removal of the needle stimulus, suggesting longer term plastic changes in motor cortical excitability.

Clinical reasoning model: the layering method

Clinical reasoning within acupuncture intervention requires that the clinician ask a series of questions as to what is required from the needle. The question provides a problem-solving pathway as to effects on pain and tissue mechanisms presented, appropriate points and stimulation parameters chosen, in an effort to provide an optimum intervention. The clinical reasoning questions can be seen in the flowchart in Fig. 1.2.

Local effects

Healing

If healing or treating scar tissue is the aim of therapy, blood flow can be improved by eliciting local effects of acupuncture, using local acupuncture

Table 1.1 Suggested points to stimulate blood flow to hypothalamus

Meridian	Points
Large intestine	LI4
Lung	LU5
Gall bladder	GB34, GB40
Spleen	SP6
Stomach	ST36
Liver	LIV3

Biella et al (2001); Fang Kong et al (2004); Hsieh et al (2001); Hui et al (2000); Wu et al (1999, 2002); Yan et al 2005; Zhang et al (2003)

Table 1.2 Suggested points for deactivation of limbic system

Meridian	Points
Large intestine	LI4
Gall bladder	GB34
Spleen	SP6
Stomach	ST36
Liver	LIV3

Hsieh et al (2001); Hui et al (2000, 2005); Kong et al (2002); Wu et al (1999,2002); Zhang et al 2003

points, or by putting the needle directly into the damaged tissue. Lundeberg (1998) recommended needling close to the injured tissue with LI stimulation to encourage peripheral neuropeptide release. However, in the early stages of an injury the increase in blood flow, substance P, and other inflammatory agents are potentially detrimental and have the effect of overloading, leading to increased pain and inflammatory response (Longbottom 2006a).

Segmental effects

Analgesia

Local points can induce segmental effects if desired. In acute pain, segmental blocking of painful afferent input can produce strong analgesia. Any acupuncture

The layering method

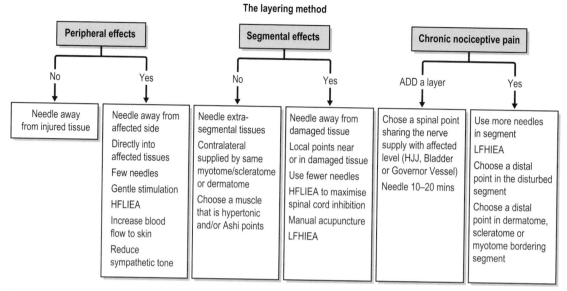

Peripheral effects		Segmental effects		Chronic nociceptive pain	
No	Yes	No	Yes	ADD a layer	Yes
Needle away from injured tissue	Needle away from affected side Directly into affected tissues Few needles Gentle stimulation HFLIEA Increase blood flow to skin Reduce sympathetic tone	Needle extra-segmental tissues Contralateral supplied by same myotome/scleratome or dermatome Choose a muscle that is hypertonic and/or Ashi points	Needle away from damaged tissue Local points near or in damaged tissue Use fewer needles HFLIEA to maximise spinal cord inhibition Manual acupuncture LFHIEA	Chose a spinal point sharing the nerve supply with affected level (HJJ, Bladder or Governor Vessel) Needle 10–20 mins	Use more needles in segment LFHIEA Choose a distal point in the disturbed segment Choose a distal point in dermatome, scleratome or myotome bordering segment

Figure 1.2 • Layering method of clinical reasoning in acupuncture.

points in tissues that share an innervation via that spinal segment can be chosen, as long as the injured tissue is avoided (Bradnam 2007). In cases of acute nociceptive pain it is advised that fewer needles be used since the dorsal horn is already sensitized. If the condition becomes chronic, more needles can be added into the segment (Lundeberg 1998). Choosing distal points, in other muscles or tissues sharing the same innervation as the injured tissue, may offer a more effective treatment (Bradnam 2007).

To progress, use a point that may influence a peripheral nerve supplying the targeted structure. An example is use of Triple Energizer 5 (TE5) into the posterior forearm (posterior interosseous nerve) to affect the muscles involved in lateral epicondylar elbow pain. The use of spinal points or Back Shu points, on the Bladder channel, and extra Huatuojiaji points, at the spinal level sharing innervation with the injured part, will access the dorsal rami, providing strong sensory stimulus to the spinal cord at the required level.

Sympathetic nervous system

For patients demonstrating clinical presentation suggestive of an overactive sympathetic nervous system (SNS) with oedema, sweating, and severe pain (Longbottom 2006a), acupuncture can induce specific manipulation of the ANS (Table 1.3). This may also be used when an increase in blood flow to a tissue

is required (Bradnam 2007). Slow-healing conditions might be related to trophic changes in tissues via inhibition of the SNS (Bekkering & van Bussel 1998). The sympathetic neurons are housed in the segments of the thoracic and upper lumbar spines; needling at the appropriate spinal level will alter the outflow to that region. Hsu et al (2006) found with healthy volunteers that 2 Hz electroacupuncture (EA) applied to Bladder 15 (BL15) increased heart and pulse rate, and decreased skin conductance on the upper limb, all signs of increased sympathetic outflow. Also needling a peripheral point, using strong activation of de Qi, will stimulate afferent input into the chosen segment and will increase sympathetic outflow, and increase the blood flow to muscles (Noguchi et al 1999).

If the desired effect is inhibition of sympathetic outflow gentle stimulation to the spinal points must be given. In addition, auricular acupuncture (AA) will increase parasympathetic activity (Lundeberg & Elkholm 2001), hence reducing sympathetic outflow. According to Longbottom (2006a), points that influence the cranial sympathetic outflow Bladder (BL10) and Gall Bladder (GB20), and sacral sympathetic outflow (BL28), will also activate the parasympathetic nervous system (PNS) and can be used to dampen overactive sympathetic responses. Scalp acupuncture has also been shown to stimulate the PNS and suppress sympathetic activity in healthy volunteers compared to control subjects (Wang et al 2002).

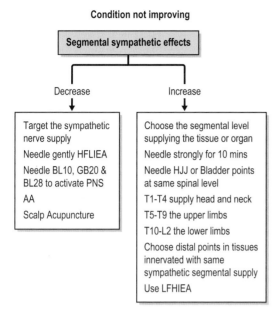

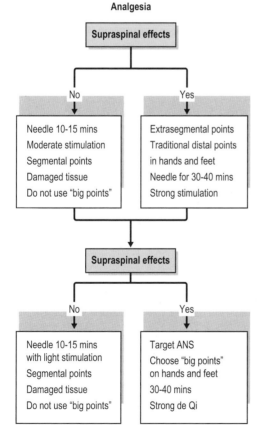

Figure 1.2 (Continued)

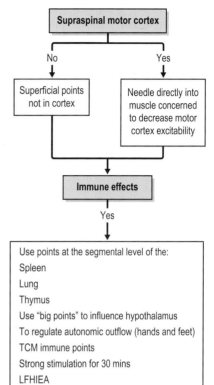

Figure 1.2 (Continued)

Table 1.3 Sympathetic supply and point suggestion		
Segmental level	**Areas supplied**	**Suggested points**
T1–T4	Head and neck	Large intestine (LI4)
T5–T9	Upper limbs	Bladder (BL15)
T10–L2	Lower limbs	Bladder (BL23)

Bekkering & van Bussel (1998).

Supraspinal effects

Analgesia

Needles left into any points in the body for 30 to 40 minutes will enhance supraspinal effects as these are time and intensity related (Andersson & Lundeberg 1995; Lundeberg 1998; Lundeberg & Stener-Victorin 2002). De Qi must be achieved to elicit brain activity; the greater the intensity of stimulation and de Qi gained, the greater the blood flow to cortical regions (Backer et al 2002; Fang et al 2004; Wu et al 2002).

Activating the DNIC by segmental acupuncture is thought to produce analgesia that is stronger than that of extrasegmental needle placement but is only short lasting (Lundeberg et al 1988a). A combination of both segmental and extrasegmental needling is commonly used in clinical practice (Barlas et al 2006). However, when trying to activate DNIC to treat acute nociceptive pain, or centrally evoked pain, it may be prudent to activate them via extrasegmental inputs to avoid overloading the sensitized spinal cord segment. The hands, and to a lesser extent the feet, have large representation on the somatosensory cortex in the brain and are considered strong points in acupuncture analgesia.

In peripheral neurogenic pain the opioid pain inhibitory systems are less effective due to increased synthesis of the neuropeptide cholecystokinin, an endogenous opioid antagonist (Wiesenfeld-Hallin & Zu 1996). Here, EA applied with a high-frequency/low-intensity (HFLIEA) paradigm, activating the noradrenergic (non-opioid) pathways in the spinal cord, should be used (White 1999).

Autonomic outflow

Autonomic outflow is under central control by the hypothalamus regulating the SNS and PNS (Kandell et al 2000). Stimulation of this system is considered non-specific and depends on intensity and length of stimulation. To effectively activate central autonomic responses, the use of strong points, similar to those used to evoke central responses, has been recommended. Acupuncture stimulation may increase or decrease sympathetic activity depending on the state of the target organ or tissue (Sato et al 1997). For optimum treatment of body organs, Stener-Victorin (2000) recommended the use of high-intensity, low-frequency EA to provide a strong stimulus to the CNS.

Motor cortex

A novel use of acupuncture may be to specifically excite and inhibit motor regions of the brain associated with overactive or inhibited muscles during a motor task. This may facilitate acupuncture to be used in the treatment of various motor control disorders. Maioli et al (2006) needled acupuncture point Large Intestine 4 (LI4), and found that the motor cortical area for the abductor digiti minimi muscle was inhibited. However, there was no observation of significant alteration in motor cortical excitability of the flexor carpi radialis muscle, suggesting that the effects are localized to the region of the body being treated. The motor cortical areas for both these muscles, and a third, the first dorsal interossei, were facilitated following needling applied to a point in the leg Stomach 38 (ST38). Furthermore, Lo et al (2005) found that acupuncture to LI10 significantly increased motor cortical excitability to the area supplying the first dorsal interossei.

Immune system

Following acupuncture beta-endorphin and adrenocorticotropic hormone (ACTH) are released in equimolar amounts from the pituitary gland into the blood stream (Lundeberg 1999). In turn, ACTH may influence the adrenal gland, increasing the production of anti-inflammatory corticosteroids (Sato et al 1997). Beta-endorphin levels may fluctuate with changes in the number and activity of T-lymphocytes and natural killer (NK) cells. These effects may optimize healing effects under slow-healing conditions associated with immune deficiency or in those individuals exhibiting high-intensity demands on the body (i.e. elite athletes). To influence the organs producing T-lymphocytes and NK cells, the thymus and spleen and lung segments, supplying both sympathetic and parasympathetic innervation, should be needled together with parasympathetic AA points, because of their potential to influence vagal parasympathetic activity (Lundberg 1999).

Conclusion

This clinical reasoning model proposes a theoretical framework for the application of Western acupuncture, using current physiological theories to underpin and inform clinical decision-making, and as a basis for treatment progression. It is recommended that clinicians measure outcomes and use reflective practice when implementing the model since it has not yet been validated by primary research in a clinical setting.

1.1   Clinical reasoning in traditional Chinese medicine

Jennie Longbottom

The diagnostic process and identification of disease categories (Bian Zheng) is an essential process of traditional Chinese medicine (TCM); indeed the traditionally trained acupuncturist cannot formulate an intervention without it. This may offer some problems with diagnostic reliability and has implications within clinical trials using TCM philosophy and interventions (Zaslawski 2003). Over the past decade there has been a proliferation in acupuncture research with increased numbers of reports offering cautious acceptance of acupuncture as a statistically proven therapeutic technique for certain conditions (Ernst 2003). Many systematic reviews and meta-analyses of acupuncture have concluded that there was insufficient evidence to determine the efficacy of acupuncture; many trials reviewed were of poor quality, and required further rigorous research. In response, a number of authors have questioned the validity of such methodologies and have emphasized a need for further investigation of the research methodologies used (Birch 2001; Cummings 2000; Ezzo et al 2001; Lao et al 2001).

Within the practice of acupuncture it is essential, whether using a Western or TCM model of intervention, to determine the diagnosis and identification of the disease or pain state (Bian Bing) in order to:

- Provide effective acupuncture intervention;
- Target the release of appropriate neurotransmitters;
- Modulate pain;
- improve well being; and
- Stimulate activity.

The pathological presentation in TCM is known as pattern identification (Bian Zheng) using a clinical reasoning model to determine the disease state and cause of the dysfunction, whether this be at a systemic organ level, presenting with the more chronic longer standing disease state (Zhang fu Bian Zheng), or superficial channel level, presenting with more acute shorter disease state (Jing Luo Bian Zheng). In Western acupuncture a parallel model of clinical reasoning, identifying the stage of the disease, and the mechanism and the source of pain presentation, is required to determine the effective stimulation of appropriate neurotransmitters in order to restore homeostasis, enhance pain modification, and

facilitate movement and rehabilitation. Once a diagnosis has been reached, the treatment principle (Zhi Ze) can be formulated and the treatment method selected (Zhi Fa) (Zaslawski 2003).

The concept of illness or pattern diagnosis (Zheng) is fundamental as this will offer the practitioner information on nature (Table 1.4), source, location, cause, and pathomechanisms involved; it will ultimately lead to the correct intervention for the management of the presenting mechanism. If, for example, a patient presents with shoulder pain, aggravated by loading specific rotator cuff muscles, worse on muscle activity but eased by unloading, careful examination and assessment may well reveal that myofascial trigger points (MTrPts) are responsible for the presenting myofascial pain mechanism. Appropriate deactivation of those responsible dysfunctional muscles, re-education of muscle imbalance, and restoration of range of movement (ROM) may resolve the pathology without the use of segmental dorsal horn inhibition or descending inhibitory techniques. A patient presenting with complex shoulder pain brought about by abnormal CNS processing and increased sympathetic excitation may well describe pain in the shoulder, but the acupuncture intervention will require a more extensive pattern identification involving the status of the SNS, emotional status, and coping mechanisms. Acupuncture intervention may well be required to stimulate parasympathetic excitation, to promote sleep and well being, whilst a more prolonged intervention using pain gate and descending inhibitory intervention may be required over a longer period of time (Spence 2004; Streng 2007).

Knowledge of the cause of the presenting condition (pathogen) is essential, whether via injury (channel and network presentation or nociceptive pain mechanisms), infection (warmth disease, circulatory dysfunction, or viral invasion), chronic development (cold invasion, Qi or blood deficiency, bi syndrome, or system dysfunction), or acute onset (heat, Qi and blood excess). Regardless of whether it is an internal organ pattern or an external superficial channel pattern, the presenting condition will have a profound effect on pain mechanisms at different levels and as such should influence the choice of needle application, length of treatment, and method of stimulation.

Table 1.4 Classification of the diagnostic system in traditional Chinese medicine

Diagnostic classification system	Guiding principles
Ba Gang Bian Zheng	Eight principles of pattern identification Yin or yang Internal or external Deficiency or excess Cold or heat
Zang Fu Bian Zheng	Viscera and bowel patterns used primarily for herbal medicine
Liu Jing Bian Zheng	Six-channel pattern identification Superficial (yang) channels to deep (yin) channels
We Qi Ying Xue Bian Zheng	Four-level pattern in superficial channels especially warmth
San Jiao Bian Zheng	Differentiation of the three compartments (jiaos)—upper, middle, and lower—and externally contracted diseases especially warm diseases
Qi Xue Bian Zheng	Qi and blood pattern identification with changes in these substances Deficiency and excess
Jin Ye Bian Zheng	Body fluid pattern identification Phlegm and fire phlegm
Wu Xing Bian Zheng	Five-phase patterns of bowels and viscera
Jing Luo Bian Zheng	Channels and musculoskeletal pattern identification

Although the language used in TCM and Western questioning may vary, the underlying principles of assessment, inquiring, and problem-solving remain an identical process. Clinical reasoning within TCM or Western acupuncture attempts to place structure and meaning to the presenting condition, derived from the clinical information presented; turning these facts into clinical decisions based upon a full knowledge of disease processes, pain physiology, and healing mechanisms is the only pathway to effective management whether via acupuncture or physiotherapy, but preferably by the integration of both.

If the primary reason for seeking intervention is pain modification, then the primary goal of intervention is to determine the presenting pain mechanism using the correct intervention. Ultimately,

resolution of the pain mechanism will lead to resolution of joint range, functional restoration, and successful rehabilitation outcomes (Lewis 2006).

It is the structure of underlying knowledge, gained through repeated problem solving, matching knowledge with experience, that provides a pathway to guide the practitioner through the many stages of the recovery process. Few research studies identify the reasoning strategies that clinical practitioners utilize in an attempt to guide the intervention. Indeed, few studies are undertaken to determine the facts underlying the choice of intervention, although a large body of evidence relating to clinical reasoning in medicine (Cox 1999; Jones & Rivett 2003), physiotherapy (Cox 1999; Higgs 1992; Higgs & Jones 1995; Jones & Rivett 2003; Pitt-Brooke 1998), and many other health care professions is now at hand. This does not appear to be the case when acupuncture is incorporated into a physical therapy management regime. As a result, a prescriptive point-selective model has been widely used which may hamper the ability to progress the treatment or re-evaluate the acupuncture should progress be slow.

The development of expertise within any clinical field relies heavily on extensive clinical practice developing a highly structured and rich knowledge base (Bordage & Lemieux 1991; Custers et al 1996), which can be attained by physiotherapists using acupuncture within manual therapy. When a clinical reasoning model is used, based upon the knowledge of the changing pain state and disease process, treatment should be mirrored by changing acupuncture point selection and methods of application. Treatments should have no constant method just as the disease state has no constant presentation. As pain and dysfunction start to resolve, acupuncture point selection should vary. Equally, if improvement and healing are not forthcoming, a reappraisal of the disease state should be undertaken and may lead to alternate pain modification techniques and point selection.

'Disease has no constant form, treatments have no constant method and practitioners have no constant formula.' (Longbottom 2007)

Acupuncture point application must reflect disease pathology and disease processes or we are in danger of utilizing acupuncture within a fixed formula without contextual thought and problem-solving skills. The result may well be a fixed formula outcome, working some of the time, at certain stages of the disease but with vastly varying outcomes. Indeed, this has huge implications for acupuncture research

(Zaslawski 2003) and clinical effectiveness. Only with this approach to acupuncture intervention will practitioners and patients gain benefit, through clinical effectiveness and improved outcomes, enhancing their own skills, justifying and reinforcing the necessity for this powerful, effective therapeutic intervention as a mainstream modality within the clinical management of pain.

Case Study 1

Efterpi Rompoti

Introduction

This case study presents a 21-year-old female with chronic knee pain following a tibial fracture during a serious jet-ski accident. This accident resulted in a brain haemorrhage and subsequent surgery, bilateral wrist fracture, menstrual irregularities (irregular frequency of menstrual cycle and amplified pain), and insomnia during menstruation. Six months after the accident, the subject presented to physiotherapy with knee pain during function and movement restriction.

The treatment administered to this patient could be described as a 'two-step' process. Initially, movement-based treatment was undertaken as peripheral, mechanical nociceptive pain was the primary mechanism driving the disorder. The treatment consisted of manual therapy techniques, exercises, and self-management through gym activities pacing. The second step involved the integration of acupuncture after 'menstrual cycle-induced central sensitization phenomena' took place, resulting in hyperalgesia and allodynia in the knee, wrists, and low back.

After 13 sessions of combined manual therapy and acupuncture, over a period of 2 months, the subject reported a 70% improvement in pain experience and functional capacity. Moreover, sleep quality during menstruation was improved and there was a return of a normal menstrual cycle.

Subjective and objective examination

A 21-year-old lady visited the clinic complaining of chronic right anterior knee pain (AKP). In August 2006 she had had a serious jet-ski accident, which resulted in 10 days in hospital and undergoing surgery for brain haemorrhage. She also fractured both wrists (distal radius) and her left tibia (undisplaced). All fractures were treated conservatively. She recovered quickly and two months later reported minimal pain in her wrists, but her knee was painful, with restricted knee extension. At the end of October 2006 she had completed 10 sessions of physiotherapy reporting moderate satisfaction in terms of pain resolution and functional limitation. Six months following this she returned with significant knee pain and lack of extension. She also stated that she was feeling tired in her legs; she had headaches 2-3 times a week and occasional bilateral wrist pain which was exaggerated during menstruation. She reported that her menstrual cycle was disrupted after the accident and irregular (every 5-6 weeks), was accompanied by low back, abdomen, bilateral wrist, and knee pain, and impaired sleep quality. Her previous history included low back pain (LBP) with referred pain to the left knee. She was working full time in a sedentary job (mainly involving a computer).

On examination the aggravating factors were:
- Menstruation;
- Deep-knee bends;
- Kneeling; and
- Climbing stairs.

The symptoms' locations, frequency, and intensity are summarized in the body chart (Fig. 1.3). Her symptoms were eased by heat. The patient reported feeling very tired all the time withy intermittent swelling of both ankles. Her sleep was disturbed and worse during menstruation (Table 1.5).

Impression

The above findings were consistent with a mechanical knee problem caused by movement impairment in extension, combined with motor control impairment of the whole lower limb chain involving quadratus lumborum, gluteus medius, vastus medialis, and tibialis posterior muscles. Additionally, her pain appeared to be augmented by menstruation that may well indicate other factors; i.e. hormonal and/or abnormal central processing is also present. Finally, if the mechanism of injury is considered, there may well be an emotional component (e.g. fear) that could well have shaped her pain experience.

Treatment and management plan

The following treatment plan was discussed with the patient:
- Reduce pain and improve mobility of the knee, and patellofemoral (PF) and tibiofemoral (TF) joints;
- Improve motor control, muscle strength, proprioception, and functional ability;
- Reduce pain and improve sleep quality during menstruation; and
- Encourage gym activities and resume general fitness activity.

Clinical reasoning and underlying mechanisms

All findings gathered from the subjective and objective examination were analysed and the following

(Continued)

Case Study 1 (Continued)

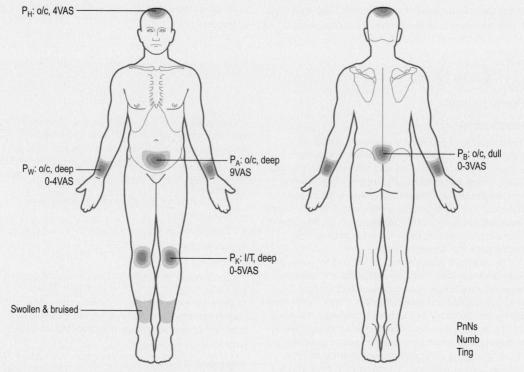

P_H: o/c, 4VAS

P_W: o/c, deep
0-4VAS

P_A: o/c, deep
9VAS

P_K: I/T, deep
0-5VAS

Swollen & bruised

P_B: o/c, dull
0-3VAS

PnNs
Numb
Ting

Figure 1.3 ● Body chart showing the areas of pain.

Table 1.5 Tests that were used to assess Lx, Hip and Knee function

Observation	↑ feet pronation (R) > (L)/(L) knee in flexion ↑ knee swelling (medial-frontal) ↓↓ (L) Quads bulk/↑ tone (L) Quadratus Lumborum (QL) (L) ASIS lower than (R)
Palpation	Tenderness over (L)　Pes Anserinus, medial Hamstrings VMO, Adductors Gluteus Medius (GM) & QL
Motion palpation	Hypomobility　Patellofemoral joint (all directions) tibiofemoral joint (in extension)
A-ROM	Knee: 18° lack of extension— ↑pain Lx & Hip: full—Ø pain
Neural function	Reflexes, sensation, key muscle testing: normal except L3 myotome: 3+ (0-5 scale)
Functional tests	Step up:↑ effort—Ø pain step down: ↑ effort—↑ pain Squat & (L) leg squat: ↑pain, knee shifts medially, Trunk shifts to the (L) and foot arch drops
Muscle tests	Quadriceps: 3+ (0-5 scale) tested in isom, ecc, con—↑ pain EOR Gluteus medius: 3+ tested in short & long lever Iliopsoas: 3 + , Gluteus maximus: 3+

Notes: ↑, increase; ↓, decrease; VMO, Vastus medialis oblique; EOR, end of range; R, right; L, left; Ø, no pain; Isom, isometric; Ecc, eccentric; Con, concentric; ASIS, anterior superior iliac spine; QL, quadratus lumborum.

mechanisms were hypothesized to be contributing to the pain and mobility dysfunction, after taking into account the relevant literature.

The major complaint of this patient was knee pain following activity; restriction of ROM affecting activities like walking, running, and wearing heels; and a feeling of tiredness. Analysing her problem it seems that peripheral, mechanical nociceptive is the dominant mechanism as pain is present after a certain amount or type of activity. The lack of knee extension has led

(Continued)

Case Study 1 (Continued)

to abnormal biomechanics to PF and TF joints which in turn has caused deconditioning (decreased strength and/or tender points) of the quadriceps, iliopsoas, hip adductors, gluteus maximus and medius, hamstrings, and tibialis posterior muscles.

The secondary complaint was an increase of all her joint pain during menstruation, accompanied by sleep disturbance. Here the underlying pain mechanisms are more complex and it seems that hormonal factors and/or abnormal central processing might be involved (Bajaj et al 2002; Baker & Driver 2004; Gazerani et al 2005). Pain during the menstrual cycle (primary dysmenorrhoea) is very common (French 2005) and is usually referred to the abdomen and the lower back as the uterus receives innervation from T10 to L1 nerve roots (King et al 1995). The mechanism possibly involves increased production of the inflammatory mediator prostaglandins by the endometrium that in turn increases uterine muscle contractions, leading to muscle ischemia, hypoxia, and pain (French 2005).

Recently it was found that dysmenorrhoeic women showed significantly decreased thresholds to painful pressure and to painful heat stimuli compared with non-dysmenorrhoeic women during their menstrual cycle (Bajaj et al 2002). The testing points were located, not only in areas within the area of referred menstrual pain, such as the abdomen and lower back, but also in control areas such as the thigh and the arm. It was suggested that increased release of nociceptive substances especially substance P and CGRP from the uterus may lead to central sensitization. Combined with the abrupt decrease of oestrogen during the menstrual phase, further systemic sensitization of the CNS may be observed, leading to decreased pain thresholds, outside of the referred pain areas. Bajaj et al (2002) concluded that moderate to severe menstrual pain could systemically sensitize nociceptors. This may partly explain the subject's hyperalgesia responses at the previous fracture sites, increased sensitivity in areas outside of abdominal menstrual pain area, e.g. wrists and knee, which led to a heightened pain perception during deep tissue palpation, which was otherwise causing mild discomfort.

The subject also exhibited allodynia, demonstrating abnormal processing of A-beta ($A\beta$) nerve fibres, which cannot be explained by the Bajaj et al (2002) study, as the tactile stimulation threshold was no different between dysmenorrhoeic and non-dysmenorrhoeic women. Evidence for the latter might be provided by a recent study in which experimentally induced pain by capsaicin injection to the forehead was applied to healthy, non-dysmenorrhoeic women during the menstrual and luteal phase (Gazerani et al 2005). Capsaicin can sensitize vanilloid receptors leading to substance P and CGRP release, creating neurogenic inflammation and a state of central sensitization (Ji et al 2003). The area

of brush-evoked allodynia was measured and it was found to be significantly larger in the menstrual phase than in the luteal phase, suggesting that the central sensitization phenomena were augmented by hormonal factors (Gazerani et al 2005). This may account for the fluctuating pain levels in this subject, varying with hormonal fluctuation and leading to central sensitization and allodynia at the previous fractured sites, involving the mechanism of acquired pain memory relapse.

The menstrual cycle has also been shown to affect sleep quality but not sleep continuity in healthy, non-dysmenorrhoeic women (Baker & Driver 2004). An earlier study (Baker et al 1999) demonstrated that women with primary dysmenorrhoea exhibited a more disturbed sleep and a sleep of a poorer quality when they had uterine pain, compared with non-dysmenorrhoeic women. This was accompanied by hormonal changes where oestrogen concentrations were shown to be significantly higher in the luteal phase for the dysmenorrhoeic women than that in controls.

Physiological reasoning for treatment selection

The first five treatments consisted of a hands-on approach as the patient could tolerate all manual techniques with a very good outcome; pain started to decrease, movement and motor control was improving, and she was feeling better. In order to address the nociceptive component of pain, a number of manual techniques were employed involving mobilization of PF and TF joints, together with motor control exercises of vastus medialis, gluteus medius, and tibialis posterior muscles during functional tasks, e.g. walking, step up/down, and squatting. Post-isometric muscle relaxation techniques to the adductors, quadriceps, and hamstring muscles were also used and she was advised to resume her gym activities within tolerance.

The subjective examination on the sixth session revealed that it was the second day of her menstrual cycle and without any other apparent/mechanical reason such as increase in her activities, her knee pain was worse and the pain in her wrists had returned. She had experienced sleep disturbance and she was quite distressed. Joint movement and deep tissue palpation, which had previously caused mild discomfort, were now very painful and her wrists and knees were hypersensitive to touch. Acupuncture was introduced at this point because it was considered to be more beneficial for the patient with this widespread symptomatology, evident signs of central sensitization, and relapse of previously acquired pain memory.

Using a clinical reasoning model it is believed that acupuncture has a local, segmental, and supraspinal effect on the CNS, which can lead to short- or long-term pain relief, depending largely on the dominant pain mechanisms (Carlsson 2002). Melzack et al (1977)

(Continued)

Case Study 1 (Continued)

proposed that acupuncture-induced pain relief shares similar mechanisms with transcutaneous, electrical, nerve stimulation (TENS) (Chen & Chen 2004). Animal experiments (Sandkuhler 2000a) showed that dorsal root stimulation of A-delta (Aδ) fibres at 1 Hz could decrease the synaptic strength of previously sensitized C-fibres, which clinically manifests as hyperalgesia. In some cases, this type of stimulation could not only decrease the synaptic strength but also reverse this long-term potentiated state (LTP) of the membrane, leading to long-term depression (LTD), clinically manifested as long-lasting analgesia. This form of anti-nociception probably involves spinal dorsal horn glutamate receptors, such as a-amino-3-hydroxy-5-methyl-4-isoxazolepropionic acid receptor (AMPA) and *N*-methyl d-aspartate receptor (NMDA) that appears to be modulated by supraspinal descending inhibitory pathways (Sandkuhler 2000a). Importantly, LTP has been shown to be one of the common mechanisms shared by pain and memory (Ji et al 2003; Sandkuhler 2000b), providing a rationale for pain recurrence after an injury has been healed.

A number of recent fMRI studies have shed more light on the brain structures activated or deactivated during acupuncture. Amongst other areas, manual acupuncture at LI4 and LIV3 caused deactivation of some prefrontal cortex and anterior cingulate cortex (ACC), respectively (Yan et al 2005). In an earlier study, the aforementioned areas were activated following experimental mechanical nociceptive pressure in healthy volunteers (Creac'h et al 2000). This may well imply that LI4 and LIV4 acupoints have pain-modulating effects. Evidence for bilateral deactivation of areas such as the amygdala following EA was provided by a study investigating the stimulation of ST36, SP6, GB34, and BL57 points (Zhang et al 2004). As reviewed recently, amygdala takes part in the acquisition, storage, and expression of conditioned fear memory and LTP is often proposed as the underlying mechanism of associative fear memory. Also, the interaction of prefrontal cortex and amygdala can lead to conditioned fear extinction (Kim & Jung 2006). If acupuncture at specific points can deactivate areas of the aforementioned structures, then it could possibly play a role in conditioned fear extinction and thus in extinction of some chronic pain states.

Specifically for the treatment of primary dysmenorrhoea, only two recent experimental studies were found that investigated the use of acupressure in pain relief (Chen & Chen 2004, Jun et al 2007). The first study showed that acupressure at Spleen 6 (SP6) acupoint (bilaterally) for 20 minutes significantly reduced pain during menstruation compared to the control group. The results were attributed to the spinal gate mechanism, where stimulation of Aβ fibres inhibit painful stimuli transmission and also lead to activation of the endogenous opioid system. The second study examined the effects of acupressure at the same point SP6, in pain ratings and temperature changes at suprapubic Conception Vessel 2 (CV2) point. The control group received light touch at SP6. It was found that acupressure for 20 minutes significantly reduced pain ratings and increased temperature at CV2 point, immediately and for two hours post treatment. The temperature increase was attributed to increased uterine blood flow, as CV2 point lies over the uterus and is cited as beneficial for Qi flow and is linked to the uterus according to TCM.

Finally, a recent systematic review (Proctor et al 2007) investigating the effects of TENS and acupuncture showed that there is not sufficient evidence for efficacy of acupuncture and the only good design trial that showed beneficial effects had a small sample size.

There is some evidence that acupuncture can be beneficial in treating insomnia, although no report was found to test insomnia following dysmenorrhoea. Recently, in an open trial it was found that 5 weeks of acupuncture (2 sessions per week) could normalize melatonin secretion (measured in urine) and could produce significant improvement in sleep quality (Spence et al 2004). However, this study failed to mention the acupuncture points utilized. Significant decrease in insomnia was reported in a study investigating the results of acupuncture in pregnancy after eight treatment sessions (da Silva et al 2005). Pregnant women treated with acupuncture showed significant improvement in insomnia scores compared with a group that received only sleep hygiene advice. The points used in this study were Heart 7 (HT7), Pericardium 6 (PC6), extra points Amnian (used bilaterally) and Yintang, Governor Vessel 20 (GV20), and Conception Vessel 17(CV17) (Table 1.6).

Outcome measurements and results

The outcome measures used were active knee extension in standing measured with a manual goniometer, subjective pain and difficulty (effort) during squats, step-down, and deep knee bends measured on a 0–10 verbal scale (0: no pain/effort and 10: maximum pain/effort) (Table 1.7). A total of thirteen treatments were administered with manual therapy techniques and exercises were used in the first 5 sessions, acupuncture in the sixth (during menstruation), and a hands-on approach was followed by acupuncture sessions thereafter. Although this patient reported marked improvement in pain scores (wrists, knee, abdomen, and low back) and sleep quality after the first acupuncture session, acupuncture was continued for the following four weeks in order to assess its efficacy in normalizing timing of menstruation. Interestingly, 5 weekly acupuncture treatments showed a tendency for menstrual cycle normalization as the second menstruation happened after 4 weeks and 6 days (the frequency of her most recent menstrual cycle before visiting the clinic was 6 weeks). During the last

(Continued)

Case Study 1 (Continued)

Table 1.6 Acupuncture point rationale

Day	Treatment aim	Points used
1	General & abdominal analgesia	LIV3[B], LI4 [B], SP9[L], SP10[L] Rationale LIV3 & LI4: major analgesic points SP9, SP10: abdominal blood flow increase, dysmenorrhoea
8	Local & abdominal analgesia, regulation of menstruation	SP9[L], SP10[L], SP6[L], Heding[L] Rationale: SP6: regulates uterus and menstruation Heding [L]: knee pain and motor control impairment
15	Regulation of menstruation, knee ROM increase	SP9[L], SP10[L], SP6 [L], KID10[L] Rationale KID10: menstrual disorders, medial knee pain
22	Regulation of menstruation, knee ROM increase	SP9[L], SP10[L], SP6[L], KID10[L], LIV2[L] Rationale LIV2: menstrual disorders
30	Regulation of menstruation, knee ROM increase	SP9[L], SP10[L], SP6[L], KID10[L], LIV, KID Rationale KID3: menstrual disorders & insomnia
36	General & abdominal analgesia	LIV3[B], LI4[B], SP6[B], SP9[B], SP10[L]

Notes: The 1st and 6th treatments were during the second day of patient's menstrual cycle. B, Bilateral; L, Left.

Table 1.7 Summary of the outcome measures

Treatment	First	Last
Knee extension (standing)	−4° (R), 18° (L)	−4° (R), 5° (L)
Squats (pain/effort)	3NRS/2	0NRS/0
Step down (pain/effort)	4NRS/6	1NRS/1
Deep knee bend (pain/effort)	5NRS/7	1NRS/1

Notes: NRS, numerical rating scale.

acupuncture session (second menstrual cycle), the patient complained mainly of LBP and knee pain. After this treatment she reported decrease in both pains and better sleep at night.

Overall there was a 70% improvement in functional capacity, including daytime tiredness and ankle swelling. Knee pain was minimal and she gradually resumed her previous gym, cycling, and swimming activities.

Limitations

Undoubtedly, there are limitations as only one objective outcome measure was used (angle measurement) and any decision-making regarding treatment selection was based mainly on the subject's subjective pain scores. Secondly, ovulation could not be confirmed in the present study; therefore the relationship between pain, menstrual phase, and hormonal secretion, e.g. oestrogen, should be interpreted with caution as

20% of menstrual cycles are non-ovulatory (Sherman & Korenman cited in Bajaj et al 2002). Finally, the acupuncture protocol used in this study has not been validated previously, as no study was found to investigate acupuncture efficacy in complex menstrual pain and irregularities.

Discussion

This case study attempted to analyse and present the physiotherapy management of a patient complaining of knee pain following a serious accident. Treatment options were considered and a hypothesis of intervention was arrived at after taking into account the underlying pain mechanisms, the chronicity of the disorder, the mechanism of injury, the relationship between presenting pain and menstrual cycle, and also her functional demands, in total using a clinical reasoning approach.

Initially a hands-on approach was the treatment of choice as movement-based treatment and management has been shown effective in dealing with chronic, mechanical, nociceptive pain (Dankaerts et al 2007; O'Sullivan 2005). The main mechanisms that have been recently proposed for movement-based treatment efficacy are:

- Arousal of descending pain inhibitory systems through passive movement;
- Habituation through repeated stimulation; and
- Extinction of aversive memories by establishing a new association between pain and movement (Zusman 2004).

This subject demonstrated a steady improvement during the first five sessions with decrease in pain and

(Continued)

Case Study 1 (Continued)

improvement in ROM, motor control, and functional capacity. Reassurance that chronic pain does not equal tissue damage and education about the benefits of maintaining an active lifestyle further enhanced patient compliance.

The results after the first and last acupuncture sessions were very good as the patient reported a marked decrease in all pains, improved sleep at night, and decreased blood flow on the last menstrual day.

Considering the research previously quoted, concerning deactivation of the pre-frontal cortex, the amygdala, and treatment of primary dysmenorrhea, specific factors account for acupuncture-induced pain modulation. However, one should not omit to mention the non-specific factors behind the mechanisms of acupuncture analgesia, mainly associated with expectancy and belief for pain relief (Pariente et al 2005). Manual acupuncture applied to patients using real needles and Streitberger needles (needling sensation but not skin penetration) demonstrated both distinct and common areas of brain activation. Areas that have been linked with pain modulation such as the dorsolateral prefrontal cortex and the rostral part of ACC were activated under both conditions, implying that expectation of a therapeutic effect might have played a significant role. Therefore, both specific and non-specific factors might have contributed to this subject's pain relief during menstruation.

Case Study 2

Sarah Rouse

Introduction

The aim of this case study is to discuss the safe usage and effects of acupuncture during pregnancy. A 38-year-old woman presented at 24 weeks gestation with pelvic pain and low back pain and was followed through into the final weeks of her third trimester. At this stage fatigue was also a problem. Her symptoms were affecting her ability to adequately care for her family. Treatment consisted of advice, exercises, and acupuncture; a visual analogue scale (VAS) for pain and subjective reporting of functional ability were used as outcome measures. A reduction in pain and fatigue were observed, together with an increase in the patient's ability to cope with the demands of family life.

Pelvic pain (PP) and LBP are common complaints during pregnancy (Kristiansson et al 1996) with incidences of up to 75% reported in the literature (Brynhildsen 1998). Indeed, Noren et al (1997) state that the majority of pregnant women experience some kind of back pain during pregnancy. Risk factors for developing PP are a history of previous LBP, trauma to the back or pelvis, multivariate, higher stress, and low job satisfaction (Albert et al 2006). There has been some debate over aetiology; recently, the traditional explanation of hormonal influence resulting in ligamentous laxity giving rise to pain has been challenged (Bjorkland, 2000; Sandler 1996) and a more biomechanical model is becoming increasingly accepted.

Subjective and objective assessment

The subject presented at 24 weeks of gestation with mild soreness over the pubic symphysis (PS), radiating into the inner thighs and a slight ache in her lower back.

At this stage, all symptoms were worse towards the end of the day only, VAS was 20/100, and on assessment, there were few objective signs. The subject had suffered from severe PP in the third trimester of her first pregnancy; she was currently looking to prevent, as far as possible, an increase in symptoms. She was therefore provided with advice and stability exercises; she would also start wearing the maternity belt retained from her last pregnancy as she had found this to be helpful. She was reviewed one month later; her VAS was 80/100 and she was frustrated by her greatly reduced mobility. She appeared fatigued and emotional. The most significant findings on assessment were bilateral trigger points (TrPts) in the adductor muscle group and moderate tenderness over the PS; the LBP was negligible. In the light of her hugely increased VAS score and overwhelming tiredness, acupuncture was proposed as a treatment option for both its analgesic effect and from a TCM point of view, for addressing fatigue.

Acupuncture in Pregnancy

Traditionally, acupuncture has been used to treat a myriad of pregnancy-related conditions including morning sickness, migraine, constipation, haemorrhoids, and breech presentation as well as being used for the induction of labour and pain relief during labour (Budd 2006). There are a growing number of studies that suggest that acupuncture is safe and effective in the treatment of PP and LBP during pregnancy. In a randomized controlled trial (RCT) of 72 pregnant women with LBP and PP, Kvorning et al (2004) found that VAS scores of pain intensity decreased in 60% of patients in the acupuncture group compared to only 14% in the control group. Importantly, no serious adverse effects

(Continued)

Case Study 2 (Continued)

were found in the patients and no adverse effects at all in the infants. Though this study can be criticized for its small sample size, the indications are that acupuncture is a useful pain-relieving tool at a time when other forms of analgesia are very limited. Similarly, in a larger RCT, Elden et al (2005) compared the effects of acupuncture and stabilizing exercises to standard treatment in 386 pregnant women with PP. Acupuncture was found to be superior to stabilizing exercises in reducing pain. Again, no serious complications occurred during treatment. Further RCTs (da Silva et al 2004; Wedenberg et al 2000) as well as case study reports (Cummings 2003, Forrester 2003) and a retrospective study of 167 pregnant women treated with acupuncture (Ternov et al, 2001) indicate that acupuncture appears to safely alleviate LBP and PP during pregnancy as well as increasing the capacity for functional activity.

Although, as always, more research is needed, such studies lend support generally to the use of acupuncture in obstetrics and specifically to the case study in question. Traditionally, however, few physiotherapists use acupuncture within obstetrics (Swan & Cook 2003) and indeed at AACP foundation training level, use of acupuncture within the first trimester is discouraged. It would therefore seem prudent to consider possible contraindications to treatment with acupuncture in pregnancy.

Forrester (2003) suggests that it may be wise to avoid acupuncture during the first trimester as this is a frequent time of natural, spontaneous miscarriage; thus the pregnancy loss may well be blamed on the acupuncture. Indeed, none of the previously cited studies used pregnant women in their first trimester. However, Smith et al (2002) in an RCT of 593 women with nausea and vomiting in early pregnancy (mean gestational age 8.5 weeks) demonstrated that there were no differences between study groups (patients received traditional acupuncture, formula acupuncture, sham acupuncture, or no acupuncture) in the incidence of perinatal outcome, congenital abnormalities, pregnancy complications, and other infant outcomes.

Other contraindications may include gestational diabetes, incompetent cervix, pre-eclampsia, and uncontrolled epilepsy (Longbottom 2006b). One should also be aware of the following signs: severe morning sickness, profuse bleeding, severe abdominal pain, urinary tract infection, and intense itching of the skin (obstetric cholestasis) (West 2001). In all of these instances, acupuncture should not be used and the patient should be referred for further monitoring.

Leading on from this discussion is the subject of 'forbidden points' during pregnancy. Much controversy exists regarding this subject and forbidden points vary according to different authors (Forrester 2003). West (2001) lists LI4, SP6, ST36, GB21, BL67, and abdominal points as best to be avoided. West (2001) also advises avoidance of BL31 and BL32 before 37 weeks gestation.

All of these points are hypothesized to induce labour. However, it seems worth remembering that many and varied points have been used in the literature including the above, without adverse effect.

Based upon the aforementioned studies, the subject was considered a suitable candidate for acupuncture; she was entering her third trimester as treatment began and had no contraindications. Assessment showed little indication for manual therapy, as there were no signs of biomechanical dysfunction around the pelvis.

Acupuncture physiology

Acupuncture was chosen for its analgesic effect. The physiological rationale for selection of acupuncture to reduce pain can be broken down into several parts.

Alterations in blood flow

Increases in blood flow to painful areas should theoretically aid healing mechanisms, bringing in nutrients and oxygen, removing metabolites, and speeding homeostasis. Acupuncture has been demonstrated to affect blood flow (Sandberg 2003). The author found that De Qi stimulation (a sensation of distension, soreness, heaviness or numbness) resulted in the most pronounced increase in skin and muscle blood flow.

Pain gate effect

Stimulation of mechanoreceptors (Aβ fibres) by acupuncture needles brings about a pain gate effect on both Aδ (fast) and C (slow) pain fibres in the posterior horn of the spinal cord. This reduces the excitability of these cells to pain-generated stimuli. This is referred to as pre-synaptic inhibition (Stux & Pomeranz 1991).

Encephalin mechanism in the posterior horn

Stimulation of the Aδ pain receptor fibres by needling creates a morphine-type effect on the C fibres by encephalin-producing interneurons in the substantia gelatinosa of the posterior horn (Low & Reed 1994).

Encephalin mechanism in the descending pathway

Again, stimulation of the Aδ pain receptor fibres (as above) creates a morphine-type (encephalin) effect on the C fibre system, but this time via centres in the mid-brain involving serotonin as a neurotransmitter (Low & Reed 1994).

Stimulation of the hypothalamic–pituitary–adrenal (HPA) and sympathetic–adrenal–medullary (SAM) axes

It is also highly likely that acupuncture will have strong effects on the thoughts and emotions of the patient. This affects the HPA axis, which in turn leads to acetylcholine (ACh) and beta endorphin production and consequential cortisol production) as well as the SAM causing release of catecholamine (adrenalin and noradrenalin) hormone. These systems have important (albeit not very well

(Continued)

Case Study 2 (Continued)

understood) effects on pain, cardiovascular and immune system functioning (Alford 2006; Haker 2000).

Effect on myofascial trigger points

MTrPts are tender, focal, hyperirritable spots located in a taut band of skeletal muscle (Alvarez et al 2002). They are thought to be the result of excessive release of acetylcholine in abnormal motor endplates. Physical overload (such as in pregnancy), overwork fatigue, and trauma have been proposed as causative factors (Travell & Simons 1983, cited by Filshie and Cummings 1999). Needling is thought to deactivate the abnormal motor endplate by providing a localized stretch to the affected area as well as increased blood flow to the hypoxic tissue. It is likely that many TrPts are tender, irritable Ah Shi acupuncture points.

Outcome and Results

The subject responded well to acupuncture; her initial subjective reporting of reduced PP was borne out in a VAS score that decreased from 80/100 to 30-40/100 (Table 1.8). De Qi was obtained when the needles were inserted at the majority of points. It was after the inclusion of the Ah Shi points over the PS that the subject considered herself to be much improved. Biweekly treatment meant that this subject was more able to cope with the rigours of family life (a 3-year-old daughter and two step children who lived in the family home during the latter part of the week). Tenderness over the PS and adductor muscle was reduced and stability exercises (transversus abdominus, pelvic floor, and static gluteal contractions) were continued throughout the treatment.

Discussion

The acupuncture regime chosen for this subject demonstrated encouraging results; her PP gradually decreased and her tiredness also became less of a problem. On reflection, a distal point could have been used to enhance the analgesic effect though this would have taken the total number of acupuncture points over the suggested 6 to 8 in pregnancy (Smith et al 2002; West 2001). However, in other studies larger numbers of needles were used; da Silva et al (2004) used an average of 12 needles and Wedenberg et al (2000) up to 10 needles. Though sample sizes were relatively small in the acupuncture groups in theses studies, there were no serious adverse effects reported. It seemed wise, however, in the current case study to err on the side of caution in the light of one's relative inexperience of acupuncture in pregnancy.

As well as variation in the number of needles used, the literature also showed diversity in the range of points chosen and stimulation techniques employed. West (2001) suggests that very gentle techniques are employed in pregnancy. Hence, an even technique was used, De Qi was obtained, and then the needle was left in situ. Early treatments lasted 15 minutes, again as advocated by West (2001), increasing to up to 25 minutes. In contrast, Kvorning et al (2004) used 2 stimulations (including periosteal stimulation) to obtain De Qi with very minimal treatment times. Wedenberg (2000) also used 2 stimulations but needles were left in for 30 minutes for all treatments. Elden et al (2005) left needles in situ for 30 minutes and stimulated every 10 minutes. Smith et al (2002) used a variety of needling techniques (tonification, even, and sedation). Furthermore, Lund et al (2006) compared two different acupuncture modes. The pregnant women in one group received subcutaneous needling with no stimulation whilst the second group received intramuscular

Table 1.8 Acupuncture Regime

Session	Points used	Duration	Outcome
1	2 TrPts to adductor muscles LU7[B]	15 minutes Even technique	Subjective reporting of decreased fatigue and pain. No adverse effects
2	3 TrPts to adductor muscles LU7[B]	15 minutes Even technique	Good pain relief for 2 days post treatment
3	2 Ah Shi points—TrPts to adductor muscles 2 TrPts over pubic symphysis		
LU7[B]	20 minutes Even technique	Generally feeling more energy	
4–9 biweekly	2 TrPts to adductor muscles 2 TrPts over pubic symphysis LU7[B]	25 minutes Even technique	VAS: 30-40/100

Note: B, bilateral.

(Continued)

Case Study 2 (Continued)

treatment with repeated stimulation. Significant decreases in pain were evident and though this study can be criticized for its small sample size (47 women completed the trial), there was no observable difference in pain reduction between the two groups.

This lack of standardization amongst the treatment approaches observed in the literature continues into the realms of point selection (as mentioned in the Introduction). A plethora of acupuncture points have been used including ear acupuncture (Thomas & Napolitano 2000; Wedenberg et al 2000), classical acupuncture (da Silva et al 2004; Lund et al 2006), segmental acupuncture (Forrester 2003), needling of MTrPts (Cummings 2003; Kvorning 2001), and also points based on TCM diagnosis (Smith et al 2002). As can be seen, it is virtually impossible to use the research in order to select appropriate points. Individual diagnosis and knowledge of forbidden points must therefore be employed. In the current case study the majority of points used were Ah Shi points (tender points). These could be interpreted as MTrPts, as palpable taut bands in the muscles were identified. Two further Ah Shi points were used directly over the PS as suggested by West (2001). Acupuncture point Lung 7 (LU7) was used bilaterally, based on a very superficial TCM diagnosis. The subject appeared tired, pale, anxious, and tearful; this may have indicated a Lung Qi deficiency (Longbottom 2006b, Course Manual). Had these symptoms not improved, BL13 could also have been considered. From a more Western interpretation,

this calming effect could be attributed to activation of oxytocin pathways by acupuncture (Uvnas 2003, cited by Forrester 2003). Of course, these symptoms may also have improved due to the decrease in pain. One should also consider the placebo effect: the subject attended twice a week over several weeks wherein a relatively close patient–therapist relationship was formed involving much humour and discussion; these effects of this on recovery should not be underestimated.

Conclusion

Obstetric acupuncture within physiotherapy is still in its infancy, a small but growing number of RCTs show promising results in terms of pain reduction and improved function. Though a wide range of treatment protocols have been utilized within the studies, which makes standardization difficult, it should be emphasized that there were no significant adverse effects either in the mothers who took part or in their infants. Though a single case study design is limited in its application, the results of this report are in keeping with those in the research. In China, acupuncture is commonly used in pregnancy; Forrester (2003) suggests that in Britain, fear of litigation (should acupuncture be blamed for pregnancy loss) may be more influential than a discerning review of the literature. It cannot be denied, however, that further large RCTs would be useful in increasing the confidence of physiotherapists embarking on their obstetrics acupuncture journey.

References

Albert, H.B., Godskesen, M., Korsholm, L., et al., 2006. Risk factors in developing pregnancy related pelvic girdle pain. Acta Obstet. Gynecol. Scandinavia 85 (5), 539–544.

Alford, L., 2006. Psychneuroimmunology for physiotherapists. Physiotherapy 92, 187–191.

Alvarez, D., Rockwell, P., 2002. Trigger points: diagnosis and management. Am. Fam. Physician 65 (4), 653–660.

Andersson, S., Lundeberg, T., 1995. Acupuncture—from empiricism to science: functional background to acupuncture effects in pain and disease. Med. Hypotheses 45 (3), 271–281.

Backer, M., Hammes, M.G., Valet, M., et al., 2002. Different modes of manual acupuncture stimulation differentially modulate cerebral blood flow velocity, arterial blood pressure and heart rate in human

subjects. Neurosci. Lett. 333 (3), 203–206.

Baja, P., Baja, P., Madsen, H., et al., 2002. A comparison of modality-specific somatosensory changes during menstruation in dysmenorrhoeic and nondysmenorrhoeic women. Clin. J. Pain 18, 180–190.

Baker, F.C., Driver, H.S., 2004. Self-reported sleep across the menstrual cycle in young, healthy women. J. Psychosom. Res. 56, 239–243.

Baker, F.C., Driver, H.S., Rogers, G.G., et al., 1999. High nocturnal body temperatures and disturbed sleep in women with primary dysmenorrhoea. Am. J. Physiol. Endocrinol. Metab. 277, 1013–1021.

Barlas, P., Ting, S., Chesterton, L.S., et al., 2006. Effects of intensity of electroacupuncture upon experimental pain in healthy human

volunteers: a randomised, double-blind, placebo-controlled study. Pain 122 (1-2), 81–89.

Bekkering, R., van Bussel, R., 1998. Segmental acupuncture. In: Filshie, J., White, A. (Eds.), Medical acupuncture: a western scientific approach. Churchill Livingstone, Edinburgh, pp. 105–135.

Biella, B., Sotgiu, M.L., Pellegata, G., et al., 2001. Acupuncture produces central activations in pain regions. Neuroimage 14 (1), 60–66.

Birch, S., 2001. Systematic reviews of acupuncture: are there problems with these? Clinical Acupuncture. Oriental Medicine 2, 17–22.

Bjorkland, K., Nordstrom, M., Ulmsten, U., 2000. Symphyseal distension in relation to serum relaxin levels and pelvic pain in pregnancy. Acta Obstetrics and gynecology Scandinavia 79, 269–275.

Bordage, G., Lemieux, M., 1991. Semantic structures and diagnostic thinking of experts and novices. Academic Med. Suppl., S70–S72.

Bradnam, L., 2007. A proposed clinical reasoning model for Western acupuncture. J. Acupunct. Assoc. Chart Physiotherapists, 21–30.

Brain, S., 1997. Sensory neuropeptides: Their role in inflammation and wound healing. Immunopharmacology 37 (2-3), 133–152.

Brynhildsen, J., Hansson, A., Persson, A., et al., 1998. Follow up of patients with low back pain during pregnancy. Obstet. and Gynaec. 91 (2), 182–186.

Budd, S. 2006. Briefing Paper No 12, Obstetrics (2) pregnancy and labour. The evidence for the effectiveness of acupuncture. Acupuncture Research Resource Centre, British Acupuncture Council.

Carlsson, C., 2002. Acupuncture mechanisms for clinically relevant long-term effects: reconsideration and a hypothesis. Acupunct. Med. 20 (2-3), 82–99.

Chan, A.K., Vujnovich, A.L., Bradnam-Roberts, L., 2004. The effect of acupuncture on alpha-motoneuron excitability. Int. J. Acupunct. Electrother. Res. 29 (1-2), 53–72.

Chen, H.M., Chen, C.H., 2004. Effects of acupressure at the Sanyinjiao point on primary dysmenorrhoea. J. Adv. Nurs. 48 (4), 380–387.

Cox, K., 1999. Doctor and patient: exploring clinical thinking. University of South Wales Press, Sydney.

Creac'h, C., Henry, P., Caille, J.M., et al., 2000. Functional MR imaging analysis of pain-related brain activation after acute mechanical stimulation. Am. J. Neuroradiol. 21, 1402–1406.

Cummings, M., 2000. Teasing apart the quality and validity of systemic reviews of acupuncture. Altern. Ther. Health. Med. 18 (2), 104–107.

Cummings, M., 2003. Acupuncture for low back pain in pregnancy. Acupunct. Med. 21 (1-2), 42–46.

Custers, E., Regehr, G., Norman, G., 1996. Mental representations of medical diagnostic knowledge: a review. Academic Med. Suppl. 71 (0), S55–S61.

Dankaerts, W., O'Sullivan, P.B., Burnett, A.F., et al., 2007. The use of a mechanism-based classification system to evaluate and direct management of a patient with non-specific chronic low back pain and motor control impairment—a case report. Man. Ther. 12 (2), 181–191.

da Silva, J., Nakamura, M., Cordeiro, J., et al., 2004. Acupuncture for low back pain in pregnancy—a prospective, quasi-randomised, controlled study. Acupunct. Med. 22 (2), 60–67.

da Silva, J.B., Nakamura, M.U., Cordeiro, J.A., et al., 2005. Acupuncture for insomnia in pregnancy—a prospective, quasi-randomised, controlled study. Acupunct. Med. 23 (2), 47–51.

Elden, H., Ladfors, L., Olsen, M., et al., 2005. Effects of acupuncture and stabilizing exercises as adjuncts to standard treatment in pregnant women with pelvic girdle pain: randomized single blind controlled trial. Br. Med. J. 330 (7494), 761.

Ernst, E., 2003. Acupuncture research: the first 10 years in Exeter. Acupunct. Med. 21 (3), 100–104.

Ezzo, J., Lao, l., Berman, B., 2001. Clin acupunct: Sci Basis. Springer, Berlin.

Fang, J.L., Krings, T., Weidemann, J., et al., 2004. Functional MRI in healthy subjects during acupuncture: different effects of needle rotation in real and false acupoints. Neuroradiology 46 (5), 359–362.

Filshie, J., Cummings, M., 1999. Western medical acupuncture. In: Ernst, E., White, A. (Eds.), Acupuncture: a scientific appraisal. Butterworth-Heinemann, Oxford, pp. 31–59.

Forrester, M., 2003. Low back pain in pregnancy. Acupunct. Med. 21 (1-2), 36–41.

French, L., 2005. Dysmenorrhoea. Am. Fam. Physician 71 (2), 285–291.

Gazerani, P., Andersen, O.K., Arendt-Nielsen, L., 2005. A human experimental capsaicin model for trigeminal sensitisation. Gender-specific differences. Pain 118 (1-2), 55–163.

Haker, E., Egekvist, H., Bjerring, P., 2000. Effect of sensory stimulation (acupuncture) on sympathetic and parasympathetic activities in healthy subjects. J. Auton. Nerv. Syst. 79 (1), 52–59.

Hecker, H.-U., Steveling, A., Peuker, E., et al., 2001. Color atlas of acupuncture. Thieme, Stuttgart.

Higgs, J., 1992. Developing clinical reasoning competencies. Physiotherapy 78 (8), 575–581.

Higgs, J., Jones, M., 1995. Clinical reasoning in the health professions. Butterworth Heinemann, Oxford.

Hsieh, J.C., Tu, C.H., Chen, F.P., et al., 2001. Activation of the hypothalamus characterises the acupuncture stimulation at the analgesic point in human: a positron emission tomography study. Neurosci. Lett. 307 (2), 105–108.

Hsu, C.C., Weng, C.S., Liu, T.S., et al., 2006. Effects of electrical acupuncture on acupoint BL15 evaluated in terms of heart rate variability, pulse rate variability and skin conductance response. Am. J. Chin. Med. 34 (1), 23–36.

Hui, K.K., Liu, J., Makris, N., et al., 2000. Acupuncture modulates the limbic system and subcortical gray structures of the human brain: evidence from fMRI studies in normal subjects. Hum. Brain. Mapp 9 (1), 13–25.

Hui, K.K., Liu, J., Marina, O., et al., 2005. The integrated response of the human cerebro-cerebellar and limbic systems to acupuncture stimulation at ST 36 as evidenced by fMRI. Neuroimage 27 (3), 479–496.

Ji, R.R., Kohno, T., Moore, K.A., et al., 2003. Central sensitisation and LTP: do pain and memory share similar mechanisms? Trends Neurosci 26 (12), 696–705.

Jones, M., Rivett, D., 2003. Clinical reasoning for manual therapists. Elsevier Science, Edinburgh.

Jones, M., Rivett, D., 2004. Introduction to clinical reasoning. In: Jones, M., Rivett, D. (Eds.), Clinical reasoning for manual therapists. Butterworth Heinemann, Oxford.

Jun, E.-M., Chang, S., Kang, D.-H., et al., 2007. Effects of acupressure on dysmenorrhoea and skin and temperature changes in college students: A non-randomised controlled trial. Int. J. Nurs. Stud. 44 (6), 973–981.

Kandell, E., Schwartz, J., Jessell, T., 2000. Principles of neural science, 4th edn. McGraw-Hill, New York.

Kim, J.J., Jung, M.W., 2006. Neural circuits and mechanisms involved in Pavlovian fear conditioning: a critical review. Neurosci. Biobehav. Rev. 30, 188–202.

King, P.M., Ling, F.W., Myers, C.A., 1995. Examination in physical therapy practice: screening for medical disease, 2nd edn. Churchill Livingstone, Philadelphia.

Kong, J., Ma, L., Gollub, R.L., et al., 2002. A pilot study of functional magnetic resonance imaging of the brain during manual and electroacupuncture stimulation of acupuncture point (LI-4 Hegu) in normal subjects reveals differential brain activation between methods.

J. Altern. Complement Med. 8 (4), 411–419.

Kristiansson, P., Svardsudd, K., von Schoultz, B., 1996. Back pain during pregnancy: A prospective study. Spine 21 (6), 702–708.

Kvorning, N., Holmberg, C., Grennert, L., et al., 2004. Acupuncture relieves pelvic and low back pain in late pregnancy. Acta Obstet Gynecol Scandinavia 83, 246–250.

Lao, l., Ezzo, J., Berman, B., et al., 2001. Assessing clinical efficacy of acupuncture: considerations for designing future clinical acupuncture trials. In: Stux, G., Hammerschlag, R. (Eds.), Clinical acupuncture: scientific basis. Springer, Berlin.

Lewis, J. (2006). Acupuncture Association of Chartered Physiotherapists Annual Conference. Personal communication.

Lewith, G.T., White, P.J., Pariente, J., 2005. Investigating acupuncture using brain-imaging techniques: the current state of play. Evid. Based Complement Alternat. Med. 2 (3), 315–319.

Lo, Y.L., Cui, S.L., Fook-Chong, S., 2005. The effect of acupuncture on motor cortex excitability and plasticity. Neurosci. Lett. 384 (1-2), 145–149.

Longbottom, J., 2006a. Not so simple pain: the complexity of chronic pain management. J Acupunct Assoc Chart Physiotherapists, 16–24.

Longbottom, J. (2007) Clinical reasoning in acupuncture. AACP Conference. Unpublished work.

Low, J., Reed, A., 1990. Electrotherapy explained—principles and practise. Butterworth Heinemann, Oxford.

Lund, I., Lundeberg, T., Lonnberg, L., et al., 2006. Decrease of women's pelvic pain after acupuncture: a randomized controlled single-blind study. Acta Obstet Gynecol Scandinavia 85 (1), 12–19.

Lundeberg, T., 1999. Effects of sensory stimulation (acupuncture) on circulatory and immune systems. In: Ernst, E., White, A. (Eds.), Acupuncture: a scientific appraisal. Butterworth-Heinemann, Oxford, pp. 93–106.

Lundeberg, T. (2006). The physiological basis of acupuncture. MANZ/PAANZ Annual Conference, Christchurch, New Zealand.

Lundeberg, T., Ekholm, J., 2001. Pain—from periphery to brain. J. Acupunct. Assoc. Chart. Physiotherapists, 13–19.

Lundeberg, T., Stener-Victorin, E., 2002. Is there a physiological basis for the use of acupuncture in pain? In: Sato, A., Li, P., Campbell, J.L. (Eds.), Acupuncture: is there a physiological basis? Elsevier, Amsterdam, pp. 3–10.

Lundeberg, T., Hurtig, T., Thomas, M., 1988a. Long-term results of acupuncture in chronic head and neck pain. Pain Clinic 2, 15–31.

Lundeberg, T., Kjartansson, J., Samuelsson, U., 1988b. Effect of electrical nerve stimulation on healing of ischaemic skin flaps. Lancet ii, 712–714.

Maioli, C., Falciati, L., Marangon, M., et al., 2006. Short- and long-term modulation of upper limb motor-evoked potentials induced by acupuncture. Eur. J. Neurosci. 23 (7), 1931–1938.

Napadow, V., Makris, N., Liu, J., et al., 2005. Effects of electroacupuncture versus manual acupuncture on the human brain as measured by fMRI. Hum. Brain Mapp 24 (3), 193–205.

Noguchi, E., Ohsawa, H., Kobayashi, S., et al., 1999. The effect of electro-acupuncture stimulation on the muscle blood flow of the hind limb in anaesthetised rats. J. Auton. Nerv. Syst. 75 (2), 78–86.

Noren, L., Ostgaard, S., Nielsen, T., et al., 1997. Reduction of sick leave for lumbar back and posterior pelvic pain in pregnancy. Spine 22 (18), 2157–2160.

O'Sullivan, P., 2005. Diagnosis and classification of chronic low back pain disorders: maladaptive movement and motor control impairments as underlying mechanism. Man. Ther. 10, 242–255.

Pariente, J., White, P., Frackowiak, R.S., et al., 2005. Expectancy and belief modulate the neuronal substrates of pain treated by acupuncture. Neuroimage 25, 1161–1167.

Pitt-Brooke, J., 1998. Rehabilitation of movement: theoretical basis of clinical practice. Elsevier Health Sciences, Edinburgh.

Proctor, M.L., Smith, C.A., Farquhar, T., et al., 2007. Transcutaneous electrical nerve stimulation and acupuncture for primary dysmenorrhoea (review). The Cochrane Library (Issue 2).

Refe, S., 2001. Systematic reviews of acupuncture-are there problems with these?. Clinical Acupunct Orient. Med. 2, 17–22.

Sandberg, M., Lundeberg, T., Lindberg, L.G., et al., 2003. Effects of acupuncture on skin and muscle blood flow in healthy subjects. Eur. J. Appl. Physiol. 90 (1-2), 114–119.

Sandkuhler, J. (2002a). Proceedings of the 9th world congress on pain. Progress in Pain Research and Management 16.IASP Press, Seattle

Sandkuhler, J., 2000b. Learning and memory in pain pathways. Pain 88, 113–118.

Sandler, S.E., 1996. The management of low back pain in pregnancy. Man Ther 1 (4), 178–185.

Sato, A., Sato, Y., Schmidt, R., 1997. The impact of somatosensory input on autonomic functions. Springer-Verlag, Berlin.

Sato, A., Sato, Y., Shimura, M., et al., 2000. Calcitonin gene-related peptide produces skeletal muscle vasodilation following antidromic stimulation of unmyelinated afferents in the dorsal roots in rats. Neurosci. Lett. 283, 137–140.

Smith, C., Crowther, C., Beilby, J., 2002. Pregnancy outcome following women's participation in a randomized controlled trial of acupuncture to treat nausea and vomiting in early pregnancy. Complement Ther. Med. 10, 78–83.

Spence, D.W., Kayumov, L., Chen, A., et al., 2004. Acupuncture increases nocturnal melatonin secretion and reduces insomnia and anxiety: a preliminary report. J. Neuropsychiatry Clin. Neurosci. 16 (1), 19–28.

Stener-Victorin, E., 2000. Acupuncture in reproductive medicine. Göteborg University, Göteborg.

Streng, A., 2007. Summary of the randomised controlled trials from the German model projects on acupuncture for chronic pain. J. Chin. Med. 83, 5–10.

Stux, G., Pomeranz, B., 1991. Basics of acupuncture, 2nd edn. Springer-Verlag, Berlin.

Swan, P., Cook, T., 2003. Acupuncture in obstetric care. J. Assoc Chart. Physiotherapists in Women's Health 92, 63–68.

Ternov, N., Grennert, L., Aberg, A., et al., 2001. Acupuncture for lower back and pelvic pain in late pregnancy: a retrospective report on 167 consecutive cases. Pain Medicine 2 (3), 204–207.

Thomas, C., Napolitano, P., 2000. Use of acupuncture for managing chronic pelvic pain in pregnancy. J. Reprod. Health 45 (11), 944–946.

Travell, J.G., Simons, D.G., 1983. Myofascial pain and dysfunction: the trigger point manual, vol. i: Upper Limb. Williams and Wilkins, Baltimore.

Wang, J.D., Kuo, T.B.J., Yang, C.C.H., 2002. An alternative method to enhance vagal activities and suppress sympathetic activities in humans. Auton. Neurosci. 100 (1-2), 90–95.

Wedenberg, K., Moen, B., Norling, A., 2000. A prospective randomized study-comparing acupuncture with physiotherapy for low back and pelvic pain in pregnancy. Acta. Obstet. Gynecol. Scandinavia 79, 331–335.

Weider, C., Klede, M., Rukwied, R., et al., 2000. Acute effects of substance P and calcitonin gene-related peptide in human skin—a microdialysis study. J. Invest. Dermatol. 115, 1015–1020.

West, Z., 2001. Acupuncture in pregnancy and childbirth. Churchill Livingstone, London.

White, A., 1999. Neurophysiology of acupuncture analgesia. In: Ernst, E., White, A. (Eds.), Acupuncture: a scientific appraisal. Butterworth-Heinemann, Oxford, pp. 60–92.

Wiesenfeld-Hallin, Z., Zu, X., 1996. Plasticity of messenger function in primary afferents following nerve injury: implications for neuropathic pain. Prog. Brain Res. 110, 113–124.

Wu, M.T., Hsieh, J.C., Xiong, J., et al., 1999. Central nervous pathway for acupuncture stimulation: localisation of processing with functional MR imaging of the brain—preliminary experience. Radiology 212 (1), 133–141.

Wu, M.T., Sheen, J.M., Chuang, K.H., et al., 2002. Neuronal specificity of acupuncture response: an fMRI study with electroacupuncture. Neuroimage 16 (4), 1028–1037.

Yan, B., Xu, J., Wang, W., et al., 2005. Acupoint-specific fMRI patterns in human brain. Neurosci. Lett. 383 (3), 236–240.

Zaslawski, C., 2003. Clinical reasoning in traditional Chinese medicine: implications for clinical research. Clin. Acupunct. Orient. Med. 4 (2-3), 94–101.

Zhang, W.T., Jin, Z., Cui, G.H., et al., 2003. Relations between brain network activation and analgesic effect induced by low vs. high frequency electrical acupoint stimulation in different subjects: a functional magnetic resonance imaging study. Brain Res. 982 (2), 168–178.

Zhang, W.T., Jin, Z., Luo, F., et al., 2004. Evidence from brain imaging with fMRI supporting functional specificity of acupoints in humans. Neurosci. Lett. 354, 50–53.

Zusman, M., 2004. Mechanisms of musculoskeletal physiotherapy. Phys. Ther. Rev. 9, 39–49.

The temporomandibular joint

2

Allison Middleditch

CHAPTER CONTENTS

Introduction

The temporomandibular joint (TMJ) is formed by the articulation of the mobile condyle of the mandible with the glenoid fossa of the temporal bone.

The mandibular condyle and glenoid fossa are separated by a cartilaginous disc that is aneural and avascular, except at its periphery in the non-load-bearing areas. The disc aids in cushioning and dissipating joint loads, promotes joint stability when chewing, lubricates and nourishes the joint surfaces, and enables joint movements.

Medial and lateral ligaments secure the disc to the condyle. Anteriorly the disc is attached to the capsule and the superior fibres of the lateral pterygoid muscle. Posterior to the disc is the retrodiscal area that contains synovial membrane, blood vessels, nerves, loose connective tissue, fat, and ligaments. The retrodiscal ligaments help to maintain the condyle–disc relationship. The retrodiscal tissues are susceptible to high or repetitive loads such as may occur in prolonged dental work. This loading can cause inflammation of the retrodiscal tissues.

The TMJ is a source of head and facial pain; evidence suggests that the majority of patients improve with non-interventional treatment (Toller 1973; Sato 1998, 1999). The term temporomandibular disorder (TMD) is used to describe a variety of medical and dental conditions relating to TMJ dysfunction (TMJD), such as true pathology of the TMJ and involvement of the muscles of mastication.

Four categories of TMD are recognized:

- A myofascial component, the commonest form of TMD, in which there is pain or discomfort in the muscles that control the jaw, neck, and shoulder;

- An internal derangement of the joint evident with the presence of a mechanical disorder, such

DOI: 10.1016/B978-0-443-06782-2.00002-5

as jaw dislocation, disc displacement, or injury to the condyle;

- Degenerative joint disease of the joint space, such as OA or rheumatoid arthritis of the TMJ; and
- An inflammatory component caused by inflammation of the joint space due to a systemic inflammatory condition or trauma.

History and physical examination

There is considerable overlap in the clinical presentation of head, neck, and TMJ disorders, and many patients present with more than one condition contributing to their problem. It is essential that a detailed history is taken, and in addition to examining the TMJ, a thorough evaluation of the head, neck, and upper thoracic spine must be included in the assessment of TMJD.

Clinical presentation

Although pain is the commonest symptom of TMJD there are a variety of associated symptoms:

- Pain in the area of the joint that may radiate into the temples, ear, eyes, face, neck, and shoulder;
- Pain of TMJD origin often made worse by joint movements and activities that load the joint, such as clenching and chewing;
- Joint noises, painful clicking, popping, or grating noises that occur in the TMJ during joint movements; joint sounds in the TMJ are fairly common in asymptomatic individuals, and unless they are accompanied by pain or lack of movement, they do not usually require treatment;
- Limited movement, reduced functional range of movement (ROM), or locking of the jaw;
- Changing occlusion, a sudden change in the way in which the upper and lower jaw fit together or a change in facial symmetry;
- Muscle dysfunction, altered activity in the muscles of mastication, with spasm, tenderness, and trigger points; and
- Other symptoms, such as dizziness, headaches, earache, and hearing problems.

These symptoms may occur in isolation or any combination. When taking the history it is essential to identify factors that could be contributing to the problem and the following points should be considered:

- A detailed history of the physical factors;
- An understanding of how the problem affects normal function, e.g. talking, and eating;
- Oral and other habits (e.g. chewing gum);
- Recent dental work;
- Trauma to the joint (e.g. direct force or indirect force, such as a whiplash);
- Perception of bite discomfort; and
- Recent change in dentition (e.g. bridges, crowns, implants).

Emotional factors can contribute to head and facial pain; high stress levels have been associated with actions such as bruxism, clenching, and chewing gum that increase the loading and forces acting on the TMJ, and can also lead to muscle overuse, fatigue, and spasm. It is important to establish whether events at work or home are causing stress, and whether patients can identify a link between this and their symptoms.

Physical examination

The routine examination of the TMJ includes assessment of general posture, head and neck position, the influences of the thoracic curvature, and scapulae positions. The postural position of the mandible (PPM) is observed. This is the relaxed position of the jaw, and optimal PPM is achieved when the teeth are slightly apart and the lips together; the average space between the upper and lower teeth in the PPM is 3 mm (Beyron 1954). The tip of the tongue should be resting on the roof of the palate, just behind the central incisors, with no pressure of the tongue against the teeth. The lips should be closed and the individual should be able to breathe comfortably through their nose.

An assessment of the bony and soft tissue contours of the face is made. Symmetry of the face is examined by observing the bipupital, otic, and occlusal lines, which should all be parallel. Routine examination for malocclusion should be done and the following observed:

- Intercuspal position (when the back teeth are closed together);
- Missing teeth;

- Overbite (maxillary teeth anterior to mandibular teeth); and
- Crossbite (mandibular teeth anterior to maxillary teeth).

Movement abnormalities

Physiological movements of the cervical and thoracic spine should be tested, and any movement abnormalities and pain provocation noted. A full range of TMJ movements should be observed. The therapist observes the quality of movement, the range available, whether it is different from the patient's normal range, and deviations from symmetrical trajectories. It is useful to palpate the lateral condyle either laterally or posteriorly to feel the quality of movement. During mouth opening, a small indentation can be felt posterior to the lateral pole; in cases of hypermobility, a large indentation can be felt. If there is unilateral hypermobility, the mandible deviates towards the contralateral side of the hypomobile joint.

The ranges of movement assessed are depression, elevation, protraction, retraction, and left and right lateral movement. If the movement is limited or painful, the mandible can be gently moved passively to assess the true range of movement, and any locking or rigidity felt at the end of range can assist in clinical diagnosis. If extreme muscle spasm is present, there is a rigid end-feel, whereas opening limited by disc displacement without reduction does not have such a firm end-feel (Kraus 1994).

Joint sounds during active movements can be assessed using stethoscopic auscultation. Clicking, popping, grating, grinding, and clunking are often used to describe sounds accompanying TMJ movements. Other factors that should be taken into account are:

- Quality;
- Frequency;
- Palpability;
- Repeatability;
- Timing of joint sounds relative to movement and movement irregularities; and
- Pain with joint signs.

Joint noises are often a sign of disc displacement, but they can also be caused by joint surface irregularities of soft tissue perforation or joint fluid abnormalities (Takahashi 1992).

Accurate diagnosis of TMJD may require additional investigations, such as radiographs, three-dimensional computed tomography (CT) to assess for bony abnormalities, or magnetic resonance imaging (MRI) to assess the disc and the retrodiscal tissues. Disc position during physiological movements can be viewed using cine MRI.

Soft tissue dysfunction

Myofascial pain is a component of most types of TMJD. The major muscles of mastication are the masseter, temporalis, medial, and lateral pterygoid muscles; digastric muscle is an accessory muscle of mastication. The temporalis and masseter muscles can be observed for hypertrophy and atrophy, and should be palpated for muscle texture, tenderness, and myofascial trigger points (MTrPts). The medial and lateral pterygoid muscles are difficult to palpate, and therefore, assessment is carried out using intra-oral palpation (see Fig. 2.1). Tenderness in the facial muscles is a common finding in head and neck musculoskeletal disorders, and it is useful to palpate the muscle of mastication at rest, during muscle contraction, and when on a stretch. It is also important to assess the strength and control of the deep neck flexors and scapula stabilizers. The position of the cervical and thoracic spine affects the PPM, and cervical position has an immediate and lasting influence on mandibular position (Dombrady 1966).

Soft tissue dysfunction is treated with myofascial techniques, manual or acupuncture trigger point deactivation, muscle relaxation, and muscle re-education, where normal movement patterns are taught. Exercises to decrease masticatory muscle activity and,

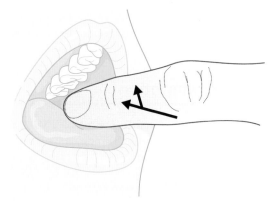

Figure 2.1 • Intra oral palpation.

hence, TMJ loading are taught (see below). These exercises also help to counteract habitual jaw bracing.

Lateral movement

The patient places the tongue in the resting position with the tip of the tongue on the roof of the palate, just behind the top teeth. The patient is instructed to keep the teeth lightly apart and gently move the jaw from side to side. Joint noises should not be heard and the tongue must remain relaxed during the jaw movements. The therapist should ensure that the patient moves the jaw and does not get just lip movement.

Open and closing movements

The patient places the tongue in the rest position, and opens and closes the mouth while holding the tongue in a relaxed position. The movement is initially performed slowly and then at speed. It is essential that the patient does not allow the back teeth to clench together during the exercise. It is suggested that this movement has a pumping effect on the joint (McCarthy et al 1992), in which intra-articular pressure is alternately increased and decreased, influencing the movement of fluid and dissolved particles in the interstitial tissues. This exercise also helps to control opening of the mouth and prevents overloading of the TMJ.

The patient should also be given exercises aimed at improving postural control including exercises for the deep neck flexors, scapular stabilizers, and thoracic extensors.

Dental appliances such as occlusal splints and night guards are commonly used to control pain arising from clenching or bruxism. These appliances may be worn during the day, but are generally worn at night, and can take several months to fully relieve the symptoms.

Joint dysfunction

Joint stiffness is a common feature of TMJD, and can be caused by capsular tightness, muscle spasm, or internal derangement of the disc. Internal derangement is the most common arthropathy and is characterized by progressive anterior disc displacement. On clinical examination joint noises are often heard. Stiffness can be treated with intra-oral passive

accessory manual mobilizations aimed at improving the gliding component of jaw motion. Joint mobilizations will not permanently relocate a displaced disc. In the first 10 to 15mm of mandibular opening, the mandibular condyle rotates beneath the disc. Forward translation of the mandible starts to occur between 10 and 15mm of mandibular opening, in conjunction with rotation; translation occurs in the upper joint space between the disc and the maxillary fossa. If translation is restricted, mouth opening may be limited to 20 to 25mm.

When TMJD is unilateral several common joint restrictions can be observed:

- During mouth opening, the mandible deflects towards the side of the affected joint and opening range is restricted;
- Restricted protrusion of the mandible and deflection of the mandible occurs towards the affected side; and
- Normal lateral movement of the jaw to the affected joint, and restricted lateral movement to the opposite side of the involved joint occurs.

Passive intra-oral joint mobilizations can be applied to the joint to increase range of movement, particularly the forward translation. These techniques are best applied with the patient in relaxed supine lying.

Distraction

This technique creates a distraction at the TMJ. The therapist stands on the opposite side of the involved joint, and using a gloved hand, places the thumb on top of the patient's molars on the affected side. The therapist's fingers are in a relaxed position on the patient's chin. The therapist's other hand stabilizes the patient's head. A gentle force is applied parallel to the longitudinal axis of the mandible; this can be a single, sustained distraction force or oscillatory movement. The mobilization can be performed as a purely passive movement, or in combination with the patient actively opening and closing his or her mouth.

Translation

The therapist uses the same hand placement as employed in the previous technique, but the force is applied so that the condyle moves in an anterior direction. This technique can also be performed as a sustained stretch, oscillatory movement and with active movement.

Lateral glide

The therapist stands on the opposite side to the joint involved, and using a gloved hand, places the thumb on the inside of the opposite molars; the other fingers are in a relaxed position over the jaw. The direction of force is lateral, towards the plinth and the patient's feet. Using a multidirectional force helps to avoid joint discomfort on the contralateral side that may occur if a purely lateral force is used (Kraus 1994).

Mobilizing joint exercises are given to help maintain the increased range of joint motion. The physiological effects of intra-oral techniques are not understood. Nitzan and Dolwick (1991) suggested that an increase in translation occurs as a result of a release of the adherence of the disc to the fossa caused by a reversible effect, such as a vacuum or viscous synovial fluid.

Conclusion

The causes of TMJD are multifactorial and, hence, treatment is individually designed. The majority of patients respond to conservative treatments and physiotherapy has an important role to play in the management of TMJD. In addition to the soft tissue and joint treatments outlined above, the physiotherapist can advise on posture, diet and stress management, and habit modification. The patient may also require treatment such as medication, maxillomandibular appliances, injections, and in rare cases surgery.

2.1 Acupuncture in the management of temporomandibular joint disorders

Jennie Longbottom

Introduction

Recent research has suggested that the TMJ and tension-type headaches overlap, sharing similar sensitization of the nociceptive pathways, dysfunction of the pain modulating systems, and contributing genetic factors. However, there are still distinct differences that need to be considered and explored further (Svensson 2007).

Acupuncture research

Uncontrolled or poorly controlled studies have suggested that acupuncture has a role in the treatment of TMJD (Corocos & Brandwein 1976; Heip & Stallard 1974; List & Helkimo 1987). A systematic review by Ernst and White (1999) of data from randomized controlled trials (RCTs) argue that acupuncture is a useful symptomatic treatment of TMJD. This analysis reported on three trials, all performed in Scandinavia, for treatment of TMJD or craniomandibular disorders. All these studies suggested that acupuncture was an effective treatment modality that seemed to be comparable with combinations of standard therapy or occlusal splints alone. The results described improvements in both pain and joint function and one study showed that the effects were sustained and noticeable even one year after therapy (List and Helkimo 1992). However, it must be noted that none of the trials were performed with blinded evaluators or gave explicit details of randomization, and more importantly, none were designed to exclude the placebo effect of acupuncture, and therefore, did not account for the patient's expectation of treatment.

More recent studies (Goddard 2002; Smith et al 2007) appear to have addressed this issue. Goddard (2002) compared the reduction of masseter myofascial pain with acupuncture and sham acupuncture. There was a statistically significant difference in pain tolerance with acupuncture ($p = 0.027$), and a statistically significant reduction in face pain ($p = 0.003$), neck pain ($p = 0.011$), and headache ($p = 0.015$) with perception of real acupuncture. Pain tolerance in the masticatory muscles increased significantly more with real than sham acupuncture.

Studies have shown that the temporalis muscle is involved in between one- and two-thirds of patients presenting with TMJ problems (Butler et al 1975; Burch 1977), whereas masseter muscle dysfunction results in severely restricted jaw movement and function (Kellgren 1938; Solberg et al 1979).

Smith et al (2007) demonstrated in double-blinded RCTs that real acupuncture had a greater influence on the clinical outcome measures of TMJ myofascial pain than sham acupuncture. This study provided clinical evidence to support the analgesic effect of acupuncture as well as of its physiological effects via the endogenous-opiate-mediated pathways. This was in direct disagreement with several meta-analyses that have indicated that acupuncture produces little more than placebo effects (Ezzo et al 2008; Mayer 2000; Smith 2000). Smith et al (2000) demonstrated that acupuncture seemed to have a positive influence on the signs and symptoms of TMJ myofascial pain.

Little research exists about the treatment of this condition by physiotherapists despite its suggested relationship with the cervical spine and the profession's involvement in the multidisciplinary management of TMJD. A systematic review of physiotherapy interventions by McNeely et al (2006) provided a broad outline of the treatment options available to a physiotherapist treating TMJ dysfunction. Most studies reviewed were of poor methodological quality, and therefore, caution was taken when interpreting their findings. Results supported the use for active and passive oral exercises, and exercises to improve posture as an effective way of reducing symptoms associated with TMJD. Studies pertaining to acupuncture intervention showed improvements in pain; however, needling was not shown to be better than sham acupuncture or occlusal splinting, and therefore, there was inadequate information to either support or dismiss the use of acupuncture in TMJD. There was poor or little evidence to support the use of other treatment modalities.

Myofascial component

Despite the inconclusive research supporting acupuncture for the TMJD, the positive results shown with acupuncture in other musculoskeletal conditions and the emerging evidence of success with TMJ management should encouraged practitioners to use acupuncture as an adjunct to manual therapy in the management of joint dysfunction.

The most common presentation of TMJ pain and dysfunction tends to emanate from the myofascial components; however, there is a strong correlation between TMJ pain, anxiety, and the presentation of visceral dysfunctions, such as irritable bowel syndrome (Spiller et al 2007), urinary dysfunction, chronic fatigue, and fibromyalgia (Spiller et al 2007), further demonstrating classical observations of high levels of sympathetic response and altered stress circuits, triggered by anxiety. It is essential that the therapist assess not only the state of the musculoskeletal presentation, but also the emotional component of the pain mechanism. It has been well documented that the hypothalamus will tune the body (homeostasis) to facilitate intention and emotional demands (van Griensven 2005). Adequate examination of signs and symptoms suggestive of hypothalamus–pituitary–adrenal axis (HPA) involvement with increased levels of corticotropin-releasing factor and adrenalergic and adrenocortical effects, stimulating anterior pituitary secretion and adrenocorticotropin hormone, reflect the pluripotent role of these neuropeptides in controlling autonomic, immunological, and emotional responses to stress (Turnbull & Rivier 1997).

Symptoms may present with segmentally related conditions suggesting involvement and hyperactivity of the sympathetic nervous system (SNS) rather than one segmental involvement, and, thus, assessment questions relating to the TMJ must involve segmental identification and cranial nerve involvement (Fig. 2.2). This may also require knowledge of other visceral symptom response, such as palpitations, headaches, swallowing changes, pain in the upper limbs, or hypochondriac pain. Patients may demonstrate exacerbation of symptoms associated with bowel or urinary function, and the more widespread the symptoms involved, the more likelihood there is that central responses may be contributing alongside the myofascial component. If patients present with these diffuse symptoms, every effort must be made to incorporate techniques that may address the initial myofascial presentation, but provide increased parasympathetic stimulation. In such cases, the use of acupuncture directly targeting known parasympathetic points (Table 2.1) or segmental points (Fig. 2.3) may be of value. These

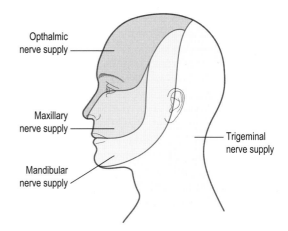

Figure 2.2 • Trigeminal nerve and dermatomal distribution.

Table 2.1 Segmental acupuncture points for TMJ

Meridian	Point	Action
Triple Energizer	TE21	Co1/Co2 segmental inhibition
Small Intestine	SI19	Co1/Co2 segmental inhibition
Gall Bladder	GB2 GB20	Co1/Co2 segmental inhibition
Bladder	BL10	Co1/Co2 segmental inhibition
Governor Vessel	GV16/15/20	Co1/Co2 segmental inhibition
TE21 + SI3 + GB2	Needled together	Parasympathetic activation

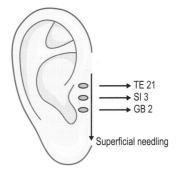

Figure 2.3 • Segmental points.

points should be used together with relaxation, cognitive behaviour therapy, hypnosis, and other such modalities to reduce sympathetic excitatory states.

If there is an inflammatory component to the pain presentation, then distal points are employed to stimulate DNIC (Table 2.2), activate the HPA axis, and reduce both pain and inflammatory cytokine activity.

The masseter and temporalis muscles are innervated by the anterior and posterior branches of the mandibular and temporal division of the trigeminal nerve (Figs 2.4 and 2.5), and are the first to contract in extreme emotional tension or stress (Laskin 1969).

It is the present author's clinical experience that the treatment of MTrPt deactivation should accompany acupuncture, often using the Shenmen auricular point (Fig. 2.6), either with needling or auricular seeds, in order to augment patient relaxation and coping strategies and empower self-management whilst stimulating the parasympathetic nervous system (PNS).

As an adjunct to MTrPt deactivation, or as an empowerment of patient management of sympathetic symptoms, auricular acupuncture may be used by the patient, in the form of auricular seeds, and by the physiotherapist to aid relaxation whilst attending to painful MTrPt deactivation.

Auricular acupuncture

Auricular acupuncture (AA) is used for various autonomic disorders in clinical practice. It has been

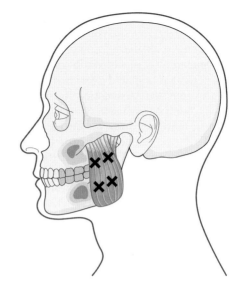

Figure 2.4 • Masseter trigger point.

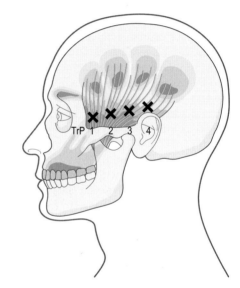

Figure 2.5 • Temporalis trigger point.

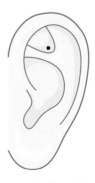

Figure 2.6 • Shenmen auricular point.

Table 2.2 Distal points for acute TMJ

Point	Rationale
LI4	Important analgesic point, influences pain and inflammation of the head region. Yuan source point, promotes Qi, discharges exogenous pathogens and heat.
LIV3	Important analgesic point. Headache and dizziness point. Shu stream point, earth point. Clears fire and heat, invigorates blood.
Masseter, temporalis, SCM, suboccipital triangle, splenis capitis, medical and lateral ptyergiod trigger points	Deactivation of the various dysfunctional motor end plates
BL10	Influences headaches and pain in the neck or shoulders, relaxes tendons, and facilitates the flow of Qi in the Bladder meridian
GB20	Influences headache, ear disorders, and dizziness. Clears the brain and relaxes the tendons

theorized that different auricular areas have a distinct influence on somatotropic and viscerotropic representation in the auricle (Gao et al 2008; Nogier 1987); hence, a disorder from a particular part of the body is treated by the corresponding point in the ear (Oleson et al 1980). Auricular acupuncture has been used for pain relief (Goertz 2006; Usichenko 2005), anxiety, and sleep disorders (Chen et al 2007) together with various autonomic disorders such as hypertension (Huang & Liang 1992), gastrointestinal disorders (Huang & Liang 1992); and urinary tract symptoms (Capodice et al 2007). However, there is very little evidence for Nogier's (1987) theory of AA; its efficacy is still a matter of conjecture.

The auricle receives innervations from both cervical and cranial nerves:

- the auricular branch of the vagal nerve;
- the great auricular nerve; and
- the auriculo-temporal nerve. (Peuker & Filler 2002)

Evidence from anatomical studies and physiological studies does not support the concept of a highly specific functional map of the ear; rather, there appears to be a general pattern of autonomic changes in response to AA, with variable intensity depending on the area of stimulation. Physiologically, the inferior concha appears to be the most powerful site (Gao et al 2008), although it is recommended that practitioners monitor the auricular areas and the responses achieved in order to determine clinical effects and effectiveness management for each pain presentation.

Traditionally, the Shenmen AA point (Fig. 2.6) has been used to calm emotions and stabilize the SNS via cranial and autonomic supply. Experimental research suggests that the PNS is activated after AA at Shenmen, while the SNS is constrained, resulting in decreased heart and pulse rates and an increase in low-frequency electroencephalograph waves (Hsu et al 2008).

A choice of AA (Table 2.1) for parasympathetic activation, local segmental points for dorsal horn and pain gate inhibitory effects, and distal points for DNIC (Table 2.2) is available. The point selection will be determined by the presenting pain and emotional status of the patient at each therapeutic interaction.

 ## Case Study 1

Brigit Murray

Introduction

The subject was a 44-year-old female, who was referred to the present author's clinic by her consultant rheumatologist for treatment of a recent flare-up of mild seronegative arthritis, which had resulted in significant neck and jaw pain. Her symptoms began one month prior to attending the clinic and had a gradual onset. Initially, jaw stiffness gradually worsened and the subject developed occipital pain and earache. A recent X-ray showed degeneration of her C2 to C3 and C3 to C4 discs.

The subject worked part-time and her lifestyle was stressful: her mother had recently had a stroke, her father was ill, and her brother was going through a divorce. The pain interfered with normal jaw activities, such as chewing, eating hard foods and talking. The subject admitted to being anxious about the persistent pain, and noted frequent oral parafunctional habits, including clenching, night grinding and sleep talking, leading to waking with a sore jaw, an inability to open her mouth wide, and pain on eating and cervical movements.

Subjective assessment

The subjective assessment revealed that the subject's bilateral jaw pain was greater on the left side than on the right. This occurred on a daily basis and was constant. The intensity varied during the course of the day, particularly after chewing and use of the jaw. Other features included:

- Constant left side earache;
- Constant bilateral occipital pain;
- Difficulty chewing;
- An inability to open the mouth wide enough in the morning to clean the teeth;
- Dizziness;
- Toothache on the left side; and
- Frequent waking during the night.

Objective examination

The following findings were noted on examination:

- The subject's head was held in slight left-side flexion;
- The left shoulder was slightly elevated;
- Cervical ROM was significantly reduced in all directions and painful, particularly with flexion and bilateral rotation;
- Neurological testing was negative;

(Continued)

Case Study 1 (Continued)

- Palpation revealed irritable joints from C0 to C4, with a particular focus at C0 to C1 and C1 to C2; the irritable joints were very stiff bilaterally;
- She was able to open her jaw by 1.5 cm actively (one finger-width between her front teeth) and her left lateral translation approximately 5 mm;
- All jaw movements were restricted and painful;
- Palpation of the TMJ on opening revealed normal translation and a fine crepitus on the left;
- Palpation of the masticatory and cervical muscles showed tenderness in her anterior, middle, and posterior masseter muscles duplicating her jaw and tooth pain;
- Palpation of the anterior temporalis muscle reproduced her ear and cheek pain;
- Palpation of the lateral and medial pterygoid muscles replicated her jaw pain; and
- On later assessment, it was discovered that palpation of the suboccipital triangle and posterior cervical muscles replicated her occipital pain.

Treatment approach

This case was treated as an acute flare-up of myofascial pain in the muscles of mastication that was associated with her underlying chronic arthritis. Factors contributing to this included oral parafunctional habits, stressful life events, a mild anxiety reaction to these events, and upper cervical stiffness. Acupuncture was used in conjunction with manual therapy initially (Tables 2.3 and 2.4), although manual therapy appeared to irritate her occipital pain and was ceased.

Treatment aims

The following aims of treatment were defined:
- Reduction of mastication pain (especially the subject's inability to eat or communicate because of her jaw pain) and occipital pain;
- Improvement of joint mobility in cervical spine;
- Restoration of her normal cervical and masticatory myofascial function and improvement of her cervical muscular stability; and
- Improvement of stress management.

The following outcome measures were chosen:
- The visual analogue scale (VAS) for masticatory pain;
- The VAS for occipital pain;
- ROM of jaw opening; and
- ROM of cervical spine.

The subject was recommended to be fitted with an occlusal splint to help reduce the effect of her night grinding and, therefore, minimize the morning stiffness (Table 2.5).

Treatment 2 (day 5)

Prior to treatment the subject had seen an orthodontist who was making her an occlusal splint. She now reported being able to sleep better and a decrease in headaches since her last session, and she felt that she was able to open her mouth wider. Therefore, treatment was repeated; however, the MTrPts in the masseter muscle were externally needled and acupressure was applied inside her mouth to the lateral pterygoid muscle.

Table 2.3 Acupoints selected during treatment programme

Meridian	Point	He Sea Point	Action
Triple Energizer	TE5	TE10	Clears inflammation and swelling Calms the spirit
Small Intestine	SI3	SI8	Clears inflammation and swelling Calms the spirit
Gall Bladder	GB41	GB34	Clears the head Benefit joints and soft tissues Clears the channel

Table 2.4 Treatment 1

Treatment no.	Points used	Needle size	De Qi	Adverse effects
1	LI4 bilaterally	30 mm	Yes	No
	LIV3 bilaterally	30 mm	Yes	No
	Masseter TrPt	Acupressure	N/A	No
Treatment guidelines	Needles in situ 20 minutes Stimulated once as strong De Qi achieved			
Other treatment modalities used	Heat and cervical mobilization			
Home exercises	Masseter stretch			

(Continued)

Case Study 1 (Continued)

Table 2.5 Outcome measurements treatment 1

Measure	Pre-treatment	Post-treatment
Masticatory pain	VAS 100/100	VAS 90/100
Occipital pain	VAS 80/100	VAS 60/100
Jaw opening	1 finger-width (1.5 cm)	1 finger-width

Table 2.6 Outcome measurements treatment 2

Measure	Pre-treatment	Post-treatment
Masticatory pain	VAS 70/100	VAS 80/100 (jaw was very achy post needling)
Occipital pain	VAS 70/100	VAS 60/100
Jaw opening	1 finger-width	2 finger-widths

Table 2.7 Outcome measurements treatment 3

Measure	Pre-treatment	Post-treatment
Masticatory pain	VAS 40/100	VAS 30/100
Occipital pain	VAS 60/100	VAS 60/100
Jaw opening	2 finger-widths tightly	2 finger-widths

The subject was taught how to apply acupressure to both muscles as a home exercise (Table 2.6).

Treatment 3 (day 8)

Pre-treatment, the subject reported some difficulty holding her head up and more problems with sleeping. She was able to eat hard foods with minimal discomfort and talk without pain. The subject also had right-sided headache and earache. On re-assessment the subject had active MTrPts in the suboccipital triangle, posterior cervical muscles and right temporalis. This was addressed with MTrPt needling (Table 2.7).

Treatment 4

Pre-treatment the subject reported no problems with sleeping and she was able to eat a normal diet. She felt that the cervical mobilization was irritating her cervical spine. Bladder 10 (BL0) and Gall Bladder 20 (GB20) were introduced bilaterally, for increased segmental and parasympathetic response, whilst Large Intestine 4 (LI4) and Liver 3 (LIV3) were used bilaterally (Table 2.8).

Treatment 5

Pre-treatment the subject reported that her jaw range of motion, activity, and pain remained settled. Cervical

Table 2.8 Outcome measurements treatment 4

Measure	Pre-treatment	Post-treatment
Masticatory pain	VAS 0/100	VAS 0/100
Occipital pain	VAS 5/100	VAS 5/100
Jaw opening	2 finger-widths	2 finger-widths

Table 2.9 Outcome measurements treatment 5

Measure	Pre-treatment	Post-treatment
Masticatory pain	VAS 0/100	VAS 0/100
Occipital pain	VAS 40/10	VAS 1/100
Jaw opening	2 finger-widths	2 finger-widths

ROM was still very stiff in all directions, but pain had settled and she felt more optimistic.

Acupuncture was used again to points BL10, GB20, LI4, and LIV3 bilaterally; however, she was positioned in sitting, leaning forward onto the plinth and supported by pillows, since she attributed some of her dizziness to being previously positioned in prone.

Addressing the major limitation of jaw range of motion and pain associated with mastication using myofascial acupuncture meant that the subject was able to talk and eat with minimum pain within one treatment session. Pain was reduced from 10/100 to 0/100 VAS within four sessions. The inclusion of an occlusion splint in treatment also appeared to have helped reduce pain, but more importantly, this reduced nocturnal teeth grinding and, therefore, prevented further aggravation of the condition (Table 2.9).

With the lessening of her pain, the subject reported a reduction of stress levels and an elevation in her mood. She felt better able to cope with the demanding events in the family and noted a decline in parafunctional habits such as jaw clenching during the day, and had activated the stress management programme.

Discussion

The majority of this subject's pain experience was myofascial, originating from MTrPts (Simons et al 1998). The underlying mechanism of this condition is unknown, but the literature best supports the theory that MTrPts result from altered activity at the motor end-plate (Whyte-Ferguson & Gerwin, 2005). The effect of this can be seen in the rapid return of jaw function and the reduction of pain during mastication achieved after successful MTrPt deactivation, providing some evidence for the clinical effectiveness of acupuncture in the management of TMJD.

References

Beyron, H.L., 1954. Characteristics of functionally optimal occlusion and principles of occlusal rehabilitation. J. Am. Dent. Assoc. 48, 648.

Bradnam, L., 2007. A proposed clinical reasoning model for Western acupuncture. J. Acupunct Assoc Chart Physiotherapists 1, 21–30.

Burch, J., 1977. Occlusion related to craniofacial pain. In: Alling, C.C., Mahan, P.E. (Eds.), Facial pain, 2nd edn. Lea & Febiger, Philadelphia, pp. 70–174.

Butler, J., Folke, L., Bandt, C., 1975. A descriptive survey of signs and symptoms associated with myofascial pain-dysfunction syndrome. J. Am. Dent. Assoc. 90, 635–639.

Capodice, Z., Jin, D., Bernis, D., et al., 2007. A pilot study on acupuncture for lower urinary tract symptoms related to chronic prostatitis/chronic pelvic pain. Chin. Med. 2, 1–2.

Chen, H., Shi, C., Ng., et al., 2007. Auricular acupuncture treatment for insomnia: A systematic review. J. Altern. Complement. Med. 13, 669–676.

Corocos, J., Brandwein, R.E., 1976. Treatment of temporomandibular joint pain by acupuncture. Am. J. Acupunct. 4, 157–160.

Dombrady, L., 1966. Investigation into the transient instability of the rest position. J. Prosthet. Dent. 16, 479.

Ernst, E., White, A., 1999. Acupuncture as a treatment for temporomandibular joint dysfunction: a systematic review of randomised trials. Arch. Otolaryngol. Head 125, 269–272.

Ezzo, J., Berman, B., Hadhazy, V.A., et al., 2008. Is acupuncture effective for the treatment of chronic pain? A systematic review. Pain 86, 217–225.

Gao, X., Zhang, S., Zhu, B., et al., 2008. Investigation of specificity of auricular acupuncture points in regulation of autonomic function in anaesthetised rats. Auton. Neurosci. 138 (1–2), 50–56.

Goddard, G., 2005. Short-term pain reduction with acupuncture for chronic orofacial pain patients. Med. Sci. Monit. 11 (2), 71–74.

Goertz, C.M.H., Niemtzow, R., Burns, S.M., et al., 2006. Auricular acupuncture in the treatment of acute pain syndromes: a pilot study. Mil. Med. 171, 1010–1014.

Heip, N., Stallard, R.E., 1974. Acupuncture: a valuable adjunct in the treatment of myofascial pain. J. Dent. Res. 53, 203–205.

Hsu, C., Weng, C., Sun, M., et al., 2008. Evaluation of scalp and auricular acupuncture on EEG, HRV and PRV. Am. J. Chin. Med. 35 (2), 219–230.

Huang, H., Liang, S., 1992. Acupuncture at otoacupoint heart for treatment of vascular hypertension. J. Tradit. Chin. Med. 12, 133–136.

Kandell, E.R., Schwartz, J.H., Jessell, T.M., 2000. Principles of Neural Science, 4th edn. McGraw-Hill, New York, pp. 482–486.

Kellgren, J., 1938. Observations on referred pain arising from muscle. Clin. Sci. 3, 175–190.

Kraus, S., 1994. History and physical examination for TMD. In: Kraus, S. (Ed.), Clinics in Physical Therapy, Temporomandibular Disorders, 2nd edn. Churchill Livingstone, New York.

Laskin, D., 1969. Aetiology of the pain-dysfunction syndrome. J. Am. Dent. Assoc. 79, 147–153.

List, T., Helkimo, M., 1987. Acupuncture in the treatment of patients with chronic facial pain and mandibular dysfunction. Swed. Dent. J. 11, 83–92.

List, T., Helkimo, M., Andersson, S., Carlsson, G., 1992. Acupuncture and occlusal splint therapy in the treatment of craniomandibular disorders: a comparative study. Swed. Dent. J. 16, 125–141.

Mayer, D., 2000. Acupuncture: an evidence-based review of clinical literature. Annu. Rev. Med. 51, 49–63.

McCarthy, M.R., O'Donoghue, P.C., Yates, C.K., et al., 1992. The clinical use of continuous passive motion in physical therapy. Phys. Ther. 15, 132.

McNeely, M.L., Armijo, O.S., Magee, D.J., 2006. A systematic review of the effectiveness of physical therapy interventions for temporomandibular disorders. Phys. Ther. 86 (5), 710–725.

Melzack, R., Wall, P., 1996. The challenge of pain. Penguin, London.

Nitzan, D.W., Dolwick, F.M., 1991. An alternative explanation for the genesis of close-lock symptoms in the internal derangement process. J. Oral. Maxillofac. Surg. 49, 810.

Nogier, P., 1987. Points Reflexes Auriculares. Maisonneuve, Moulins-les-Metz, France.

Oleson, T.D., Kroening, R.J., Bresler, D.E., 1980. An experimental evaluation of auricular diagnosis: the somatotopic mapping or musculoskeletal pain at ear acupuncture points. Pain 8, 217–299.

Peuker, E., Filler, T., 2002. The nerve supply of the human auricle. Clin. Anat. 15, 35–37.

Sato, S., Takahashi, K., Kawamura, H., et al., 1998. The natural course of nonreducing disk replacement of the temporomandibular joint: changes in condylar mobility and radiographic alterations at one-year follow-up. Int. J. Oral. Maxillofac. Surg. 27, 173.

Sato, S., Sakamoto, M., Kawamura, H., et al., 1999. Long-term changes in clinical signs and symptoms and disc position and morphology in patients with nonreducing disc displacement in the temporomandibular joint. J. Oral. Maxillofac. Surg. 57, 23.

Simons, D.G., Travell, J., Simons, L.S., 1998. Myofascial pain and dysfunction: the trigger point manual, vol. i: Upper half of body, 2nd edn. Lippincott Williams & Wilkins, Baltimore.

Smith, L.A., Oldman, D.A., McQuay, H.J., et al., 2000. Teasing apart quality and validity in systematic reviews: an example from acupuncture trials in chronic neck and back pain. Pain 86, 119–132.

Smith, P., Mosscrop, D., Davies, S., et al., 2007. The efficacy of acupuncture in the treatment of temporomandibular joint myofascial pain: a randomised control trial. J. Dent. 35 (3), 259–267.

Solberg, W., Woo, M., Houston, J., 1979. Prevalence of mandibular dysfunction in young adults. J. Am. Dent. Assoc. 98, 25–34.

Spiller, R., Aziz, Q., Creed, F., et al., 2007. Guidelines on the irritable bowel syndrome: mechanisms and practical management. Gut 56, 1770–1798.

Svensson, P., 2007. Muscle pain in the head: overlap between temporomandibular disorder and tension-type headaches. Curr. Opin. Neurol. 20 (3), 320–325.

Toller, P.A., 1973. Osteoarthritis of the mandibular condyle. Br. Dent. J. 134, 223.

Trinh, K.V., Graham, N., Gross, A.R., et al., 2007. Acupuncture for neck disorders. Spine 32 (2), 236–243.

Turnbull, A.V., Rivier, C., 1997. Corticotropin releasing factor (CRF) and endocrine responses to stress: CRF receptors, binding protein and related peptides. Proceedings of Society for Experimental Biological Science 215, 1–10.

Ulett, G.A., Han, S.P., 2002. The Biology of Acupuncture. Warren H Green, St Louis, MO.

Usichenko, T.I., Dinse, M., Lysenyuk, V.P., et al., 2006. Auricular acupuncture for pain relief after total hip arthroplasty. Acupunct. Electrother. Res. 31 (3–4), 213–221.

van Griensven, H., 2005. Pain in Practice: Theory and Treatment Strategies for Manual Therapists. Butterworth Heinemann, Oxford.

Whyte-Ferguson, L.W., Gerwin, R., 2005. Clinical Mastery in the Treatment of Myofascial Pain. Lippincott Williams and Wilkins, Philadelphia.

Cervical spine

3

Neil Tucker

CHAPTER CONTENTS

Introduction

The application of the biopsychosocial and evidence-based models directs the assessment and management of cervical spine disorders. In physiotherapy, the biopsychosocial model recognizes the presence of injury, pathology, and pain, and integrates them with psychological and social issues to manage cervical spine dysfunction and pain syndromes (Jones et al 2002). Rehabilitation of the cervical spine involves pain management, physical therapies, assurance, explanation, education, self-help strategies, ergonomics, and most importantly, exercise.

Assessment

Comprehensive history

Subjective history taking should attempt to identify the problem and its cause. Special questions of individuals with cervical spine injuries may focus on symptoms of headache and dizziness, the mechanism and intensity of trauma, symptoms suggesting cervical artery insufficiency, and interaction with upper limb activity. Clinicians must gain enough information so that they can develop an effective hypothesis that allows them to apply their own knowledge of pathobiology and effectively manage their patient. Consideration should be given to potential red flags (e.g. serious life-threatening pathology) and yellow flags (e.g. psychosocial indicators).

Objective assessment

The aim of manual assessment of the cervical spine is to identify the presence of any organic musculoskeletal physical impairment related to the patient's pain.

DOI: 10.1016/B978-0-443-06782-2.00003-7

The initial focus should be on the investigation of any subjective findings, which may indicate cervical artery insufficiency, craniocervical ligament instability, or neurological lesion. Early detection of the presence of any of these factors may impose further restrictions on examination and treatment. Any potential symptoms must be monitored carefully throughout the examination.

Cervical artery insufficiency and manipulative therapy

Research investigating what was previously called vertebral artery testing now suggests that therapists should now be aware of and incorporate the entire cervical blood flow into their diagnostic triage. Currently, there is a move away from the cardinal vertebral artery signs (Thiel & Rix 2005) and functional pre-screening tests in patients who are susceptible to a spontaneous dissection event during manual or manipulative therapy (Kerry et al 2007). Clinicians should be aware that symptoms of cervical artery dissection are diverse, and not only include the classic brainstem signs and symptoms, but can also include symptoms such as unilateral head and neck pain (Sturzenegger 1994). The latest Australian Physiotherapy Association guidelines (APA 2006; Magarey et al 2004) suggest that history taking is the best indicator to use when identifying those patients who may be at risk. Key questioning around atherosclerotic risk factors and repeated or significant trauma are two areas that may help a clinician in their clinical reasoning (Mitchell 2002).

Craniocervical ligament instability testing

As with cervical artery testing, craniocervical ligament instability testing has shown to have poor sensitivity and specificity (Cattrysse et al 1997). Therefore, a comprehensive history and a decision made from a clinician's index of suspicion should guide the management of a patient. Krakenes et al (2002) estimated a probable incidence of alar ligament injuries in 39% of patients with chronic whiplash associated disorder (WAD). A history of upper cervical pain post trauma, radiological evidence of craniocervical abnormalities, congenital craniocervical anomalies, and degenerative conditions, which may be associated with craniocervical instability, can all be indications for further investigation or testing. Symptoms of cervical artery insufficiency, cord signs, and parenthesis of the lips or tongue (compression of the hypoglossal nerve at the ventral ramus of C2) may raise the index of suspicion of craniocervical instability. The classic tests used clinically are the Sharp-Purser test (transverse ligament), the tectorial membrane flexion test, and alar ligament stress tests (Aspinall 1990).

Neurological examination

Many nerve root injuries go undiagnosed (Gifford 2001) because the nervous system often provokes vague distributions of pain as well as the classic dermatomal distributions. A good neurological examination provides key information about the structures involved, the patient's prognosis, and the efficacy of treatment. A comprehensive history, combined with neurological and musculoskeletal examination, has been shown to provide good diagnostic accuracy in patients with cervical radiculopathy (Wainner et al 2003). Detailed neurological examinations have been described in the literature (Butler 2000). Table 3.1 outlines the sensory signature zones (Butler 2000), associated muscle tests, and muscle stretch reflex for the mid- to lower cervical spine.

Adverse neural dynamics

A neural provocation or neurodynamic test is a sequence of movements designed to assess the mechanics and physiology of that part of the nervous system by elongating the length of the nerve (Coppieters et al 2002). The following tests are useful in the clinical picture of cervical spine dysfunction:

- Passive neck flexion test;
- Brachial plexus provocation test; and
- Slump tests.

Both the slump and upper limb neurodynamic test have shown to heighten responses in subjects with chronic WAD (Sterling et al 2002; Yeung et al 1997). Jull (2001) found that there was a 10% increase in the incidence of sensitized neuromeningeal structures using the passive neck flexion test in chronic headache sufferers.

Observation

Forward head posture has historically been linked with cervical dysfunction (Janda 1994). Currently,

Table 3.1 Neurological examination for the mid- to lower cervical spine

	Sensory (signature zone)	Motor	Reflex
C5	Distal 1/3 of lateral upper arm	Shoulder abduction (deltoid, C5–6)	Biceps (C5–6)
C6	Thumb	Elbow flexion (biceps brachii, C5–6)	Biceps (C5–6)
C7	Middle finger	Elbow extension (triceps, C6–8)	Triceps (C7–8)
C8	5th finger and ulnar aspect of the palm	Thumb extension (extensor pollicis longus, C7–8)	Triceps (C7–8)
T1	Proximal 1/3 of medial forearm	Finger abduction and adduction (interossei and lumbrical, C8–T1)	

the literature associating forward head posture and cervical spine pain is not strong (Dalton & Coutts 1994; Griegel-Morris et al 1992; Haughie et al 1995; Johnson 1998; Treleaven et al 1994; Watson & Trott 1993). The importance of any observations must be put into context on a multifactorial basis. Deviations may be normal variations. Postural differences may reflect structural, muscle, joint, and neural system sensitivity, be reactive to pain states, or may reflect psychological factors.

Active range of movement

There is now enough research indicating that disorders of the cervical musculoskeletal system are characterized by a reduction in range of motion (ROM) (Dall'Alba et al 2001; Hall & Robinson 2004; Zwart 1997). Deficits in ROM appear not to be pathology specific; however, assessment of active ROM may give an insight about the structures affected. Distribution of pain associated with bilateral rotation, side bend, upper cervical spine flexion, lower cervical spine flexion, and extension, plus extension rotation quadrants, should be recorded. Active tests may be progressed by:

- Applying overpressure;
- Changing the velocity or repetition of the movement; and
- Applying axial compression or distraction.

Techniques for segmental localization can also be useful; for example, rotation performed in full flexion to assess upper cervical spine rotation (C1 to C2) has been shown to be limited in the majority of cervicogenic headache sufferer (Hall & Robinson 2004). Sustained positioning can also be of benefit, especially when subtle pain originating from the nervous system is apparent. The key findings of the active movement examination should be recorded. This information should lead the practitioner in the direction for further physical examination and provide important outcome measures.

Manual assessment

Passive, manual assessment can be broken down into:

- Passive accessory intervertebral movements (PAIVMs); and
- Passive physiological intervertebral movements (PPIVMs).

PAIVMs are short lever techniques used during assessment of the cervical spine and are also beneficial in the treatment of acute conditions or in elderly patients (Hing et al 2003). PPIVMs use combined movements to access restriction in a joint using a longer lever.

The manual examination provides basic in vivo measures of pain reproduction and the elastic properties of the viscoelastic tissues of the spinal motion segment. This information should support or reject the clinician's hypothesis gleaned from the initial subjective and objective findings. A clinician's ability to detect a symptomatic segment in the cervical spine has been a point of debate, which questions the basis for the manual examination. Jull et al (1988) performed the pioneering study comparing manual examination to local segmental blocks in the cervical spine. In this study, the experienced manual therapist correctly detected all 15 symptomatic segments in patients with cervical pain. However, King et al (2007) reproduced Jull et al's study using a larger number of subjects and new local segmental blocking techniques. The results of this later study showed significantly lower levels of accuracy in the manual examination. There continues to be discussion about whether the local segmental block is an accurate diagnostic tool and about other methodological differences published in the studies. The manual examination has also been shown to have poor inter-tester and intra-tester reliability with regard to detecting stiffness (Maher & Adams 1994).

Motor and sensory assessment

There is now a significant amount of research demonstrating that there are impairments to the motor system associated with cervical spine dysfunction that do not spontaneously resolve (Falla et al 2004; Jull 2000; Tjell & Rosenhall 1998; Tjell et al 2003). This research has shown that there is impairment to the deep stability muscles of the cervical spine and shoulder girdle, and in some instances, oculomotor and global proprioceptive strategies.

Asking the patient to sit up and assume what they perceive is correct posture may be a useful way for assessing the patient's ability to assume a normal upright position. Clinically, if there is an obvious postural dysfunction, it is useful to alter the apparent problem and assess whether it affects the patient's symptoms. Consideration should be given to the appropriate sitting, standing, or functional positions. Special attention should be given to the interaction of the shoulder girdle and cervical spine. Loss of the feed-forward postural mechanisms associated with upper limb movement (Falla et al 2004) and low-load holding capacity of the deep cervical flexors and scapulothoracic muscles (Grant et al 1997) have been associated with chronic cervical spine dysfunction. Assessment of shoulder elevation and simple workstation tasks can be clinically useful in detecting dysfunction. The two most common postural dysfunctions affecting the upper limb and cervical spine are a downwardly rotated scapular and a protracted, elevated scapula (Janda 1994; Sahrmann 2002).

Specific analysis of the deep flexors of the cervical spine can be done by looking at a patient's active cervical spine extension and the craniocervical flexion test (C-CFT). Active cervical spine extension tests a patient's ability to eccentrically use the deep flexors muscles. Dysfunction is commonly seen either when a patient will not allow the head centre of rotation to pass behind the frontal plane or when they perform a compensatory strategy, therefore loading the osseoligamentous structures of the cervical spine (Jull et al 2004). The recovery from this position is also useful to show compensatory motor strategies. The C-CFT, as described by Jull et al (2004), uses a pressure biofeedback unit (Pressure Biofeedback Unit, Chattanooga Group, Hixon, USA). This tool will augment the skills of a clinician in movement and muscle analysis in order to assess the function of the deep stability muscles of the neck. The aim of the test is twofold: first, to assess the movement pattern by asking the patient to progressively move the needle up in 2 mmHg increments from 20 to 30 mmHg so as to assess the use of superficial neck muscles and the patient's kinaesthetic sense; and secondly, to look at the holding capacity for the muscles starting at 22 mmHg for 10-second periods. This test gives key information in the implementation of a patient's home exercise programme. The postural control system for the body receives important information from cervical spine afferents. The deep muscles of the upper cervical spine have a high number of muscle spindles, which are responsible for the complex interaction between the cervical spine, ocular motor, proprioceptive balance control, and vestibular systems. Dizziness and unsteadiness are the next most frequent complaints (after pain) in subjects with WAD (Treleaven et al 2003, 2005). Tests for balance, proprioception, and eye movement control are described elsewhere in the literature to which readers are referred (Jull et al 2004).

Diagnosis

Making a diagnosis is essential for goal setting and the clinician's evaluation of treatment. The diagnosis should consider the tissue affected; the time frame of tissues healing, and the apparent pain mechanisms. This will guide a clinician through the appropriate clinical reasoning and evidence-based pathway for management. Assessment is an ongoing, progressive task that must accompany the treatment. Red flag conditions should be identified and referred on to the appropriate health professional immediately. Early identification of yellow flags and patients who may benefit from cognitive behavioural therapy (CBT) is essential for the effective management of this patient group. Outcomes such as visual analogue score (VAS) for pain, function, and performance can then be used to record the outcomes of treatment. The Neck Disability Index (NDI) (Vernon & Moi 1992) and the Patient-Specific Functional Scale (PSFS) (Westerway et al 1998) are two other commonly used outcome measures. Common cervical spine problems seen within a musculoskeletal clinic include:

- Cervical postural dysfunction;
- Acute wryneck (apophyseal/discogenic);
- Acceleration/deceleration injury (WAD);
- Radiculopathies (discogenic/spondylotic);
- Stingers (brachial plexus trauma); and
- Osteoarthritis.

Treatment

The aims of physiotherapy treatment are:

- To normalize afferent input;
- To restore ROM;
- To regain optimal motor function;
- To regain optimal proprioceptive function; and
- To address any changeable predisposing factors.

A multimodal treatment approach involving manual therapy and a therapeutic home exercise programme (including cervical stability and proprioceptive training) have been shown to be of benefit in the treatment of both traumatic and idiopathic cervical spine pain (Allison et al 2002; Cleland et al 2007a, b; Jull et al 2002).

Modalities such as acupuncture, electrotherapy, and soft-tissue mobilization are effective adjuncts to manual therapy, and are good for reducing pain, reducing soft tissue sensitivity, and promoting relaxation.

Spinal manual and manipulative therapy

Although there is ongoing discussion about the safety issues associated with manipulation of the cervical spine, manual and manipulative spinal therapy (DeFabio 1999) continue to be widely used in the treatment of cervical spine dysfunction. The exact mobilization and manipulation mechanisms that provide therapeutic benefit are not known. Research indicates there is a multisystem response from the motor, sensory, and sympathetic nervous systems (Sterling et al 2000; Vernon et al 1990; Wright 1995; Wright & Vincenzino 1995). Importantly, it also appears that manual therapy may also improve the performance of the therapeutic exercise programme (Sterling 2000). Most theoretical models of manual therapy use manual assessment (active ROM, PPIVM, and PAIVM) and apparent pathological state to determine grade and direction of movement. For simple mechanical cervical spine pain, the sequence of palpation, mobilization, and manipulation of a spinal segment is logical and simple in clinical application. The most common clinical dysfunctions usually involve ipsilateral rotation and side bend dysfunctions. The graded application of palpation, mobilization, and manipulation to restore a mid-cervical spine dysfunction is shown in Fig. 3.1. The techniques are progressed as the patient's symptoms allow and the tissue-healing model indicates. With more complex pathologies (e.g. acute traumas,

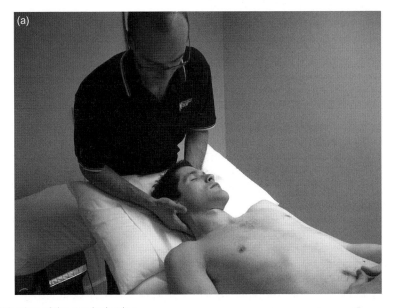

Figure 3.1 • (a) Palpation of the cervical spine.

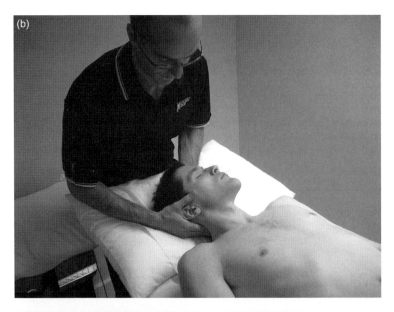

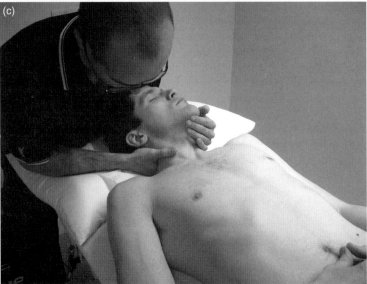

Figure 3.1 (Continued) • (b) Passive physiological intervertebral movement and right side bend. (c) Side bend mobilization/manipulation.

nerve root irritation, segmental instabilities and arthropathies) more care is needed in the selection of manual therapy techniques and their application. Tables 3.2 and 3.3 suggest some indications, precautions, and contraindications to cervical spine mobilization and manipulation (adapted from Aspinall 1989; Bogduk 1994; Gibbons & Tehan 2000; Gross et al 1996; Kerry & Taylor 2006; McCarthy 2001; Magarey et al 2004; Maitland 2000; Mitchell 2002; Rubinstein et al 2005; Shekelle & Coulter 1997; Sran 2007).

Therapeutic exercise program

A good therapeutic exercise programme reinforces a clinician's manual therapy treatment, and addresses the motor control and proprioceptive requirements of the patient. The patient participation is essential; patients must perceive that they get symptomatic benefit from it. Therefore, education and, if possible, a clear demonstration that the therapeutic exercise gives them analgesic or mechanical

Table 3.2 Indications, precautions, and contraindications to cervical mobilization

Indications	• Organic musculoskeletal dysfunction of reproducible pattern

Precautions	• Severe pain
	• Irritable conditions
	• Certain involvements of the nerve root:
	   ○ Acute nerve root pain
	   ○ Signs and symptoms of increasing neuropathy
	   ○ Nerve root irritation
	• When spinal movements and/or palpation reproduced distal pain
	• Any patient's condition which is worsening
	• Dizziness, aggravated by neck rotation
	• Rheumatoid arthritis
	• Osteoporosis
	• Spondylolisthesis
	• Previous malignant disease, extra spinal

Contraindications	• Malignancy involving the vertebral column • Physical involvement of the central nervous system • Spinal cord compression • Cauda equina lesions • Neurological disease • Inflammatory and infective arthritis (e.g. rheumatoid arthritis, cervical spine, active phase) • Ankylosing spondylosis—active phase • Bone disease (osteoporosis is not contraindicated provided that extreme care is used) • Recent fractures

Table 3.3 Indications, precautions and contraindications to cervical spinal manipulation

Indications	• Informed consent gained • Acute facet dysfunction with limited muscle guarding and only two linked biomechanical directions of movement loss • Pain with a regular and recognizable biomechanical pattern • No contraindications to manipulation present • The patient has progressed through mobilization procedures, but has a plateau in progress
Precautions	• Pregnancy and post partum period • Craniovertebral anomalies • Congenital absence of the odontoid process • Spinal deformity caused by old pathology • Scoliosis • Kyphosis caused by adolescent osteochondritis • Congenital generalized hypermobility • Ehlers Danlos syndrome • Patients in whom indications for high-velocity thrust techniques are not present
Contraindications	• Lack of provision of informed consent by patient. • Malignancy: primary or secondary where there is risk of involvement of the tissues of the vertebral column • Inflammatory and infective arthritis • Bone disease: osteomyelitis, tuberculosis, Paget's disease, osteoporosis • Cranial artery insufficiency; arteriosclerosis; history of vascular disease

(*Continued*)

Table 3.3 (Continued)

- Physical involvement of the central nervous system:
  ○ Spinal cord compression
  ○ Cauda equina lesions
  ○ Neurological disease (e.g. transverse myelitis)
- Gross foraminal or spinal canal encroachment on X-ray: advanced degenerative disease
- Acute and severe nerve root pain, irritation or compression
- Presence of involvement of more than one nerve root
- Recent major trauma
- Segmental instability: unstable spondylolisthesis, traumatic or degenerative instability. Never manipulate through spasm protecting spinal region
- Post-surgical spinal fusion
- Advanced diabetes when tissue vitality may be low
- Drug use: long-term steroids
- Patients on anticoagulant medication or haemophilia

benefit is important. There is now over 15 years of research showing the benefit of a therapeutic exercise programme for patients with both idiopathic and traumatic cervical spine pain (Allison et al 2002; Beeton & Jull 1994; Cleland et al 2005, 2007a, b; Jull et al 2002, 2004). These programmes usually incorporate ROM exercises/mobilization techniques, deep-flexor (cervical stabilization) strength training, and ergonomic and postural advice.

Cervical spine articular dysfunction, tight suboccipital muscles, or neural hypersensitivity will often prevent the patient from performing cervical stabilization exercises. Therefore, specific mobilization of the upper cervical spine and neural structures is the starting point for treatment and the home exercise programme. Lateral glide techniques have been shown to be of benefit in patients with neural hypersensitivity (Allison et al 2002, Cleland et al 2005), and specific mobilization techniques for the upper cervical spine can be found elsewhere in the literature (Hing et al 2003). Two useful, patient-directed upper cervical spine mobilization exercises are shown in Figs. 3.2 and 3.3. Neurodynamic mobilization, as described by Butler (2000), is also useful.

The aims of a cervical stabilization programme are to provide specific low-load stimulus to the deep stabilizers of the neck and shoulder girdle. A holding capacity at 28-30 mmHg without patients using their superficial musculature will improve their tonic endurance and is a good initial outcome from treatment. Application to the postural and functional requirements of the individual is essential. Falla et al (2007a, b) found an increase in deep cervical flexor recruitment of the cervical spine with correct versus incorrect sitting postural strategies, and then showed that patients with chronic cervical spine pain improved their ability to hold an upright sitting posture with deep cervical flexor training and a home exercise programme. Incorporating graded interaction with the cervical extensors; superficial neck musculature, and shoulder girdle muscles are common progressions to return a patient to functional tasks. When a patient is able to perform isometric holds of their cervical spine flexors and extensors, kinaesthetic training and balance retraining (in some cases of WAD) may start. Revel et al (1994) performed a randomized controlled trial and found that the addition of proprioceptive and kinaesthetic exercises improved cervical spine position sense, pain, and cervical spine disability. Depending on the physical findings (e.g. cervicogenic dizziness, unsteadiness and balance disturbance), exercises involving cervical spine relocation, gaze stability, eye follow, head-and-eye coordination, and balance can be incorporated into cervical stability exercises. The addition of these exercises may also improve motor function in those patients who are struggling to progress beyond the cognitive training phase of the therapeutic exercise programme.

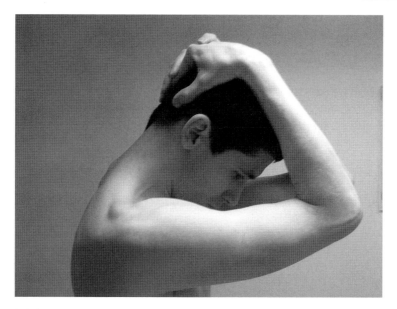

Figure 3.2 • Hang stretch.

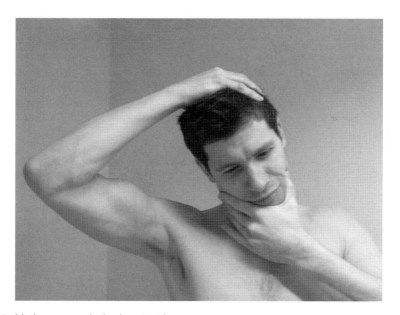

Figure 3.3 • Right-sided upper cervical spine stretch.

3.1   Acupuncture intervention in cervical spine dysfunction

Jennie Longbottom

Research background

The use of acupuncture for the treatment of cervical spine pain is not universally supported. White and Ernst (1999) concluded from their systematic review that equal amounts of data existed to both support and refute acupuncture as an effective modality for neck pain. The practitioner is hindered further in making a reasoned choice by the varying quality of these papers, a point well made by Smith et al (2000). Despite these initial difficulties, a growing body of evidence lays claim to the short-term benefits of acupuncture for neck pain. Nabeta and Kawakita (2002) found clinically significant results in a study of cervical spine pain and stiffness, albeit that the benefits were not maintained at the one-month follow-up. These findings were mirrored by Irnich et al (2001) with the ceiling of their reassessment being at 3 months. White et al (2004) extended the follow-up period in their more recent investigation; although acupuncture was found to be statistically significant at reducing chronic neck pain and subsequent analgesia administration, these results failed to reach a clinically pertinent level. Despite these perhaps modest claims to utilize acupuncture, collections of authors have stated more robust arguments. Trinh et al (2007) found moderate evidence in both short- and long-term trials that acupuncture was effective in reducing chronic neck pain. David et al (1998) suggests from their research that acupuncture is perhaps most appropriate for those with high baseline pain scores. Irnich et al (2002) suggested more specifically that motion-related pain in the cervical spine was effectively treated by acupuncture; it was also found to be superior to a sham procedure and dry needling.

As advancements in medical scanning technology have been made, a refinement in the physiological processes instigated by acupuncture has followed. Hsieh et al (2001) and Hui et al (2000) both used positive emission tomography imaging (PET) to confirm that only the de Qi sensation at LI4 activated the hypothalamus and subsequently produced a significant analgesic affect. Using the same imaging method, Alavi et al (1997) and Biella et al (2001) confirmed that acupuncture activated the same areas of the brain responsible for acute and chronic pain. Later studies by Newberg et al (2005) found an asymmetry in the thalamus of chronic pain sufferers before needling; this thalamic variation disappeared after one acupuncture treatment.

This collection of studies suggests that similar central pathways are shared by nociceptive and acupuncture signals, but that the central nervous system (CNS) responds in an opposite manner to each (Wang et al 2008). A less well-researched hypothesis for acupuncture is scrutinized by Cho et al (2006), who propose that via the hypothalamus–pituitary–adrenal axis (HPA), there is not only central descending pain inhibition, but also communication with possible anti-inflammatory and neuroimmunity pathways. It is postulated that acupuncture suppresses the release of inflammatory cytokines via the autonomic nervous system (Kavoussi & Evan-Ross 2007); this cholinergic suppression is believed to be a crucial component in the analgesic qualities of acupuncture.

The growing weight of favourable evidence for acupuncture application gives a practitioner confidence, whilst offering a potential quandary about how best to implement the most effective programme. The following case studies used a clinical reasoning model in point choice for the management of pain and emotional presentation, in order to provide best practice to support the use of acupuncture, within a multifactorial physiotherapeutic management approach.

 ## Case Study 1

Charlie Plummer

Introduction

A 49-year-old man presented with cervical spine pain radiating into his right shoulder. The subject's injuries had occurred following an occupational accident one month earlier whilst he was pushing a stock crate up a slope.

The crate had moved awkwardly, hitting him in the right clavicular region. The subject was immediately aware of right-sided neck pain and over the following week, this radiated into his right shoulder. Two days prior to his

(Continued)

Case Study 1 (Continued)

initial assessment, he became troubled by intermittent paraesthesia into the dorsum of his right hand. As a direct result of this accident, the subject was restricted to light duties at work and had been unable to ride his motorcycle ever since. As the assessment progressed it became clear that this accident had adversely influenced his mood, a finding further consolidated when he voiced grave concerns about his physical capability to move house as planned in 2 weeks.

Clinical impression

The findings of the objective and subjective assessments were consistent with a cervical spine facet joint dysfunction with C6 to C7 nerve root irritation (Table 3.4). The hypomobile cervical spine segments coupled with the cervical nerve root triad of symptoms confirmed this diagnosis because:
- Spurling's test was positive;
- There was less than 60° cervical rotation on the side with pain; and
- Brachial plexus provocation test (BPPT) was positive.

Treatment goals

The following goals were discussed with the subject:
- Reduction of cervical spine pain;
- Increasing active ROM in the cervical spine;
- Decreasing paraesthesia in the right hand; and
- Allowing the subject to return to full duties at work.

Treatment

On initial assessment, what was striking was the severity of the subject's neck pain and its obvious effect on his mood. These two problems crucially needed to be addressed within the opening treatment. Bradnam (2003) stated that fewer needles should be used in cases of intense, acute nociceptive pain. Despite the subject having these symptoms for almost a month, the pain remained acutely prominent, and thus applying acupuncture points locally into the neck was ill advised (Table 3.5). Bradnam (2003) highlighted that the segment will already be sensitized by the painful afferent input caused by the injury and that needling local to the origin of the pain may exacerbate symptoms. Once pain improves this route becomes more feasible. As a result of these findings, more distal points were utilized. Lung 7 (LU7) used bilaterally, which is indicated for neck pain and stiffness (Deadman et al 1998), was targeted in an effort to influence spinal mechanisms. LU7 lies in the same dermatome as C6 and thus needling at this point attenuates the nociceptive input to the dorsal horn. Lundeberg (1998) and Sato et al (1997) found that low-intensity or non-painful acupuncture could reduce sympathetic outflow from the area and could elicit immediate and powerful analgesic results. Irnich et al (2001, 2002) used LU7 to good effect in treating neck pain. Inhibition of the dorsal horn is stimulated by an increase in serotonin, a reduction in dopamine, and a release of gamma-aminobutyric acid (GABA). Increased enkephalins and dynorphin result in, among other effects, improved analgesia and well being (Lundeberg 1998). The introduction of Governor Vessel 20 (GV20) was to augment LU7 in enhancing the patient's mood, a method used by Irnich et al (2002). Application of the extra point, Luozhen (Fig. 3.4), used bilaterally, was combined with this initial treatment regime.

The aim was to activate descending inhibitory pathways from the brain, including the hypothalamus, as outlined earlier in a case study by Wang et al (2008). Bradnam (2003) suggested that, when treating acute nociceptive pain, evoking these supraspinal effects with needles extrasegmentally, such as in the hands with their somatosensory representation, is preferable to avoid

Table 3.4 Subjective and objective examination

Aggravating factors		Cervical rotation right, cervical extension, sitting beyond 10 mins (paraesthesia caused), right-side lying.
Easing factors		Co-codamol (slight improvement)
Lsp red flags		Nil
24-hour pattern-	AM	Cervical spine stiff when first moving, no shoulder pain or paraesthesia.
	PM	Worst part of day—increasing cervical spine pain radiating into right shoulder. Intermittent.
	Night	Disturbed, especially if sleeping right-side lying. Paraesthesia into right hand more prominent.
Past medical history		Nil
Medication		Co-codamol (when pain extreme).

(Continued)

Case Study 1 (Continued)

Table 3.5 Acupuncture point rationale

Session	Day	Points used	Needle size	De Qi	Outcome measure	Allied therapies
1	1	GV20, LU7 (bilat), Luozhen (bilateral)	40 mm	Yes	Pre-Rx VAS 80/100; Post Rx VAS 50/100	Heat, taping, postural correction
2	8	LI4 (bilat), LU7 (bilat), Luozhen (bilat)	40 mm	Yes	Pre-Rx VAS 60/100 Post Rx VAS 40/100	Heat, DNF in supine, R upper traps/ neural stretch
3	15	HJJ @C7 (bilat), Bailao C7 (bilat), GV14— segmental block	40 mm	Yes	Pre-Rx VAS 5/100 Post Rx VAS 20/100	DNF in sitting

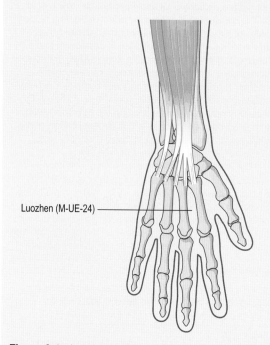

Luozhen (M-UE-24)

Figure 3.4 • Luozhen point.

pain exacerbation. A series of 20-minute sessions were administered and effective analgesia was achieved, all of which were tolerated well by the subject.

The use of acupuncture was supported by other treatment modalities; for example, heat was used to aid relaxation and reduce overactivity in the right upper trapezius. Birch and Jamison (1998) found that acupuncture and heat treatment contribute to modest reductions in neck pain. Postural correction exercises and taping the right proximal humerus into a more superior position in order to relieve strain on the cervical nerve roots were also included in the therapy.

Acupuncture made a marked improvement in the pain levels reported by the subject and subsequently to his ROM and mood. Consequently, the second acupuncture session focused exclusively on reducing further the remaining moderate pain levels. Large Intestine 4 (LI4), a cardinal analgesia point in the dermatome of C6 and an important mediator of neck pain, was introduced. The aim was to facilitate further spinal and supraspinal affects. Because the subject had not received acupuncture before and this point has strong effects, it was felt prudent not to apply LI4 initially. Coupled with this, a deep neck flexor exercise in supine and a right upper trapezius stretch were added to improve stability and muscle length, respectively.

By the final acupuncture treatment, the acute nociceptive pain had abated, leaving a dull, intermittent ache. A C6 segmental approach was implemented with core stability exercises in sitting, inducing the release of sensory neuropeptides, such as substance P, bradykinin, and histamine, and resulting in local vasodilation and mediation of local immune reactions (Lundeberg 1998).

Although this regime proved highly effective in this instance, other possible points for consideration existed. Had the neck symptoms been chronic, GB20 or BL10 could have been utilized. BL60, used bilaterally, could also have been an effective distal point, lying along the same meridian. Perhaps more debatable was the exclusion of the LI4 and LIV3 combination, particularly since pain was so problematic. The decision was made not to include this, as these are such sensitive points. With the subject's mood particularly vulnerable to reacting adversely to any setback, it was felt that other points were more appropriate and carried less risk of antagonizing his symptoms.

(Continued)

Case Study 1 (Continued)

This subject improved noticeably over the one-month period during which treatment was administered. Pain reduced from 8/10 on the numerical pain rating scale (NPRS) initially, to 2/10 after the final acupuncture session. Cervical spine ROM also demonstrated similar dramatic alteration. On discharge, the subject had regained full, pain-free ROM with normal upper limb neural provocation test correlating with a return to full function. The subject was limited to weekly treatments because of his shift patterns; however, some studies imply that multiple weekly sessions are optimal (Irnich 2002; Lundeberg 1998). Practitioners are also limited by the quality of research and its focus on investigating chronic neck pain, resigning a therapist to extrapolate these findings to acute cases. This case study has clearly demonstrated the effective application of acupuncture within a multifaceted treatment regime.

Case Study 2

Rose Sutcliffe

Introduction

A 51-year-old man with chronic neck pain and left arm pain was referred to physiotherapy having been assessed for the chronic pain rehabilitation programme and been accepted. Referral was made to physiotherapy to address muscle shortening in the left shoulder and neuromuscular imbalance as well as lack of core and overall fitness. The problem had started after a road traffic accident 5 years ago. The subject now considered himself permanently damaged, with a withered non-functional left arm. Previous treatments had consisted of cervical traction, manipulation, and both private and National Health Service physiotherapy and psychotherapy and he attended the pain clinic for spinal injections, all of which had only resulted in short-term benefits. His self-efficacy score rated 2/60 on referral. He was assessed subjectively and objectively according to local and national guidelines (Tables 3.6 and 3.7).

Clinical impression

The initial clinical impression was a chronic presentation of radicular pain of cervical origin C6 to C7 with associated neuromuscular and articular changes affecting the cervical spine, thoracic spine, and left shoulder complex. The subject also suffered from comorbidities, lack of sleep, depression, and anxiety.

Multidisciplinary treatment plan

The following treatment plan was drawn up and discussed with the subject:
- Pain clinic review and repeat of magnetic resonance imaging;
- Hydrotherapy to commence a paced exercise programme with active assisted movements;
- Progression of a home-based, paced exercise programme to increase cardiovascular work, core control, and left arm functional movement;
- Manual mobilization of the left glenohumeral joint and stretching the left upper trapezius.

- Acupuncture for pain control;
- Trigger point release with dry needling;
- Attendance at the chronic pain programme with review; and
- Acupressure and transcutaneous electrical nerve stimulation (TENS) for home use.

Clinical trials that attempt to establish the relative effectiveness of acupuncture against other treatments often score low on methodological quality because of the blinding of treatment groups (Johnson 2006), and effectiveness is difficult to assess with different treatment techniques being run concurrently. Neck pain is a common complaint, and in many cases, symptoms persist, causing severe discomfort and disability, and inability to work (Smith et al 2000). Chronic neck pain is a major medical and social problem, and in many cases, it is correlated with limited cervical mobility (Hagen et al 1997). Evidence is hard to find for the efficacy of procedures. Table 3.8 highlights recent research supporting the use of acupuncture for chronic neck pain.

Physiological reasoning for acupuncture selection

Chronic pain is a complex multifactorial condition; its cause may not be clearly identifiable, and imaging and assessment may not fully explain the pain presentation or accompanying disability (Watson 2007). Pain is not just described as a sensation: there are also affective and emotional aspects of the stimulus that have a major impact on the sufferer, producing comorbidities. The most common clinically described comorbidities are anxiety, sleep disorder, and depression (Dickenson 2007). Although the sensory and psychological aspects are separable, the neural pathways that contribute to these aspects of pain are interlinked and therefore certain spinal neurons project to the thalamus and cortex, and generate the sensory aspects of pain, whilst others project in parallel to the limbic areas (Suzuki et al 2004). Whilst the physiological

(Continued)

Case Study 2 (Continued)

Table 3.6 Subjective assessment

Present pain	70/100 (VAS) in the cervical spine centrally referring sharp shooting electric shocks into the left arm and hand accompanied by a stinging nettle feeling in the arm and hand.
History	RTA 5 years ago immediate pain onset of cervical and left arm seen in A/E X-rays NAD. 1 year later 1st MRI following failed physiotherapy and then subsequent spinal injections in the pain clinic.
Current medication	Pregablin and Tramadol. Pregablin had reduced then stopped and an increase of Tramadol to 100 mg q.d.s had begun. Also stopped the Lamotrigine due to drowsiness.
Special questions	Nausea with the Tramadol and a sensation of light-headedness at times thought to be related to the medication. Feels blurred vision at times driving no drop attacks.
Social history	Lives with his wife no children. PADL can be achieved and ADL very restricted. On incapacity benefits now. Social activities much reduced. Goes to bed early due to tiredness. Poor relationship with his wife due to this.
Job and hobbies	No job for over four years, was an IT manager. No hobbies now, these had included rock climbing, gardening, and cycling.
24-hour pattern	Disturbed, only sleeps for 2-3 hours per night. Wakes in pain and is stiff, easing very slowly by mid-morning, aggravated by mechanical movement of the left arm and cervical spine.
Aggravating factors	Turning his head particularly to the left and elevation of the left arm above 20°. Prolonged sitting or lying for more than 30 mins.
Easing factors	Heat and medication; pain once aggravated lasts for days.
Mood	Depressed due to the limitations of pain. Loss of enjoyment and sense of achievement. Loss of self worth and confidence. Lack of sleep.
Belief	Damaged withered left arm will it ever change?
Expectations of treatment plan	Wants to restart the left arm and regain a fitness level to begin enjoying some cardiovascular exercise outside.

Table 3.7 Objective assessment

Present condition	Pain ↑ due to sitting 90/100, irritability high, and severity high.
Observation	Stands and sits with Cx held in a flexed position 10°. Increased Thx lordosis. Left shoulder elevated with tight upper band of trapezius.
Range of movement	AROM Cx Flexion 1" = P ↑ 80/100 referred 90/100 L arm. AROM L Cx Rotation 4" = P ↑ 80/100 referred 90/100 L arm. AROM L arm elevation in scaption 60° P ↑ 90/100, attempted AAROM with short lever into scaption L no ease found. Accessory glide of the glenohumeral joint L tight on AP/caudal translation.
Neurological assessment	Pain inhibition prevented muscle strength tests. Reflexes 6/6 found L brisk compared to the right. Dermatomes increased sensation L C4, ↓C6 slight, C7 slight.
Muscle length assessment	Shortened upper fibres of L trapezius. Tight rectus abdominus flexed head posture leading to associated muscle imbalance.

(Continued)

Case Study 2 (Continued)

Table 3.7 Continued

Neural Provocation tests	BPPT 1, 2a & b, 3, modified due to irritability, increased symptoms at 10° of elevation L arm.
Other joints	AC/SC Joint glide 0/100 R, poor scapula depression on the left no pain ↑. R arm normal movement. Lx AROM average with poor core control. Thx AROM poor in all directions.

Table 3.8 Recent trials for acupuncture and neck pain

Trial	Numbers and results
Ammendolia, Furlan, Imamura et al 2008	Systematic review (SR) of randomized controlled trials (RCTs) evaluating the effects of acupuncture for chronic low back pain, containing RCTs that looked at spinal pain. Concluded that the most consistent evidence found to support the use of acupuncture was for the addition of this therapy with other therapies to treat one condition. This demonstrated more effective benefit in pain relief and functional improvement when compared to the same treatment without acupuncture. Statistical data for the proportion of each therapy to the condition evaluated is not found for obvious reasons.
Vickers and Wilson et al 2008	SR. The most problematic area being chronic pain where there is a large body of data with conflicting opinion. Similarly there is enough evidence to suggest that attempts to curtail acupuncture would be unjustified.
Trinh, Graham, Gross et al 2007	SR 10 trials. For chronic neck disorders with ridiculer symptoms there was moderate evidence that acupuncture was more effective than a wait-list control at short-term follow-up.
White P 2006	Review only. Considered safe (caution with anticoagulants) and should be considered as a part of any pain management programme.
Irnich, Behrens et al 2001	RCT. $N = 177$. Conclusions were drawn after only 5 weeks of treatment. The acupuncture group showed a significantly greater improvement in motion-related pain than massage ($p = 0.00052$) but not compared with sham laser ($p = 0.327$). The difference between the groups was more significant in the subgroup that had had pain for more than 5 years. No mention of clinical significance.
Smith, Oldman, McQuay et al 2000	SR to assess the analgesic efficacy and adverse effects of acupuncture and develop an outcome measure. Although they concluded they found no convincing evidence for the analgesic effect of acupuncture for either back or neck pain; the authors highlighted the lack of insufficient data collection a current theme on data research.

mechanisms of acupuncture are closely related to the pain pathways of the CNS, its mechanism of action remains obscure. Lo and Cui (2003) were able to find an effect of acupuncture using transcranial magnetic stimulation (TMS), and a reduction in motor cortex excitability was achieved in comparison with a sham needle insertion. The treatment goals were to relieve pain, improve the function of the left arm, alleviate the destructive environment, improve the subject's mood, and increase his well being. Centrally evoked pain involves altered CNS circuitry and processing, a feature in this chronic pain presentation (Coderre et al 1993). The subject has exhibited a poor response to treatment and medication so far (Gifford & Butler 1997). The slow healing process under this condition points to inhibition of the sympathetic nervous system (SNS), which can lead to trophic changes to target tissue (Bekkering & van Bussel 1998; Lundeberg & Ekholm 2001). Advances in the understanding of pain neurophysiology and acupuncture mechanisms have suggested that there is a valid scientific basis for Western acupuncture and would appear to support its use in the treatment of chronic pain, as exemplified by this case study (Table 3.9).

(Continued)

Case Study 2 (Continued)

Table 3.9 Acupuncture point rational including outcome measures and results

Treatment session[a]	Points	Outcome measures[b]	Outcome post Rx
1. Assessment. Discussion. Hydrotherapy to run concurrently once x weekly with a home exercise plan and acupuncture.		PSEQ score = 2/60	
2. Two hydrotherapy sessions attempted > pain levels therefore acupuncture commenced at this stage.	HT7 LI4 + LIV3	90/100 Cx L rotation = 4" L arm flexion 10°	40/100 Felt in a relaxed state reduced tension.
3. Acupuncture – pain levels had reduced for 4 days. Nausea due to Pregablin, changes to gabapentamin.	HT7 LI4 + LIV3 PC6	70/100 Cx L rotation = 4" L arm flexion 30° Sleep pattern improving Nausea	30/100 Again reduced tension and relaxed state Some relief of nausea Taught acupressure on PC 6 for home use.
4. Maintained reduced pain TNS on LIV3 + LI4. Stop the Gabapentin due to nausea. Continue with the beneficial effects of acupuncture.	HT7 LI4 +LIV3 BL11 BL13 GV14 HJJ points @ C7, T1	Reduced hand pains VAS 40/100 Cx rotation = no change L arm flexion 40° Sleep pattern changeable	20/100 Relaxed state Cx L rotation = 6" L arm flexion = 60° Mood change much more positive.
5. Acupuncture needle points increased and upper trapezius stretches commenced due to remaining palpable band of tightening	HT7 LI4 + LIV3 HJJ, C7, T1 BL11 BL13 Release trigger point in L upper trapezius	90/100 Cx L rotation = 4" L arm flexion 40°	50/100 Relaxed ++ Cx L rotation = 6" L arm flexion now 100° Good response to local needling to release palpable muscle band local twitch stopped now able to tolerate AIR stretches to the upper trapezius and added to the HEP
6. Lasting effect of muscle release 4 days felt so well spent 3 hours at the computer and suffered setback to muscle release. On palpation muscle band tension felt at GB21 and B43 repeat the analgesic the acupuncture session and add BL 43 to release the upper trapezius tension. Use of own TNS LI 4 + LIV	H7 LI4 + LIV3 GV14 + HJJ @ C7, T1 BL11 BL13 GB21 BL43 Release trigger point in L upper trapezius	30/100 > to 90/100, due to over pacing at the computer. Cx L rotation = 4" L arm flexion 90°	Relaxed 20/100 pain experienced Cx L rotation = 7" L arm flexion 140° with wall support to activate the rotator cuff Referral of arm pain only at end range to the elbow 4/10 No tension band experienced in trapezius

(Continued)

Case Study 2 (Continued)

Table 3.9 Continued

Treatment session[a]	Points	Outcome measures[b]	Outcome post Rx
7. Maintained pain control now able to add CV work for the legs on static bike. EOR arm elevation still painful. Finding the use of acupressure at night on Ying Tang relaxing. Use of TNS at the LI4 + LIV	HT7 LI4 + LIV3 GV14 + HJJ @ T1 BL11 BL13 GV14 LI15 TW14 LI14	60/100 L arm flexion 90° Minimal Cx pain Cx L rotation = 5" Upper trapezius tension minimal on palpation	Relaxed and happy. L arm flexion = 120° with wall support 140° 3/10 arm elevation EOR pain now able to repeat arm and AIR trapezius stretch and continue to maintain Cx Increased ROM. Positive thoughts re ↑ activity outside at home. Ordered a pedometer to measure daily strides.
8. Release of posterior capsule of the shoulder joint following acupuncture using SI11. Accessory glides to the left glenohumeral joint with stretches x 5 then added to HEP.	HT7 LI4 + LIV3 GV14 HJJ @ T1 BL11 BL13 GV14 LI15 TW14 L 14 SI11	20/100 Cx and shoulder pains Cx L rotation = 7" L arm flexion = 90°	No report of pain at rest EOR P on arm elevation 20/100 No referral to the arm at rest still 40/100 EOR arm elevation no P/N at160° with wall support. AROM without wall support 110°. PSEQ score = 29/60

[a] Sessions 2 to 5, twice-weekly treatment; sessions 6-8, weekly treatment.

[b] VAS 0-100. Cx L rotation = measured in inches. L arm flexion measured with inclinometer (Green et al 1998), pain self-efficacy questionnaire (PSEQ) (Nicholas 1989).

Discussion

Supraspinal and spinal effects were considered together since prolonged pain, as in this case presentation, may indicate a change in both the CNS and SNS. Bekkering & van Bussel (1998) considered that the distal points used in the extremities have a significant sympathetic innervation and would be useful in manipulating sympathetic responses, as would needling at a point sharing the spinal level supplying the target tissue or region. In this case, LI4 is located in the adductor pollicis muscle and has T1 innervation. Therefore, needling LI4 may activate the sympathetic lateral horn at the T1 level, and alter the sympathetic outflow to the head and neck (Bradnam 2007). Combining this with Liver 3 (LIV3) and Heart 7 (HT7) may increase the extrasegmental outflow of both CNS and SNS, and could activate descending inhibitory mechanisms in this subject. Combining acupuncture with hydrotherapy and a simple exercise regime to stimulate core control and arm movement was the initial treatment choice for this patient. De Qi was considered necessary to achieve efficacious acupuncture. Abad-Alegria and Pomaron (2004) concluded that a clear relationship between the intensity of the acupuncture neuroreflex stimulus and the response gained was the de Qi effect. The subject experienced a reduction in pain, in a positive non-uniform pattern with the use of self-acupressure and TENS used over these points. Kotze and Simpson (2007) suggested that TENS had benefits over acupuncture points, but pointed out that studies to prove these benefits are minimal. Pericardium 6 (PC6), which was used to overcome the nausea, caused by the change in medication, was difficult to equate: once the medication effects had worn off no nausea was felt, although nausea was reduced at the time of needling. After treatment 4, progress had been

(Continued)

Case Study 2 (Continued)

satisfactory with regard to reduction in pain and arm movement. Progression of the acupuncture was made by the introduction of spinal points close to the spinal level that share innervation with the injured part. Governor Vessel 14 (GV14), under the spinous process of C7, was chosen because of its close affinity with the spinal cord and spine, and since it addresses the segmental stiffness. Corresponding Huatuojiaji (HJJ) points at C7 and T1 were added to influence the posterior rami at this level, along with Bladder channel points BL11 and BL13 (Bradnam 2007). With the presence of a shortened band in the upper fibres of trapezius, sensitivity and pain to touch, and a taut band of skeletal muscle, trigger point (TrPt) deactivation was used to disrupt the dysfunctional motor endplate (Cummings & White 2001; Simons et al 1998). Further use of the Large Intestine meridian provided the analgesic effect, especially in the upper part of the body, whilst acupuncture points Small Intestine 11 (SI11), LI14, and Triple Energizer (TE14) were incorporated to improve circulation and mobilize the posterior glenohumeral joint. By treatment 8 the patient considered himself to feel better than he had for 5 years. His pain self-efficacy questionnaire (PSEQ) score rose from 2/60 to 29/60. With the use of the inclinometer without wall support, his left arm elevation was 110° and the VAS of pain report was 22/100 and nil at times post-treatment. On palpation of the upper fibres of left trapezius these were relaxed. Left cervical rotation had increased from 10.2 to 17.8 cm. The subject's mood was relaxed, his sleep pattern was improving, and he undertook regular cardiovascular training with the use of a pedometer and a static pedal set at home.

The subject had only had a short-term response to the treatment previously and now, 5 years post-trauma, he was in considerable pain. His desire to change remained and support for the inclusion of a multidisciplinary approach to treatment was present; in particular, he was willing to try acupuncture intervention to complement the goals of treatment progression identified at his assessment. Post-treatment, it was possible to assess and evaluate the treatment goals chosen (Table 3.10) for the short term. Over 3 months progress was favourable and this supported the acupuncture intervention.

Table 3.10 Pre- and post treatment outcome measurements

Pre-treatment	Post treatment
PSEQ = 2/60	PSEQ = 29/60
VAS = 90/100	VAS = 20/100
Cervical rotation to the left = 7"	Cervical rotation to the left = 4"
Left arm flexion = 10°	Left arm flexion = 110°
Subjectively negative about life state	Subjectively positive, had commenced cardiovascular training, improving sleep pattern with increased functional use of the left arm.

References

Abad-Algeria, F., Pomaron, C., 2004. About the neurobiological foundation of the De-Qi—stimulus–response relation. Am. J. Chin. Med. 32 (5), 807–814.

Alavi, A., LaRiccia, P., Sadek, Ah et al., 1997. Neuroimaging of acupuncture in patients with chronic pain. J. Altern. Complement. Med. 3, 41–53.

Allison, G.T., Nagy, B.M., Hall, T., 2002. Randomised clinical trials of manual therapy for cervico-brachial pain syndrome—a pilot study. Man. Ther. 7 (2), 95–102.

Ammendolia, C., Furlan, A.D., Imamura, M., et al., 2008. Evidence-informed management of chronic low back pain with needle acupuncture. Spine 8 (1), 160–172.

Aspinall, W., 1989. Clinical testing for cervical mechanical disorders, which produce ischaemic vertigo. J. Orthop. Sports. Phys. Ther. 11, 176–182.

Aspinall, W., 1990. Clinical testing for craniovertebral hypermobility syndrome. J. Orthop. Sports. Phys. Ther. 12 (2), 47–53.

Australian Physiotherapy Association (APA). 2006. Clinical guidelines for assessing vertebrobasilar insufficiency, in the management of cervical spine disorders. [Online]. Available at URL: http://www.Physiotherapy.asn.au

Beeton, K., Jull, G., 1994. The effectiveness of manipulative physiotherapy in the management of cervicogenic headache: a single case study. Physiotherapy 80, 417–423.

Bekkering, R., van Bussel, R., 1998. Segmental acupuncture. In: Filshie, J. White, A. (Eds.), Medical acupuncture: a western scientific approach. Churchill Livingstone, Edinburgh, pp. 105–135.

Biella, G., Sotgiu, M.L., Pellegata, G., et al., 2001. Acupuncture produces central activations in pain regions. Neuroimage 14, 60–66.

Birch, S., Jamison, R., 1998. Controlled trial of Japanese acupuncture for chronic myofascial neck pain: assessment of specific and non-specific effects of treatment. Clin. J. 14 (3), 248–255.

Bogduk, N., 1994. Cervical causes of headache and dizziness.

In: Boyling, J.D., Palastanga, N. (Eds.), Grieve's modern manual therapy, the vertebral column, 2nd edn. Churchill Livingstone, Edinburgh, pp. 317–331.

Bradnam, L., 2003. A proposed clinical reasoning model for Western acupuncture. New Zealand J. Physiother. 20, 83–94.

Bradnam, L., 2007. A proposed clinical reasoning model for western acupuncture. Journal of the Acupuncture of Chartered Physiotherapists 1, 21–30.

Butler, D.S., 2000. The sensitive nervous system. Noigroup Publications, Adelaide.

Campbell, A., 2006. Point specifity of acupuncture in the light of recent clinical and imaging studies. Acupunct. Med. 24 (3), 118–122.

Cattrysse, E., Swinkles, R.H.A.M., Oostendorp, R.A.B., et al., 1997. Upper cervical instability: are clinical tests reliable? Man. Ther. 2 (2), 91–97.

Cho, Z.H., Hwang, S.C., Wong, E.K., et al., 2006. Neural substrates, experimental evidences and functional hypothesis of acupuncture mechanisms. Acta Neurologica Scandinavica 113, 370–377.

Cleland, J.A., Whitman, J.M., Fritz, J.M., et al., 2005. Radiculopathy: a case series. J. Orthop. Sports. Phys. Ther. 35, 802–811.

Cleland, J.A., Childs, J.D., Fritz, J.M., et al., 2007a. Development of a clinical prediction rule for guiding treatment of a subgroup of patients with neck pain: use of thoracic spine manipulation, exercise, and patient education. Phys. Ther. 87 (1), 9–23.

Cleland, J.A., Glynn, P., Whitman, J.M., et al., 2007b. Short-term effects of thrust versus nonthrust mobilization/ manipulation directed at the thoracic spine in patients with neck pain: a randomised clinical trial. Phys. Ther. 87 (4), 431–440.

Coderre, T., Arroyo, J., Champion, G., 1993. Contribution of central neuroplasticity to pathological pain: A review of clinical and experimental research. Pain 52, 259–285.

Coppieters, M., Stappaerts, K., Janssens, K., et al., 2002. Reliability of detecting 'onset of pain' and 'submaximal pain' during neural provocation testing of the upper quadrant. Physiother. Res. Int. 7 (3), 146–156.

Cummings, T.M., White, A.R., 2001. Needling therapies in the management of myofascial trigger point pain: a systematic review. Arch. Phys. Med. Rehabil. 82, 986–992.

Dall'Alba, P., Sterling, M., Treleaven, J., et al., 2001. Cervical range of motion discriminates between asymptomatic and whiplash subjects. Spine 26, 2090–2094.

Dalton, M., Coutts, A., 1994. The effect of age on cervical posture in a normal population. In: Boyling, P.J.D., Palastanga, N. (Eds.), Grieve's modern manual therapy, the vertebral column, 2nd edn. Churchill Livingstone, London, pp. 361–370.

David, J., Modi, S., Aluko, A.A., et al., 1998. Chronic neck pain: A comparison of Acupuncture treatment and physiotherapy. Br. J. Rheumatol. 37, 1118–1122.

Deadman, P., Al-Khafaji, M., Baker, K., 1998. A manual of acupuncture. Journal of Chinese Medicine Publications.

DeFabio, R.P., 1999. Manipulation of the cervical spine risks and benefits. Phys. Ther. 79 (1), 50–65.

Dickenson, A., 2007. The neurobiology of chronic pain states. Anaesthesia and Intensive Care Medicine 9 (1), 8–12.

Ezzo, J., Berman, B., Hadhazy, V.A., 2000. Is acupuncture effective for the treatment of chronic pain? A systematic review. Pain 93 (2), 198–200.

Falla, D., Jull, G., Hodges, P.W., 2004. Feedforward activity of the cervical flexor muscles during voluntary arm movements is delayed in chronic neck pain. Exp. Brain Res. 157 (1), 43–48.

Falla, D., O'Leary, S., Fagan, A., Jull, G., 2007a. Recruitment of the deep cervical flexor muscles during a postural correction exercise performed in sitting. Man. Ther. 12, 139–143.

Falla, D., Jull, G., Russell, T., et al., 2007b. Effect on neck exercise on sitting posture in patients with chronic neck pain. Phys. Ther. 87 (4), 408–417.

Gifford, L., 2001. Acute low cervical nerve root conditions: symptom presentations and pathobiological reasoning. Man. Ther. 6 (2), 106–115.

Gifford, L.S., Butler, D.S., 1997. The integration of pain sciences into clinical practice. J. Hand Ther. 10 (2), 87–95.

Goldstein, A., 1976. Opioids peptides (endorphins) in the pituitary and brain. Science 193, 1081–1086.

Grant, R., Jull, G., Spencer, T., 1997. Active stabilization for screen based keyboard operators—a single case study. Aust. J. Physiother. 43 (4), 235–242.

Green, S., Buchbinder, R., Forbes, A., et al., 1998. A standardised protocol for the measurement of the range of movement of the shoulder using the pluviometer-V inclinometer and assessment of its interrater reliability. Arthritis Care Res. 11 (1), 43–52.

Griegel-Morris, P., Larson, K., Mueller-Klaus, K., et al., 1992. Incidence of common postural abnormalities in the cervical, shoulder, and thoracic regions and their association with pain in two age groups of healthy subjects. Phys. Ther. 72 (6), 425–431.

Gross, A.R., Aker, P.D., Quartly, C., 1996. Manual therapy in the treatment of neck pain. Rheumatic Disease Clinics of North America 22 (3), 579–598.

Hagen, K.B., Harms-Ringdahl, K., Enger, N.O., et al., 1997. Relationship between subjective neck disorders and cervical spinal mobility and motion related pain in male machine operators. Spine 13, 1501–1507.

Hall, T., Robinson, K., 2004. The flexion-rotation test and active cervical mobility- a comparative measurement study in cervicogenic headache. Man. Ther. 9, 197–202.

Haughie, L.J., Fiebert, I.M., Roach, K.E., 1995. Relationship of forward head posture and cervical backward bending to neck pain. J. Man. Manip. Ther. 3 (3), 91–97.

Hing, W.A., Reid, D.A., Monaghan, M., 2003. Manipulation of the cervical spine. Man. Ther. 8 (1), 2–9.

Hsieh, J.C., Tu, C.H., Chen, F.P., et al., 2001. Activation of the hypothalamus characterises the acupuncture stimulation at the analgesic point in a human: a positron emission tomography study. Neuroscience Letters 307, 105–108.

Hui, K.K.S., Liu, J., Makris, N., et al., 2000. Acupuncture modulates the limbic system and subcortical gray structures, of the human brain; evidence from fMRI studies in normal subjects. Human Brain Mapping 9, 13–25.

Irnich, D., Behrens, N., Molzen, H., et al., 2001. Randomised trial of acupuncture compared with conventional massage and sham, laser acupuncture for treatment of chronic neck pain. Br. Med. J. 322, 1574–1580.

Irnich, D., Behrens, N., Gleditsch, J.M., et al., 2002. Immediate effects of dry needling and acupuncture at distant points in chronic neck pain: results of a randomised, double-blind, sham-controlled crossover trial. Pain 1-2, 83–89.

Janda, V., 1994. Muscles and motor control in cervicogenic disorders: assessment and management. In: Grant, R. (Ed.), Physical Therapy of the Cervical and Thoracic Spine. Churchill Livingstone, New York, pp. 195–216.

Johnson, G.M., 1998. The correlation between surface measurement of head and neck posture and the anatomic position of the upper cervical vertebrae. Spine 23 (8), 921–927.

Johnson, M.J., 2006. The clinical effectiveness of acupuncture for pain-you can be certain of uncertainty. Acupuncture in Medicine 24 (2), 71–79.

Jones, M., Edwards, I., Gifford, L., 2002. Conceptual models for implementing biopsychosocial theory in clinical practice. Man. Ther. 7 (1), 2–9.

Jull, G.A., 2000. Deep cervical neck flexor dysfunction in whiplash. Journal of Musculoskeletal Pain 8 (1/2), 143–154.

Jull, GA., 2001 The physiotherapy management of cervicogenic headache: a randomised clinical trial. PhD Thesis, University of Queensland Australia.

Jull, G., Bogduk, N., Marsland, A., 1988. The accuracy of manual diagnosis for cervical zygapophysial joint pain syndromes. Med. J. Aust. 148, 233–236.

Jull, G.A., Trott, P., Potter, H., et al., 2002. A randomised controlled trial of exercise and manipulative therapy for cervicogenic headache. Spine 27 (17), 1835–1843.

Jull, G.A., Falla, D., Treleaven, J., et al., 2004. A therapeutic exercise approach for cervical disorders. In: Boyling, J.D., Jull, G.A. (Eds.), Grieve's modern manual therapy: the vertebral column, 3rd edn. Elsevier Churchill Livingstone, Edinburgh, pp. 451–470.

Kaptchuk, T.J., 2002. Acupuncture: theory, efficacy, and practice. Ann. Intern. Med. 136 (5), 374–383.

Kavoussi, B., Evan-Ross, B., 2007. The neuroimmune basis of anti-inflammatory acupuncture. Integrated Cancer Therapy 6, 251–257.

Kerry, R., Taylor, A.J., 2006. Cervical arterial dysfunction assessment and manual therapy. Man. Ther. 11, 243–253.

King, W., Lau, P., Lees, R., et al., 2007. The validity of manual examination in assessing patients with neck pain. Spine 7, 22–26.

Kotze, A., Simpson, K.H., 2007. Stimulation produced analgesia; acupuncture, TENS and related techniques. Anaesthesia and Intensive Care Medicine 9 (1), 29–32.

Krakenes, J., Kaale, B., Moen, G., et al., 2002. MRI assessment of the Alar ligaments in the late stage of whiplash-a study of structural abnormalities and observer agreements. Neuroradiology 44, 617–624.

Lo, Y.L., Cui, S.L., 2003. Acupuncture and the modulation of cortical excitability. Neurophysiology, Basic and Clinical 4 (9), 1229–1231.

Lundeberg, T., 1998 The physiological basis of acupuncture. Paper presented at the MANZ/PAANZ Annual Conference, Christchurch, New Zealand.

Lundeberg, T., Ekholm, J., 2001. Pain—from periphery to brain. Journal of the Acupuncture Association of Chartered Physiotherapists 5 (Feb.), 13–19.

McCarthy, C.J., 2001. Spinal manipulative thrust technique using combined movement theory. Man. Ther. 6 (4), 197–204.

Magarey, M.E., Rebbeck, T., Coughlan, B., et al., 2004. Pre-manipulative testing of the cervical spine review, revision and new clinical guidelines. Man. Ther. 9 (2), 95–108.

Maher, C., Adams, R., 1994. Reliability of pain and stiffness assessments in clinical manual lumbar spine examination. Phys. Ther. 74 (9), 801–809.

Maitland, G.D., Hengeveld, E., Banks, K., et al., 2000. Maitland's vertebral manipulation, 6th edn. Butterworth-Heinemann, London.

Melzack, R., Wall, P.D., 1965. Pain mechanism: A new theory. Science 150, 971–979.

Mitchell, J., 2002. Vertebral artery atherosclerosis: A risk factor in the use of manipulative therapy? Physiother. Res. Int. 7, 122–135.

Nabeta, T., Kawakita, K., 2002. Relief of chronic neck and shoulder pain by manual acupuncture to tender points- a sham-controlled randomised trial. Complement. Ther. Med. 10 (4), 217–222.

Newberg, A.B., Lariccia, P.J., Lee, B.Y., et al., 2005. Cerebral blood flow effects of pain and acupuncture; a preliminary single-photon emission computed tomography imaging study. J. Neuroimaging. 15, 43–49.

Nicholas MK, 1989. Self-efficacy and chronic pain. Paper presented at the Annual Conference of the British Psychological Society, St Andrews.

Pomeranz, B., Chiu, D., 1976. Naloxone blockade of acupuncture analgesia: endorphin implicated. Life Science 19, 1757–1762.

Porreca, F., Ossipov, M.H., Gebhart, G.F., 2002. Chronic pain and medullary descending facilitation. Trends in Neuroscience 25, 319–325.

Research Group of Acupuncture Anaesthesia PMC, 1973. The effect of acupuncture on human skin pain threshold. Chin. Med. J. 3, 151–157.

Revel, M., Minguet, M., Gregory, P., et al., 1994. Changes in cervicocephalic kinaesthesia after a proprioceptive rehabilitation program in patients with neck pain: a randomised controlled study. Arch. Phys. Med. Rehabil. 75, 895–899.

Rubinstein, S.M., Peerdeman, S.M., Van Tulder, M., et al., 2005. A systematic review of the risk factors for cervical artery dissection. Stroke 36, 1575–1580.

Sahrmann, S., 2002. Diagnosis and treatment of movement impairment syndromes. Mosby, St Louis.

Sato, A., Sato, Y., Schmidt, R., 1997. The impact of somatosensory input on autonomic functions. Springer-Verlag, Heidelberg.

Shekelle, P.G., Coulter, I., 1997. Cervical spine manipulation: summary report of a systematic review of the literature and a multidisciplinary expert panel. J. Spinal Disord. 10, 223–228.

Simons, D.G., Travell, J.G., Simons, L.S., 1998. Myofascial pain and dysfunction: the trigger point manual, vol. i: Upper half of body, 2nd edn. Williams and Wilkins, Baltimore.

Smith, L.A., Oldman, A.D., McQuay, H.J., et al., 2000. Teasing apart quality and validity in systematic reviews: an example from acupuncture trials in chronic neck and back pain. Pain 86 (1-2), 119–132.

Sran, M., 2007. Neck pain. In: Brukner, P., Khan, K. (Eds.), Clinical sports medicine. McGraw-Hill, Sydney, pp. 229–242.

Sterling, M., Jull, G.A., Wright, A., 2000. Cervical mobilization: concurrent effects on pain, sympathetic nervous system activity and motor activity. Man. Ther. 6, 72–81.

Sterling, M., Treleaven, J., Jull, G.A., 2002. Responses to nerve a tissue provocation test in whiplash-associated disorders. Man. Ther. 7 (2), 89–94.

Sturzenegger, M., 1994. Headache and neck pain: the warning symptoms of vertebral artery dissection. Headache. Journal of Head and Face Pain 34 (4), 187–193.

Suzuki, R., Rygh, L.J., Dickenson, A.H., 2004. Bad news from the brain: descending $5HT^3$ pathways that control spinal pain processing. Trends Pharmacol. Sci. 25, 613–617.

Thiel, H., Rix, G., 2005. Is it time to stop functional pre-manipulation testing of the cervical spine? Man. Ther. 10, 154–158.

Tjell, C., Rosenhall, U., 1998. Smooth pursuit neck torsion test: a specific test for cervical dizziness. Am. J. Otol. 19, 76–81.

Tjell, C., Tenenbaum, A., Sandstrom, S., 2003. Smooth pursuit neck torsion test: a specific test for WAD. J. Whiplash and Relat. Disord. 1, 9–24.

Treleaven, J., Jull, G.A., Atkinson, L., 1994. Cervical musculoskeletal dysfunction in post-concussional headache. Cephalalgia 14, 273–279.

Treleaven, J., Jull, G.A., Sterling, M., 2003. Dizziness and unsteadiness following whiplash injury: characteristic features and relationship with cervical joint position error. J. Rehabil. Med. 35 (1), 36–43.

Treleaven, J., Jull, G.A., Lowchoy, N., 2005. Standing balance in persistent whiplash: a comparison between subjects with and without dizziness. J. Rehabil. Med. 37 (4), 224–229.

Trinh, K., Graham, N., Gross, A., et al., 2007. Acupuncture for neck disorders. Spine 32 (2), 236–243.

Vernon, H., Moir, S., 1992. The neck disability index: a study of reliability and validity. J. Manipul. Physiol. Ther. 14 (17), 409–415.

Vernon, H.T., Aker, P.D., Burns, S., et al., 1990. Pressure pain threshold evaluation of the effect of spinal manipulation in the treatment of chronic neck pain: a pilot study. J. Physiol. Ther. 13, 13–16.

Vickers, A., Wilson, P., Kleijnen, J., 2008. Acupuncture. Effectiveness Bulletin [Online].

Wainner, R.S., Fritz, J.M., Irrgang, J.J., et al., 2003. Reliability and diagnostic accuracy of the clinical examination and patient self-report measures for cervical radiculopathy. Spine 29 (1), 52–62.

Wang, S.M., Kain, Z.N., White, P., 2008. Acupuncture analgesia: 1. the scientific basis. International Anaesthesia Research Society 106 (2), 602–610.

Ware, J.F., Sherbourne, C.D., 1992. The MOS 36-item short form survey (SF-36): 1. Conceptual framework and item selection. Medical Care 30, 473–483.

Watson, D.H., Trott, P.H., 1993. Cervical headache: an investigation of natural head posture and upper cervical flexor muscle performance. Cephalalgia 13 (4), 272–284.

Watson, P.J., 2007. Soft tissue pain and physical therapy. Anaesthesia and Intensive Care Medicine 9 (1), 27–28.

Westerway, M.D., Stratford, P.W., Binkley, J.M., 1998. The patient specific functional scale: Validation of its use in persons with neck dysfunction. J. Orthop. Sports. Phys. Ther. 27 (5), 331–338.

White, A.R., Ernst, E., 1999. A systematic review of randomised controlled trials of acupuncture for neck pain. Rheumatology 38, 143–147.

White, P., Lewith, G., Prescott, P., et al., 2004. Acupuncture versus placebo for the treatment of chronic mechanical neck pain. Ann. Intern. Med. 141 (2), 911–919.

Witt, C., Jena, S., Brinkhaus, B., et al., 2006. Acupuncture for patients with chronic neck pain. Pain 125, 98–106.

Wright, A., 1995. Hypoalgesia post manipulative therapy. Man. Ther. 1, 11–16.

Wright, A., Vincenzino, B., 1995. Central mobilization techniques, sympathetic nervous system effects and their relationship to analgesia. In: Shacklock, M. (Ed.), Moving on in pain. Butterworth-Heinemann, Sydney, pp. 164–173.

Yeung, E., Jones, M., Hall, B., 1997. The response to the slump test in a group of female whiplash patients. Aust. J. Physiother. 43 (4), 245–252.

Zwart, J., 1997. Neck mobility in different headache disorders. Headache 37, 6–11.

The shoulder

4

Jennie Longbottom

CHAPTER CONTENTS

Background

Musculoskeletal shoulder pain is a frequent presentation within physiotherapy, often with a multifactorial aetiology. It is a commonly treated problem in primary care: between seven and twenty five per 1000 adults consult general practitioners for shoulder problems (Lamberts et al 1991); and one in every three people experience shoulder pain at some stage of their lives. Of these, 54% of sufferers report ongoing symptoms at 3 years (Lewis & Tennent 2007). The most frequent diagnosis is that of rotator cuff disease (RCD)

(van der Windt 1995); however, there is extremely poor correlation between magnetic resonance imaging, X-ray, ultrasound findings, and symptoms (Lewis & Tennent 2007). In addition, histological research does not provide strong evidence for an inflammatory tendon component associated with this condition; rather, the evidence points to the potential role of oxidative stress and the biochemical mediation of symptoms. Cytokines, vascular endothelial growth factor, interleukin-1beta (IL-1β), tumour necrosis factor alpha (TNF-α), and the neuropeptide substance P have all been cited as potential factors involved in tendon pathology and pain (Lewis & Tennent 2007). For those whose recovery is not self-limiting, slower or incomplete, a multitude of structures can contribute to the pain mechanism that will form the foundation of the treatment hypothesis.

Donatelli (1997) refers to the shoulder as complex, which is composed of a number of joint structures and articulations that maintain the humerus in the joint space. Integrated and harmonious links between all structures are required for full mobility and function (Dempster 1965). The synchronized movement of four joints must occur for elevation to take place and for function to be achieved

- Glenohumeral;
- Scapulothoracic;
- Sternoclavicular; and
- Acromioclavicular (Fig. 4.1).

It is necessary for the manual therapist to have a comprehensive understanding of functional biomechanics, movement phases, muscle imbalance, and injury

© 2010 Elsevier Ltd.
DOI: 10.1016/B978-0-443-06782-2.00004-9

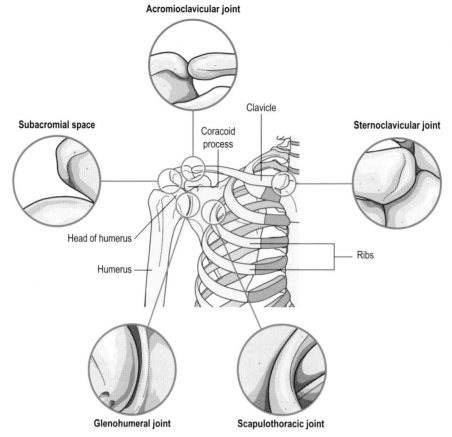

Figure 4.1 • Shoulder complex.

pathology, including trauma, microtrauma, or disease processes that may interfere with any of the movement mechanisms giving rise to pain and dysfunction:

> 'Acupuncture may be more or less effective for different pain types; therefore diagnosis of the predominant pain mechanisms should always underpin treatment decisions and prognosis.' (Lundeberg & Ekholm 2001).

It is essential that relevant pain presentation mechanisms are addressed with the help of manual therapy, electrotherapy, and acupuncture intervention; once pain is under control, functional rehabilitation is facilitated (Lewis 2007). We cannot expect patients to enter into a therapeutic alliance without understanding how and why we are trying to achieve pain modulation; similarly, we must ask whether it is correct to treat the pain presentation if we do not understand the mechanisms ourselves. Assessment of these mechanisms is crucial for the development of the hypothesis that will dictate

whether the manual or acupuncture intervention is to be effective (Lundeberg & Ekholm 2001).

Consider some of the structures involved in shoulder dysfunction:

- Anatomical abnormalities such as congenital acromial osteophyte variations;
- Poor scapula control;
- Shoulder instability whether through hypermobility, trauma, or RCD; and
- Poor glenohumeral, scapulothoracic, or shoulder girdle mechanisms.

The shoulder is an inherently mobile complex, with varying joint surfaces allowing the freedom of movement, and vast mobility occurs at the expense of stability (Donatelli 1997). Because there are over 20 muscles acting upon the joint to provide stability, the possibility of pain provoked from myofascial structures should never be overlooked. Indeed, it is recommended that this may well be the first line of investigation since restoration of full movement and full stability cannot occur if the muscle component is the pain-provoking structure (Ceccherelli et al 2001). Restoration of full muscle balance cannot occur with the presence of a dysfunctional motor end-plate, which prevents full muscle length. A shortened, abnormal muscle length will result in pain provoked by loading of the muscle, a characteristic presentation of myofascial pain involvement and resulting muscle weakness.

Mechanisms of myofascial pain

Mechanisms of myofascial pain occur as a result of nociceptor stimulation in peripheral tissues via mechanical structures associated with conditions such as:

- Impingement;
- Entrapment;
- Bony abnormalities; and
- Mechanical pressure.

The alleviation of nociceptive or myofascial pain must be directed towards the tissues causing this pain. The source of dysfunctional tissues involved can only be revealed by careful assessment and elimination; similarly, the mechanism of acupuncture can only be effective if treatment targets the structures involved. The presence of active myofascial pain can result in:

- Increased acetylcholine at the motor end plate;
- Shortened muscle fibres, ischaemic and/or mechanical pressure on associated blood vessels; or
- Increased production of cytokines and substance P within the area.

If any of the above is the cause, then the aim of acupuncture intervention must be:

- To deactivate the myofascial trigger point (MTrPt);
- To restore muscle length and relaxation;
- To restore blood flow; and
- To assist in the removal of neuropeptide-aggravating chemicals.

Patients will clearly report a myofascial component to their pain if they describe:

- Pain aggravated on muscle loading;

- Pain eased on off-loading;
- Pain eased by touch, heat or ice, indicating an ischaemic component;
- Pain referred along a given muscle referral pattern; and/or
- Reproduction of pain on palpation of tender spot or taut band.

If any of the above is involved in the pain presentation, then a full myofascial assessment with a subsequent TrPt deactivation of the myofascial component is the first requirement for the needle application whether in the rotator cuff and/or cervical muscles.

Rotator cuff disease

Rotator cuff disease (RCD) represents the most common cause of modern shoulder pain and disability. Much of the clinical literature on RCD focuses on subacromial impingement and supraspinatus tendinopathy, although other patterns of lesions are also recognized. Both extrinsic and intrinsic factors to the cuff tendon are thought to be involved in the pathogenesis, leading on to a spectrum of conditions ranging from subacromial bursitis to mechanical failure of the cuff tendon itself (Barying et al 2007). Careful history and examination followed by pertinent investigation are essential to establish the correct diagnosis. The main aim of treatment is to improve symptoms and restore the function of the affected shoulder.

There is no definitive evidence for the efficacy of physical therapy interventions in the management of RCD (Al-Shenqiti & Oldham 2005). Myofascial pain syndromes are common conditions that result from active TrPts (Sola et al. 1955). Myofascial pain has two important components: motor dysfunction of the muscle, and sensory abnormality characterized by either local or referred pain (Whyte-Ferguson & Gerwin 2005). There are a number of clinical diagnostic characteristics that may be presented during assessment that can be used to confirm and/or exclude the presence of MTrPts. The reliability of TrPt identification has been the subject of much criticism (Bohr 1996), but the reliability of physical signs is essential to obtaining meaningful clinical information (Al-Shenqiti & Oldham 2005; Nice et al 1992). These indicators include: spot tenderness, pain recognition, and referred pain pattern.

Patients demonstrating diagnostic rotator cuff tears on magnetic resonance imaging (MRI) investigation may respond favourably to the deactivation of TrPts, but it is essential to understand both the anatomical presentation of pain and the muscles commonly involved (Fig. 4.2). It is equally important to adopt rigor and standardization of assessment in order to eliminate the contributing myofascial pain component of rotor cuff pain presentation. The TrPts must be deactivated prior to shoulder stability exercise, postural and ergonomic retraining, and any future muscle imbalance and scapula retraining. The most common TrPts are found in the infraspinatus muscle, whilst the subscapularis is least affected muscle in RCD (Al Shenqiti & Oldham 2005).

Muscles involved

The supraspinatus muscle

A major function of the supraspinatus (Figs. 4.3 and 4.4) is to maintain balance amongst the other rotator cuff muscles and therefore offer stability to the joint. A common clinical symptom is 'a catch' of severe pain whilst the movement of elevation is attempted, with a positive Neer or Hawkins sign, or both. Pain is referred to the mid-deltoid region, extending to the arm and forearm if severe, especially at the lateral epicondyle of the elbow. It may often be mistaken for subdeltoid bursitis or later

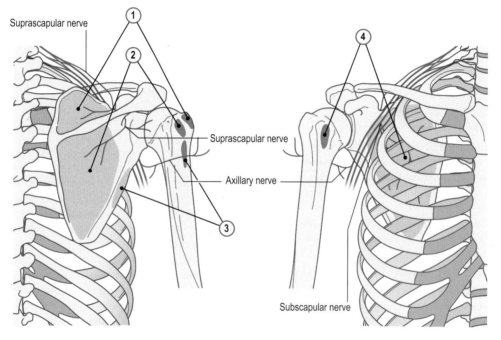

Muscle	Origin	Insertion	Action	Innervation
① **Supraspinatus**	Supraspinous fossa of the scapula	Greater tuberosity of the humerus	Abduction	Suprascapular nerve (C4–C6)
② **Infraspinatus**	Infraspinous fossa of the scapula	Greater tuberosity of the humerus	External rotation	Suprascapular nerve (C4–C6)
③ **Teres minor**	Lateral border of the scapula	Greater tuberosity of the humerus	Abduction	Axillary nerve (C5,C6)
④ **Subscapularis**	Subscapular fossa of the scapula	Lesser tuberosity of the humerus	Internal rotation	Subscapular nerve (C5–C6)

Figure 4.2 • The muscles of the rotator cuff.

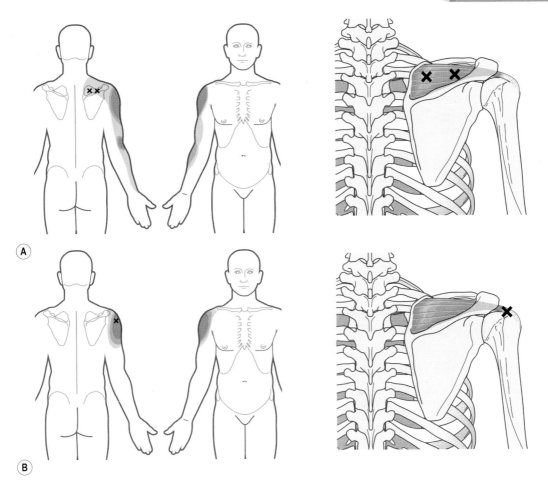

Figure 4.3 • Supraspinatus pain referral pattern.

epicondylitis (Simons et al 1999), but in reality, the supraspinatus muscle is in direct contact with the bursa and, hence, we are presented with nociceptive sensitization. It is necessary to undertake TrPt release and manage the patient with appropriate stretching and muscle re-education. This muscle should not be stretched if related RCD processes are present (Fig. 4.5).

The infraspinatus muscle

Infraspinatus injury is a common presentation characterized by deep, intense pain at the anterior edge of the shoulder within the bicipital groove, radiating down the radial aspect of arm and forearm, and it

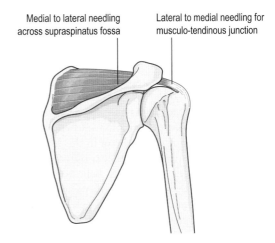

Medial to lateral needling across supraspinatus fossa

Lateral to medial needling for musculo-tendinous junction

Figure 4.4 • Direction of trigger point needling for supraspinatus muscle.

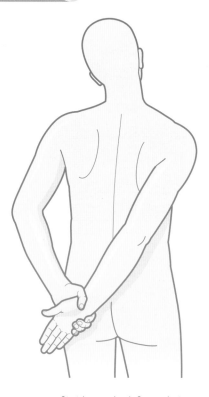

Stretch excercise 1: Supraspinatus

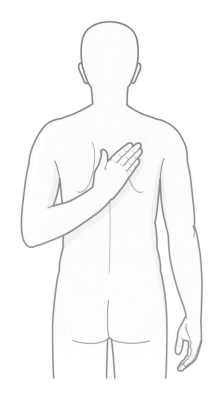

Stretch excercise 2: Supraspinatus

Figure 4.5 • Stretching exercises for supraspinatus muscle.

is identified as a major source of arm pain (Figs. 4.6 and 4.7) (Travell 1952). The pain is associated with abduction and medial rotation, and is most commonly a result of the acute overload associated with whiplash injury. If joint restriction accompanies the trigger point, then mobilization of the acromioclavicular and sternoclavicular articulations may be required. If there is suspicion of rotator cuff damage, the infraspinatus should not be stretched, but sustained myofascial contract–relax should be used (Fig. 4.8).

Isolated posterior pain is usually not involved in a single muscle pain presentation. However, if the patient complains of dysaesthesia in the fourth and fifth fingers, this may well be attributed to a single muscle element (Escobar & Ballesteros 1998). This is usually the result of overload stresses, and repetition of upward reaching and extension of the shoulder, commonly associated with window cleaning. Its action is often coupled with the infraspinatus, and it is necessary to deactivate both muscles before any muscle imbalance retraining.

The subscapularis muscle

Subscapularis trigger point pain referral presents with posterior scapula and shoulder pain in the form of a 'watchstrap band' of pain on the affected arm (Fig. 4.9) (Zohn 1988). The subscapularis medially rotates and adducts the arm and patients initially have pain on medial rotation and abduction; for example, when throwing a ball or playing golf. It can also manifest in patients following hemiplegia. Gradually abduction is restricted to below 45° and is often diagnosed as frozen shoulder. The subscapularis is often overlooked in shoulder dysfunction (Donatelli 1997; Simons et al 1999). It has a large and relatively inaccessible muscle mass that serves to sensitize the other rotator cuff muscles, which often develop latent TrPts. This leads to loss of rotation and pain patterns that may mimic joint range of movement loss, especially in lateral rotation. Management aims to identify the factors involved, whilst pain management remains a priority because pain leads to inhibition of rotator cuff

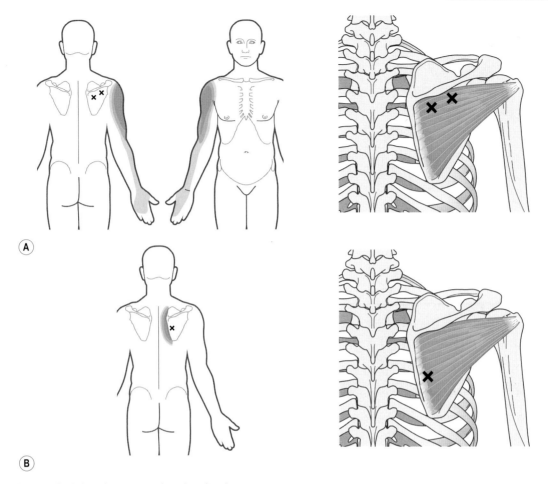

Figure 4.6 • Infraspinatus muscle pain referral pattern.

and shoulder weakness (Donatelli 1997; Itoi et al 2007). The goals of the rehabilitation process should include:

- Reduction of TrPt dysfunction;
- Return of normal shoulder movement;
- Muscle imbalance re-education;
- Re-establishment of movement synchrony; and
- Progressive return to function.

What if inflammation is present?

Although the evidence for the presentation of inflammatory processes in RCD is poor, there are some indications that these processes are present

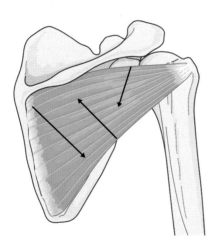

Figure 4.7 • Direction of needling for infraspinatus muscle.

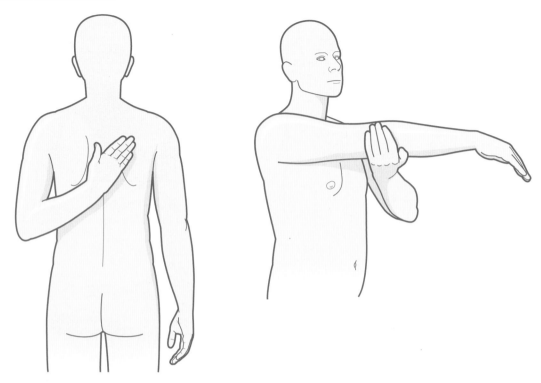

Figure 4.8 • Stretching for Infraspinatus muscle.

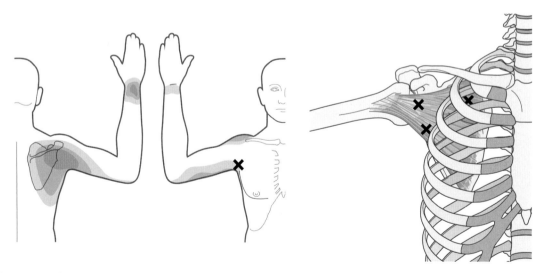

Figure 4.9 • Subscapularis pain referral pattern.

in cases of acute injury. Acupuncture is thought to have a modulating effect on both the systemic and peripheral mechanisms implicated in neurogenic inflammation (Ceccherelli et al 2002). After stimulation with acupuncture, calcitonin gene-related peptide (CGRP), substance P, and beta-endorphin are all released (Raud & Lundeberg 1991). Substance P initiates mast cells and macrophages to secrete inflammatory mediators; CGRP stimulates vasodilatation and thus induces peripheral events, improving tissue function and pain relief. If the acupuncture is too intense and too frequent, it can result in overstimulation of substance P and CGRP, causing a proinflammatory effect. Well-performed acupuncture (obtaining de Qi) that is low dose and frequently applied (two or three times per week for 10 to 20 minutes) using points distal to the injury site, at the segmental dorsal horn or on the contralateral side (Bradnam 2002) at the start of the injury process, could provoke a sustained low-dose release of CGRP with resulting anti-inflammatory effects (Sandberg et al 2004) and without activation of proinflammatory agents (Raud & Lundeberg 1991). This offers a case for promoting early acupuncture intervention at the acute stage of the inflammatory process. How often have we turned to acupuncture after three or more treatments when pain modulation has not been met? If inflammation and pain are preventing manual intervention and active return to function, then acupuncture should be considered within the first few treatments to promote cortisol release, increase blood flow, and facilitate manual intervention and rehabilitation (Tables 4.1 and 4.2). Distal points, He-Sea points, and Qi Cleft points should all be considered for the activation of Qi and blood flow and for the promotion of homeostasis and healing. Qi Cleft points are referred to in traditional Chinese medicine (TCM) for the treatment of acute conditions where inflammatory agents are causing pain, swelling, and limited movement. It is common to choose Qi Cleft points that correspond to the injury site and affected meridians.

Table 4.1 Suggested points for increased blood flow

Points	Traditional Chinese medicine	Western
SI3	Alleviates pain in arm and face Clears heat	Upper quadrant pain
LI4/5	Alleviates pain Expels pathogens	Alleviates pain and swelling in upper extremity
LI11	Arm pain Stimulates Qi flow in LI meridian	Increases blood flow in the meridian
GB20	Removes pain and heat in the area of neck and arm	Increases blood flow to head and neck
LIV3	Alleviates pain and induces relaxation	
GV14	Moves Qi and alleviates stiffness	Increases blood flow to head and neck
BL40	He-Sea point of meridian	Increases blood flow in meridian
BL60	Removes heat and activates the channel	
BL62	Activates channel and alleviates pain	
ST44	Alleviates pain and swelling	Alleviates pain and swelling in lower extremity
ST36	Tonifies Qi Nourishes blood	

Return of normal shoulder movement

Normal movement may be restored by a variety of therapeutic means, including: proprioceptive training; stretching; and a range of movement (ROM) home exercise programme.

Muscle imbalance re-education

There are no significant differences between patients who are given customized exercises and those who are given standard exercises on measures of pain, intensity, functional status, shoulder ROM, and strength (Wang 2004). The best exercise protocol for RCD or subacromial impingement syndrome (SIS) has not yet been established, although the benefit of subjecting patients to a reinforcement programme for the glenohumeral and scapulothoracic muscles to improve joint stability, reduce pain, and regain strength is generally accepted. Rehabilitative programmes based on either non-specific or specific exercises seem to give favourable results but further research is necessary in order to verify which protocol is the most effective. Stretching is often proposed to be associated with re-enforcement exercises to lengthen shortened muscular and ligamentous structures, and manual therapy has been demonstrated to be a valid instrument for reducing in the impingement syndrome. At the moment, muscular reinforcement

Table 4.2 Suggested points for enhancing acute symptom resolution

Points	Area supplied	Suggested conditions
LU6 PC4 HT6	Palmer aspect of wrist and forearm	Acute swelling and inflammation to contralateral wrist and forearm Tendinosis of wrist flexors Repetitive strain injury Distal points for shoulder/ elbow injury
LI7 SJ7 SI6	Postero-ulnar aspect of wrist and forearm	Acute swelling and injury to contralateral wrist. Extensor tendinosis Repetitive strain injury Distal points for shoulder/ elbow injury
ST34 GB36 SP8 LIV6 KID5 GB35	Acute knee injury, swelling and stiffness Sports injuries All soft tissue injuries Acute flare up of inflammatory processes	Contralateral knee if area within point location swollen May be used as distal points if outside the area of swelling
BL63 BL59 KID8 KID9	Acute ankle or lower limb injury Shin splints	Contralateral ankle if area within point location swollen May be used as distal points if outside the area of swelling hip and knee pain

is the recommended approach for an impingement syndrome and instability problems because of the dependence of the scapulohumeral girdle on the surrounding muscle (Casonato 2003).

Re-establishment of movement synchrony

Re-establishment of movement synchrony is necessary to restore the patient to previous performance and functional levels. In the case of the athlete, the development of a throwing or activity programme that pertains to the individual sport is necessary, and with this, a progressive return to function simulating sport activity in the resisted exercise programme. If a build-up of inflammatory neuropeptides aggravating the peripheral pain mechanisms is the cause, then acupuncture

using distal, He Sea, or Qi Cleft points may well provide the modulating effect to facilitate cortisol release and blood flow, thus enhancing rehabilitation. However, if the pain nature is caused by myofascial structures, a variety of other factors must be explored.

The unresolving shoulder

Patients are often referred to physiotherapy with the catch all diagnosis of frozen shoulder (FS) (Neviaser 1945), which is loosely defined as a painful, stiff shoulder, varying in duration from several weeks to several months. Pain, along with diminished function, usually motivates the patient to seek help (Cailliet 1981; DePalma 1983). It is essential to eliminate any cervical or thoracic spine involvement along with acromioclavicular, sternoclavicular, and scapulothoracic dysfunction, or first rib involvement. Although there is little agreement on treatment protocols, the goals for rehabilitation remain clear, namely, pain relief and restoration of function. Pain tends to be more long standing, radiating beyond the shoulder joint and involving sleep disruption; therefore, the aim of acupuncture intervention should be directed towards activation of descending inhibitory mechanisms involving:

- Pain modulation;
- Sleep enhancement;
- Well being; and
- Functional restoration.

Within TCM, FS is referred to as Jianning and belongs to the yin group of disease patterns known as Bi syndrome (Sun & Vangermeersch 1955), or painful obstructive syndrome (Maciocia 1994). It is mainly confined to superficial meridian or channel blockage, stagnation or obstruction caused by an attack of pathogenic factors such as cold (Han Bi), dampness (Shi Bi), or wind (Feng Bi) or a combination of all three. External pathogens will only invade the channel when defensive Qi (Wei Qi) or internal organ Qi and/or blood is weak, and cannot counteract the stronger pathogen factor. Within the flow of Qi dynamics, joints are important areas of convergence of Qi and blood. Through the joints, yin and yang Qi meet (Maciocia 1994), Qi and blood enter and exit, and pathogenic factors converge after penetrating the channels causing an obstruction to the flow, resulting in stagnation. The concept of Bi encompasses superficial disease processes in connective tissue structures paralleled in Western anatomical theory, such as tendons, ligaments, muscles, and joints. Stagnation causes pain and obstruction results in loss of normal joint range.

Within the diagnosis of FS, all three pathogens may be responsible, but cold and damp predominate. Cold freezes and contracts, leading to the intense, stabbing pain consistent with the first stages of FS. Damp will produce the numbness, loss of movement, and deep ache characteristic of the second and third stages of FS. The Large Intestine and Stomach meridians are both superficial to and cross the shoulder joint, offering vulnerable areas to the invasion of cold and damp (Needles 1982). Emotional trauma, such as anger, grief, or shock, is classed as pathogenic agents and may influence Qi and blood flow; Cyriax (1978) refers to the shoulder as the most emotional joint of the body.

The Large Intestine meridian is thought to be important for shoulder function because of its close proximity to the joint. Because Bi syndrome corresponds to a yin disease and the philosophy of TCM is to maintain a balance between yin and yang, stimulation of yang energy is desirable to address this yin excess. In classical acupuncture, stimulation of a distal yang point on the channel will open the channel (Maciocia 1994), eliminate stagnation, and promote Qi and blood flow and help to expel pathogenic factors. One channel can affect another related channel on the same polarity with opposite potential (e.g. Large Intestine and Stomach on the Yang Ming Stomach meridian intersects with the Large Intestine meridian crossing the shoulder and is known as Yang Ming in ancient Chinese literature). In order to facilitate descending inhibitory processes in pain modulation and stimulate Qi flow for restoration of function, traditional local and distal points may be used to facilitate these two objectives (Table 4.3).

Pain modulation may be enhanced by the use of transcutaneous electrical nerve stimulation (TENS) at home, or in the case of more prolonged dysfunction, electroacupuncture. Using a frequency of 2 to 4 Hz at distal points may enhance opioid and endorphin production, whilst a frequency of 80 to 100 Hz at local points may enhance production of leu-enkephalins and meta-enkephalins for segmental pain gate modulation (Han & Terenius 1982).

Table 4.3 Traditional local & distal points

Local points	Function (segmental dorsal horn inhibition)
LI15/14	Stimulate Qi within the shoulder joint
TE14	Improve blood flow
GB21	Stiffness of shoulder
Extra points	
JianQian (M-UE-48)	Stiffness of shoulder
Distal points (bilateral application)	**Function (descending inhibitory control)**
LI4	Pain above the sternum
TE5	Pain in shoulder
ST38	Activates the Large Intestine and Stomach channels to move Qi
GB34	Action on soft tissue structures He-Sea point
Extra points	
Yintang (M-HN-3)	Sleep enhancement
Amnian (N-HN-54)	Activates melatonin within pineal gland

Chronic shoulder pain and stiffness

There is no clear evidence to support one or a combination of treatments for the patient with FS; reports of success in the literature are equally outnumbered by research to the contrary (Hunt 2005). Frozen shoulder affects 2 to 5% of the general population (Kordell 2002). The exact mechanism of the onset is unknown, but changes to the capsule are thought to be similar to that of Dupuytrens contracture (Bunker et al 2000). The diagnosis is based on detailed history and assessment with decreased ROM (up to 50%) with:

- Stiff end feel;
- Negative instability tests; and
- Normal X-ray to rule out bony injury or calcification of the rotator cuff tendons (Lundeberg 1969).

As stated, the primary aim of treatment should be pain relief. It is likely to increase patient compliance with his rehabilitation programme, and affect any pain-related muscle inhibition and abnormal biomechanics.

Case Study 1

Dan Franklin

A 39-year-old male lawyer presented with a 5-week history of right shoulder pain; he had woken with the pain one morning, but had not been able to attribute it to any incident or activity. The subject rested his shoulder, and when the pain did not abate after 3 weeks, sought advice from his general practitioner, who prescribed ibuprofen; there were no further investigations. The medication helped somewhat, and three days before presentation to physiotherapy, the subject decided to test his shoulder with a social game of tennis; it soon became obvious that he could not continue, and therefore he rested again and made a physiotherapy appointment for further input. The subject described sharp and localized right shoulder pain over the lateral aspect of the deltoid that occurred in conjunction with arm movements, especially abduction or fast movements in any direction. The subject was not able to lie on his right side, but did not report any sleep disturbances; there were no neural signs and there was no concurrent neck pain. Previous medical history revealed that he had twice dislocated his right shoulder while playing rugby; the last episode had occurred over 15 years previously and he had experienced no further problems until this recent episode of pain.

Examination findings

On examination, the subject was found to have an increased middle and upper thoracic kyphosis, and a protracted cervical spine. Both scapulae were also protracted, the right more so than the left, and his right humeral head was observed to be sitting anteriorly in the glenoid relative to the left side. Cervical spine movements were slightly reduced in all directions from what the present author would expect in a subject of this age group, and his cervical paraspinal muscles were a little tender on palpation, but neither reproduced his shoulder pain. The subject's thoracic spine was stiff in extension, and posteroanterior mobilizations of the spinous processes and costovertebral joints at thoracic levels 1 to 4 (T1 to T4) and ribs 2 to 4 on the right revealed hypomobility and reproduced local pain. The subject's right shoulder demonstrated flexion to 170°, with slight pain at the end of ROM. Abduction revealed a painful arc between 80° and 120° before resistance and the return of pain at 170°. Poor scapulohumeral rhythm was present in flexion and more obviously in abduction. This included a reduced glenohumeral contribution to flexion and abduction in mid-ranges, and a compensatory increase in scapular elevation and upward rotation. The hand-behind-back movement, a combination of shoulder extension, adduction, and internal rotation, was painful and restricted. Resisted external rotation on the right was weak compared with the left, but range was full and pain-free bilaterally. Resisted isometric flexion, abduction, adduction,

extension, and internal rotation with the right shoulder in neutral were of full strength and pain-free.

The subject underwent three tests indicative of impingement, as described by Brukner and Khan (2002): Neer test, the Hawkins–Kennedy test, and the 'empty can test' (resisted abduction in 90° abduction, with 30° horizontal flexion. Speed's (biceps) test and O'Brien's superior labrum anteroposterior lesion test were both negative. An apprehension test was painful, but not positive. A diagnosis of SIS was made on the basis of the above examination. MRI provides an accurate anatomical image of the subacromial space and is the current gold standard in the diagnosis of SIS (Silva et al 2008). Actual shoulder diseases can be differentiated aetiopathologically according to a primary and secondary impingement syndrome. Narrowing of the subacromial space, which is caused by an osseous shape variant, leads to primary impingement. Secondary impingement develops when the subacromial space is reduced by swollen tissue below the osseous shoulder roof (Adamietz et al 2008). Factors that needed to be addressed by the treatment included:

- Improvement of the glenoid alignment of the humeral head;
- Strengthening of and coordination work for the rotator cuff, especially the external shoulder rotators;
- Mobilization to restore extension range throughout the upper thoracic spine and lower cervical spine;
- Improvement of right-sided scapulohumeral rhythm;
- Achieving pain relief as quickly as possible to ease discomfort; and
- Reduction of antalgic biomechanics and promotion of compliance with further treatment.

A visual analogue scale (VAS) for pain was completed at the time of the initial assessment, and this, along with flexion and abduction ROM measures, was used throughout treatment to assess progress.

Treatment

The primary treatment goal for the first session was pain relief. It was also felt that pain relief would be likely to increase the subject's compliance with his rehabilitation programme, and affect any pain-related muscle inhibition and abnormal biomechanics. The first treatment choice to achieve this aim was acupuncture, given its accepted analgesic effects. Treatment consisted of:

- Grade II anterior–posterior mobilization of the glenohumeral joint;
- Grade III posterior–anterior mobilization of the T1 to T4 spinal segments, right costovertebral joints, and ribs 2 to 4;
- Soft-tissue massage to the upper trapezius, posterior shoulder muscles, and pectoralis muscles of the right side;

(Continued)

Case Study 1 (Continued)

- Gentle horizontal or cross-flexion stretches for the posterior of the right shoulder; and
- Taping to encourage better alignment of the right humeral head in the glenoid fossa.

Three days later, the subject reported aggravation of his symptoms, possibly as a result of the initial examination and treatment. Distal acupuncture points were chosen during this second session, because of their strong analgesic potential. Manual techniques had potentially aggravated the subject's condition previously and local acupuncture would also have the potential to aggravate the injury (Lundeberg & Ekholm 2001). Because the subject demonstrated an acute to subacute presentation, it was decided to needle the contralateral shoulder, thereby triggering the pain-gate mechanism at the correct spinal segment without risking an inflammatory response in the affected shoulder. For the local shoulder points, Large Intestine 15 (LI15) and Triple Energizer 14 (TE14) were chosen because these points are in the same dermatome as the shoulder and are known to be effective in the treatment of shoulder pain (Hecker et al 2001; Kleinhenz et al 1999; White & Ernst 1999). Large Intestine 4 (LI4) was used bilaterally because it is also a well-recognized point for shoulder dysfunction (Hopwood et al 1997; He et al 2005; Hecker et al 2001; Kleinhenz et al 1999), and is acknowledged to be one of the strongest points in the body for analgesia since it is a strong instigator of opioid release and descending inhibition (Table 4.4) (Carlsson 2002; He et al 2005; Hecker et al 2001; Hopwood et al 1997; Kleinhenz et al 1999).

The subject had improved objectively by the time of the third treatment in terms of VAS score and ROM, although he still felt subjectively worse than prior to the first treatment. Two treatments per week were booked since this may be more effective than less frequent sessions (White & Ernst 1999), and because there had been an objective improvement but no subjective recovery, it was decided to change the distal point from LI4 to Stomach 38 (ST38), one which is more specific to shoulder injury (Hecker et al 2001; Hopwood et al 1997). Having increased the subject's pain with the first treatment using manual therapy a concern remained about the potential irritability of the condition, and therefore the present author was not prepared to risk needling locally, preferring to continue with contralateral needling of the shoulder and arm instead.

Fourth session

The subject felt much improved by the fourth session, but he still had pain on sudden movements and any abduction with an internal rotation component. With his pain now significantly reduced, a change was made to the treatment, which now included ipsilateral local needling at LI15 and TE14, as well as LI11. Additional manual therapy was used during this session.

Table 4.4 Case study 1: treatment choice justification

Day	VAS	ROM pre-treatment	Treatment	ROM post treatment
1	37/100	Flexion 170° R2, P1 Abduction 80° P1 170° P2	Mobilization T/S GHJ, massage, taping	Flexion 170° Abduction: 70-120° P1 170° P2
2	65/100	Flexion 60° P2 Abduction 60° P2	LI15, TE14, LI11[C] LI4[B] Mobilization GHJ Pendular exercises	Flexion 130° P1 Abduction 70° P1
3	65/100	Flexion 175° Abduction 175°	LI15, TE14, LI11[C], ST38[B] Scapula stability Retraction exercises	Flexion 130° Abduction 70°
6	43/100	Flexion 175° Abduction 175°	LI15, TE14, LI11[C] St 38[B] Scapula stability LI15 TE14, LI11[R]	Flexion 170° Abduction 170°
9	27/100	Flexion 175° Abduction 175°	T/S, STM post shoulder Neer test positive Rotational exercises	Flexion 175° Abduction 175°

Notes: ROM, range of motion; C, contralateral; B, bilateral; R, right; VAS, visual analogue scale; R2, end of ROM caused by resistance rather than pain; P1, the point in a ROM where pain is felt for the first time, but does not cause cessation of movement; P2, end of ROM because of resistance (pain also present at this point, but not restrictive of movement); mobilization T/S, posterior/anterior mobilization centrally and unilaterally (right) of thoracic spine segments T1–T4; mobilization GHJ, anteroposterior mobilization of the glenohumeral joint; STM, soft-tissue massage.

Discussion

While it was disappointing that the first manual therapy treatment appeared to aggravate the subject's condition, his improvement following the commencement of acupuncture was encouraging. Unfortunately,

(Continued)

Case Study 1 (Continued)

acupuncture was not used during the initial treatment session because he disclosed that he had not eaten all day, and it is accepted that acupuncture can have an effect on blood glucose levels (Carlsson 2002; Chen et al 1994). Once he had experienced the acute exacerbation of his condition after the first treatment session, descending inhibition of pain might have been enhanced by including Liver 3 (LIV3) with LI4 (the four

gates), which are known for their very powerful central effects (Carlsson 2002). Small Intestine 3 (SI3), which aids the release of cortisol, could also have been chosen to reduce inflammation (Roth et al 1997; Toyama et al 1982). One point that will be included in this subject's future treatments is Gall Bladder (GB21) because it has been incorporated in successful studies of acupuncture in shoulder pain (He et al 2005).

 Case Study 2

Kevin Hunt

A 40-year-old female shop assistant presented with a 3-month history of pain in her right shoulder that had become worse in 3 weeks prior to her assessment. The pain pattern was distributed over the anterior and posterior aspects of the shoulder, radiating to the deltoid insertion in a band around the deltoid muscle (Fig. 4.10).

The subject's VAS was 40/100 at best and 90/100 at worst with movement (A). Pain along the lateral border of the scapula (B) was 90/100. Pain along the anterior chest in line with the axilla (C) was rated 90/100 and the patient was very anxious about whether this might be associated with a more serious pathology. There had been a previous injury to her right shoulder 2 years before that had required 6 months of physiotherapy for subacromial dysfunction. The subject had been prescribed co-codamol (30/500 mg q.d.s) and X-ray showed no bony changes. The treatment plan is shown in Table 4.5.

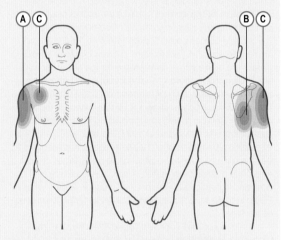

Figure 4.10 • Case Study 2 pain presentation.

Clinical reasoning

The deactivation of the subscapularis trigger point and the consistent pain pattern from an active trigger point at B resulted in a dramatic increase in ROM (flexion increased from 84° to 140°; abduction from 82° to 140°). MRI findings to subscapularis tendons in FS show that there are synovitis-like abnormalities relating to the superior border (Mengiardi et al 2004; Pearsall et al 2000). The improvement in pain and ROM after deactivation of subscapularis trigger point is consistent with those following surgical release (Pearsall et al 2000). The subject reported improved sleep, reduced anxiety levels, and resolution of pain B. Subsequent treatments involved acupuncture to improve the cumulative pain management. Acupuncture stimulation releases endorphins and enkephalins such as adrenocorticotrophic hormone into the blood stream, providing further systemic pain inhibition as well as the potential for sympathetic nervous system inhibition (Ma 2004). Other hormones and neurotransmitters, such as serotonin, catecholamines, inorganic chemicals, and

amino acids (e.g. glutamate and aminobutyric acid), have been proposed as mediators of certain analgesic effects of acupuncture, and research is ongoing into their contributing effect. Recent functional MRI (fMRI) trials have demonstrated an effect on limbic and paralimbic structures involved in the modulation of pain that is strongest when de Qi is elicited by peripheral acupuncture stimulation (Brooks & Tracey 2005; Hui 1995; Tracey 2007).

As the treatment progressed, local tender and joint acupuncture points were added especially Lung 1 (LU1); however, this also corresponds to the TrPt presentation of the pectoralis major muscle and a greater release of pain and ROM might have been achieved by adding the pectoralis TrPt, if positive (Fig. 4.11).

Conclusion

The subject reported an improvement of 70% in her condition, ceased taking medication; slept through the night again, and was able to perform normal activities of daily living. The pain reduction achieved in the present

(Continued)

Case Study 2 (Continued)

Table 4.5 Treatment summary of patient with secondary frozen shoulder

Day	VAS	ROM pre-treatment	Treatment	ROM post treatment
0	A 90/100 B 90/100 C 90/100	Flexion: 84° Abduction: 82°	Subscapularis Trigger point deactivation	Flexion: 140° Abduction: 104°
5	A 70/100 B 0/100 C 70/100	Flexion: 125° Abduction: 100°	LI4 [B] LI11, 14,15 [R] LI4 [B]	Flexion: 125° Abduction: 100°
13	A 80/100 B 0/100 C 70/100	Flexion: 120° Abduction: 90°	SI9, 11. 12[R] GB21 [R]	Flexion: 120° Abduction: 90°
18	A 40/100 B 0/100 C 70/100	Flexion: 140° Abduction: 110°	LI4 [B] LU1 [R] SI9, 11, 12 [R] GB21 [R]	Flexion: 120° Abduction: 90°
23	A 40/100 B 0/100 C 70/100	Flexion: 150° Abduction: 110°	LI4 [B] SI9, 11, 12 [R] GB21 [R]	Flexion: 150° Abduction: 110°

Notes: C, contralateral; B, bilateral; R, right; A, B, C: see Fig. 4.10.

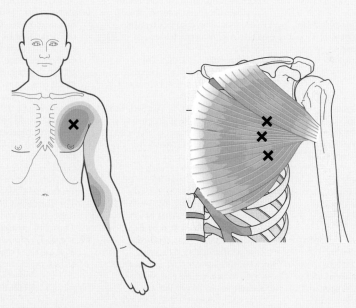

Figure 4.11 • Pain presentation in the pectoralis major muscle.

small case report was consistent with that found in other studies using acupuncture for pain modulation and as a precursor to active rehabilitation (Lin et al 1994; Tukmachi 1999), and as a postoperative pain modulator following acromioplasty (Gilbertson et al 2003). More frequent treatment involving an increased use of distal and bilateral points could have enhanced the effect reported in the present study (Guerra et al 2003).

References

Adamietz, B., Sauer, R., Keilholz, L., 2008. Radiotherapy for shoulder impingement. Strahlenther Onkol. 184 (5), 245–250.

Al-Shenqiti, A.M., Oldham, J.A., 2005. Test–retest reliability of myofascial trigger point detection in patients with rotator cuff tendonitis. Clin. Rehabil. 19 (5), 482–487.

Barying, T., Emery, R., Reilly, P., 2007. Management of rotator cuff disease: specific treatment for specific disorders. Best practice and research. Clin. Rheumatol. 21 (2), 279–294.

Bohr, T., 1996. Problems with myofascial pain syndrome and fibromyalgia. Neurology 46, 593–597.

Bradnam, L., 2002. Western acupuncture point selection: a scientific clinical reasoning model. J. Acupunct. Assoc. Chartered Psychother. 1, 21–29.

Brooks, J., Tracey, I., 2005. From nociception to pain perception: imaging the spinal and supraspinal pathways. J. Anat. 207 (1), 19–33.

Brukner, P., Khan, K., 2002. Clinical Sports Medicine, 2nd edn. McGraw-Hill, New York.

Bunker, T.D., Reilly, K.S., Hambleden, D.L., 2000. Express of growth factors, cytokines and matrix metalloproteinases in frozen shoulder. J. Bone Joint Surg. 82, 768–773.

Cailliet, R., 1981. Shoulder Pain, 2nd edn. FA Davis, Philadelphia.

Carlsson, C., 2002. Acupuncture mechanisms for clinically relevant long-term effects- reconsideration and a hypothesis. Acupunct. Med. 20 (2–3), 82–99.

Casonato, O., 2003. The role of therapeutic exercise in the conflicting and unstable shoulder. Phys. Ther. Rev. 8 (10833196), 69–84.

Ceccherelli, F., Bordin, M., Gagliardi, G., et al., 2001. Comparison between superficial and deep acupuncture in the treatment of the shoulder's myofascial pain: a randomised and controlled study. Acupunct. Electrother. Res. 26 (4), 229–238.

Ceccherelli, F., Gagliardi, G., Ruzzanti, L., et al., 2002. Acupuncture modulation of capsaicin-induced inflammation: effect of intraperitoneal and local administration of naloxone in rats.

A blinded controlled study. J. Altern. Complement. Med. 8 (3), 341–349.

Chen, D., Gong, D., Zhai, Y., 1994. Clinical and experimental studies in treating Diabetes Mellitus with acupuncture. J. Tradit. Chin. Med. 14 (3), 163–166.

Cyriax, J., 1978. Textbook of Orthopaedic Medicine, 7th edn. Bailliere Tindall, London.

DePalma, A., 1983. Surgery of the Shoulder. JB Lippincott, Philadelphia.

Dempster, W., 1965. Mechanism of shoulder movement. Arch. Phys. Med. Rehabil. 46A (49), 49–70.

Donatelli, R., 1997. Physical Therapy of the Shoulder, 3rd edn. Churchill Livingstone, Edinburgh.

Escobar, P., Ballesteros, J., 1998. Teres minor: source of symptoms resembling ulnar neuropathy or C8 radiculopathy. Am. J. Phys. Med. Rehabil. 67 (3), 120–122.

Gilbertson, B., Wenner, K., Russell, L.C., 2003. Acupuncture and arthroscopic acromioplasty. J. Orthop. Res. 21, 752–758.

Guerra, J., Bassas, E., Andres, M., et al., 2003. Acupuncture for soft tissue shoulder disorders: a series of 201 cases, including commentary by White AR. Acupunct Med. 21 (1-2), 18–22.

Han, J., Terenius, L., 1982. The neurochemical basis of acupuncture analgesia. Annu. Revis. Pharmacol. Toxicol. 22, 91–104.

He, D., Hostermark, A.T., Veirsted, K.B., et al., 2005. Effects of intensive acupuncture on pain related social and psychological variables for women with chronic neck and shoulder pain-an RCT with six months and three year follow up. Acupunct Med. 23 (2), 52–61.

Hecker, H.U., Steveling, A., Peuker, E., et al., 2001. Color Atlas of Acupuncture: Body Points, Ear Points, Trigger Points, 2nd edn. Thieme Publishing, Stuttgart.

Hopwood, V., Lovesey, M., Makone, S., 1997. Acupuncture and Related Techniques in Physiotherapy. Churchill Livingstone, Edinburgh.

Hui, H., 1995. A review of treatment for diabetes by acupuncture during the post forty years. J. Tradit. Chin. Med. 15 (2), 145–154.

Hunt, K., 2005. Acupuncture in a female patient with secondary frozen shoulder. J. Acupunct. Assoc. Chartered Psychother. (Jan.), 50–55.

Itoi, E., Managawa, H., Sato, T., et al., 2007. Isokinetic strength after tears of the suraspinatus tendon. J. Bone Joint Surg. 79B (1), 77–82.

Kleinhenz, J., Streitberger, K., Windeler, J., et al., 1999. Randomised clinical trial comparing the effects of acupuncture and a newly designed placebo needle in rotator cuff tendinitis. Pain 83 (2), 235–241.

Kordell, T., 2002. Frozen shoulder and diabetes. Diabetes Forecast 55 (8), 60–64.

Lewis. J., 2007. Rotator cuff pathology. Personal Communication, AACP Conference.

Lewis, J., Tennent, T., 2007. How effective are our diagnostic tests for rotator cuff pathology?. In: MacAuley, D., Best, T.M. (Eds.) Evidence-Based Sports Medicine, 2nd edn. Blackwell, Oxford.

Lin, M.L., Huang, C.T., Lin, J.G., et al., 1994. A comparison between the pain relief effect of electroacupuncture, regional nerve block and electroacupuncture plus regional nerve block in frozen shoulder. Acta Anaesthesiol. Sin. 32 (4), 237–242.

Lundeberg, B.J., 1969. The frozen shoulder. Clinical and radiographical observations. The effect of manipulation under general anaesthetic. Structure and glycosaminoglycan content of the joint capsule. Local bone metabolism. Acta Ophthalmol. Scand. Suppl. 19, S1–S59.

Lundeberg, T., Ekholm, J., 2001. Pain—from periphery to brain. J. Acupunct. Assoc. Chartered Psychother. (Feb.), 13–19.

Maciocia, G., 1994. Painful obstruction syndrome. In: The Practice of Traditional Chinese Medicine: The Treatment of Diseases with Acupuncture and Chinese Herbs. Churchill Livingstone, Edinburgh.

Mengiardi, B., Pfirmann, C.W., Gerber, C., et al., 2004. Frozen shoulder: MRI arthrographic findings. Radiology 233 (2), 486–492.

Needles, J., 1982. Bi syndrome. J. Chin. Med. 10 (1), 1–4.

Neviaser, J., 1945. Adhesive capsulitis of the shoulder; study of pathological findings in periarthritis of the shoulder. J. Bone Joint Surg. 27, 211.

Nice, D., Riddle, D., Lamb, R., et al., 1992. Inter-tester reliability of judgements of the presence of trigger points in patients. Arch. Phys. Med. Rehabil. 73, 893–898.

Pearsall, A.W., Holovacs, T.F., Speed, K.P., 2000. The intra-articular component of the Subscapularis tendon: anatomic and histological correlation in reference to surgical release in patients with frozen-shoulder syndrome. Arthroscopy 16, 236–242.

Raud, J., Lundeberg, T., 1991. Potent anti-inflammatory action of calcitonin gene-related peptide. Biochem. Biophys. Res. Commun. 180, 1419–1435.

Roth, L., Maret-Maric, A., Adler, R., et al., 1997. Acupuncture points have subjective (needling sensation) and objective (serum cortisol increase) specificity. Acupunct. Med. 15 (1), 2–5.

Sandberg, M., Lindberg, L., Gerdle, B., 2004. Effects of acupuncture on skin and muscle blood flow in healthy subjects. Eur. J. Pain. 8 (2), 163–171.

Silva, L., Andréu, J., Muñoz, P., et al., 2008. Accuracy of physical examination in subacromial impingement syndrome. Rheumatology 47 (5), 679–683.

Simons, D.G., Travell, J., Simons, L.S., 1999. Myofascial Pain and Dysfunction: The Trigger Point Manual, 2nd edn. Lippincott Williams & Wilkins, Baltimore.

Sola, A., Rodenberger, M., Gettys, B., 1955. Incidence of hypersensitive areas in posterior shoulder muscles. Am. J. Phys. Med. 34, 585–590.

Sun, P., Vangermeersch, L., 1955. Classification of Bi syndrome. J. Chin. Med. 47, 8–14.

Toyama, P., Popell, C., Evans, J., et al., 1982. Beta endorphin and cortisol measurements following acupuncture and moxibustion. J. Holistic Med. 4 (1), 58–67.

Tracey, I., 2007. Objectifying pain: lessons from imaging somatic and visceral pain in humans using FMRI. Cephalalgia 24 (9), 722.

Travell, J., 1952. Ethyl chloride spray for painful muscle spasm. Arch. Phys. Med. Rehabil. 33, 291–298.

Tukmachi, E.S., 1999. Frozen shoulder: a comparison of Western and traditional Chinese approaches and a clinical study of its acupuncture treatment. Acupunct. Med. 9 (1), 9–21.

Wang, S.S., 2004. Comparison of customised versus standard exercises in rehabilitation of shoulder disorders. Isokinet. Exerc. Sci. 12 (2), 135–141.

White, A.R., Ernst, E., 1999. A systematic review of randomised controlled acupuncture trails for neck pain. Rheumatology 38 (2), 143–147.

Whyte-Ferguson, L., Gerwin, R., 2005. Clinical Mastery in the Treatment of Myofascial Pain. Lippincott Williams and Wilkins, Baltimore.

Zohn, D., 1988. Musculoskeletal Pain: Diagnosis and Physical Treatment, 2nd edn. Little, Brown, Boston.

The elbow

5

Jo Gibson

Introduction

Epidemiological studies have reported that incidence of elbow pain in the general population is between 8 and 12% (Korthals-de Bos et al 2004). The elbow has proved to be the poor relation in terms of academic investigation as, other than in tennis elbow (TE), there is a paucity of literature regarding evidence-based management of elbow pathology. In considering the role of manual therapy in the treatment of elbow pathology, the therapist must often rely on what is understood regarding the pathophysiology of common elbow conditions, rather than evidence-based treatment strategies; these continue to remain elusive in the majority of elbow conditions. This may reflect the relatively low incidence of elbow pathology in comparison to conditions affecting the spine, knee, and shoulder, and the natural history of many elbow conditions. Elbow fractures account for only 7% of all fractures and reports suggest that half of all cases of cubital tunnel syndrome and ulnar neuropathy will resolve spontaneously (Walker-Bone et al 2004). However, the socioeconomic implications of conditions such as TE cannot be underestimated, and an emphasis must be placed on the importance of both understanding and optimizing the role of the manual therapist in managing this type of condition. Whilst there is currently limited evidence to support the efficacy of manual therapy in most elbow pathologies, modern advances in pain science and an increased understanding of the physiological effects of manual therapy techniques will guide future research.

Tennis elbow or lateral epicondylalgia (LE) is the second most frequently diagnosed musculoskeletal disorder of the neck and upper limb in a primary care setting, with an annual incidence of 4 to 7 cases per 1000 patients in general practice (Smidt et al 2003). Whilst over 40 different conservative treatment approaches have been described in the literature, the medical fraternity still tends to adopt a wait-and-see policy (Smidt et al 2002). This results from the failure of methodologically rigorous trials to demonstrate any long-term benefit of conservative interventions (Smidt et al 2003). There is, however, good evidence to support a short-term benefit from conservative interventions (Bisset et al 2005); from both a physiotherapist and patient perspective, this is significant in terms of return to function and reducing

DOI: 10.1016/B978-0-443-06782-2.00005-0

the socioeconomic impact of this challenging condition. The lack of consensus regarding nomenclature in LE reflects our increasing understanding regarding the underlying pathophysiological processes. Authors have reported the absence of inflammatory mediators in patients with LE (Alfredson et al 2000), thus emphasizing the importance of moving away from misleading terminology, such as LE, and questioning the role of anti-inflammatory modalities. Furthermore, the appreciation that a key aspect of this condition is an underlying tendinopathy in the common extensor tendon suggests that terms such as lateral epicondyle tendinopathy may be more appropriate (Coombes et al 2009). However, it is clear from what we currently understand regarding LE pathophysiology in terms of local tendon pathology, abnormalities in the pain system (peripheral and central), and impairments in the motor system (local and global) that the modern manual therapist is well placed to implement effective treatment strategies.

Manual therapy for the relief of pain

High levels of pain and functional disability have been reported in patients with LE and are the principal reasons that they seek treatment (Alizadehkhaiyat et al 2007a). Clinical trials commonly measure pain-free grip strength and pressure-pain thresholds as markers of improvement in pain levels in this patient group. Pain-free grip has been shown to be a valid and sensitive marker in measuring outcome in patients with LE, and correlates well with patients' perceived outcome (Pienimaki et al 2002). Active trigger points have been well described in the forearm muscles of patients with LE and are believed to be indicative of peripheral sensitization; however, the presence of latent trigger points in the unaffected side of patients with unilateral LE is also suggestive of central sensitization processes (Fernández-Carnero et al 2008a).

The link between the cervical and thoracic spine and LE remains controversial. Authors have suggested that the pain associated with LE may relate to altered neuronal afferent input to the spine (Fernández-Carnero et al 2008b). It is difficult to elucidate the true nature of this relationship because many studies of LE exclude patients with significant cervical spine signs; however, investigations

of study methodologies often reveal that this exclusion is based on reported symptomology rather than objective findings. In their study of patients with LE and a control group, Berglund et al (2008) reported that 70% of subjects with lateral elbow pain indicated pain in the cervical or thoracic spine, as compared to 16% in the control group. These patients also had a significantly increased frequency of pain response to the neurodynamic test of the radial nerve ($p < 0.001$). The above authors concluded that the cervical and thoracic spine should be included in the assessment of patients with lateral elbow pain.

The role of manual therapy techniques directed to the cervical spine in order to address pain in patients with LE remains unclear. Studies commonly fail to control for the natural history of the disorder and therefore compromise extrapolation of meaningful results. However, several studies have reported that mobilization techniques applied to the cervical spine in patients with LE produce a significant hypoalgesic effect and a concomitant sympathoexcitatory response at the elbow when compared to placebo or control groups (Vicenzino et al 2007). A pilot study by Vicenzino et al (1996) showed that patients treated with mobilization of the cervical spine, versus local elbow treatment, showed superior results in terms of pain-free grip strength and Disabilities of the Arm, Shoulder and Head (DASH) (Gummesson et al 2003) scores. A retrospective review by Cleland et al (2004) suggested that patients who received cervicothoracic mobilization, in addition to local treatment, require significantly fewer visits to achieve similar success rates in terms of pain relief and pain-free grip strength. In terms of specific manual therapy techniques, the cervical lateral glide technique has been shown to achieve significant improvements in pressure-pain threshold and an increase in pain-free grip strength, as well as the production of a sympathoexcitatory response across sudomotor, cutaneous, and vasomotor functions (Fig. 5.1). To date, this has only been demonstrated immediately after application of the technique (Vicenzino et al 2001).

The role of locally directed manual therapy techniques, such as mobilizations with movement (MWM) (see Fig 5.1), in the management of LE have been explored in several studies (Abbott et al 2001; Paungmali et al 2003). To perform the MWM technique, the therapist identifies a pain-provoking activity, which commonly involves the patient clenching their fist. This is then repeated while the

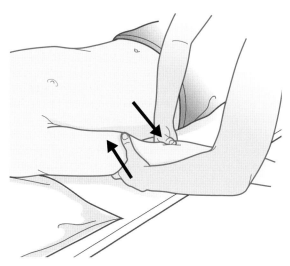

Figure 5.1 • Lateral elbow glide.
Pressure is applied in a posterior, lateral direction.

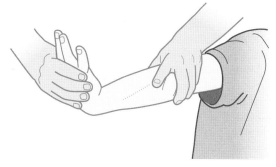

Figure 5.2 • Mills manipulation (1).
The patient is taken into:
• Passive shoulder extension;
• Full-range passive shoulder extension; and
• Passive wrist flexion.

therapist performs a laterally directed glide to the elbow. The direction in which the lateral glide is applied and the force with which it is applied are important in maximizing the hypoalgesic effect. Studies reporting the efficacy of this technique stress the importance of the procedure being performed as part of a home exercise programme between treatments (Bissett et al 2006a). A single MWM treatment has been shown to result in an immediate increase in pain-free grip strength. An initial reduction in pressure-pain thresholds over the lateral epicondyle and evidence of sympathetic excitation have also been reported. There is good evidence that MWM combined with an exercise programme has superior short-term effects in terms of pain, as measured by a visual analogue scale (VAS) versus exercise alone (Vicenzino et al 2007). This treatment approach (i.e. a combination of MWM and exercise) appears to be more effective than corticosteroid injection and crucially, wait-and-see over a 12-month period. In Bisset et al's (2006a) study, pain-free grip was optimally improved over the entire year; patients were apparently more satisfied and reported fewer recurrences. This was the first study to demonstrate a significant difference in longer term outcomes using a combination of exercise and manual therapy.

Whilst MWM combined with exercise has been the most researched manual therapy technique in

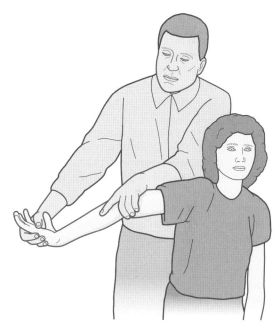

Figure 5.3 • Mills manipulation (2).
A downward pressure is exerted on:
• The radioulnar olecranon complex; and
• An upward high-velocity thrust with elbow extension and wrist flexion, shoulder extension.

LE, Cyriax (1945) claimed substantial success in treating TE using deep transverse friction (DTF) in combination with Mill's manipulation (Verhaar et al 1995) (Figs 5.2 and 5.3).

Cyriax (1945) stressed that in order to be considered a Cyriax intervention, the two components must be used together in the correct order and that patients must follow the protocol three times a week for 4 weeks. Despite this clear stipulation, only one study has been reported in which true Cyriax physiotherapy was used in the management of TE. Verhaar et al (1995) compared the effects of corticosteroid injections with Cyriax physiotherapy in treating patients with this condition. The results showed that the corticosteroid injection was significantly more effective on the outcome measures (i.e. pain, function, grip strength, and global assessment) than Cyriax physiotherapy at the end of the treatment, but at the follow-up one year after the end of treatment, there were no significant differences between the two treatment groups. Other studies have only examined the efficacy of one aspect of the Cyriax approach and have failed to demonstrate any significant treatment effect.

Current evidence suggests that manual therapy techniques such as cervical lateral glide and MWM have short-term efficacy in improving pain-free grip strength and pressure-pain threshold (Vicenzino et al 2007). There is limited evidence that manual therapy combined with exercise may have better long-term outcomes than injection or exercise alone. Vicenzino et al (2007) suggested that manual therapists should consider whether patients have greater deficits in pain-free grip measurements or pressure-pain threshold, during patient assessment. Those patients with greater deficits in pain-free grip strength may be the most appropriate candidates for MWM techniques directed at the elbow, since this is where they have been shown to have their greatest effect. Conversely, the above authors suggested that subjects with greater pressure-pain threshold deficits, relative to pain-free grip force deficits, should be treated with techniques directed at the cervical spine. Whilst this proposed classification system is based on current evidence, it requires further validation, but it does emphasize the importance of a thorough assessment that includes the cervical and thoracic spine, together with specific local palpation and testing in LE.

Manual therapy to improve joint movement

Consideration of the role of manual therapy in the management of the post-traumatic elbow has been hindered historically by the long-held belief that inappropriate mobilization can predispose the joint to the development of heterotrophic ossification (HO).

A review of the literature advocating that passive mobilization should not be performed reveals that most opinion has been based on animal studies that employed forcible passive mobilization (Casavant & Hastings 2006); this is not reflective of manual therapy techniques performed by therapists on this type of patient. Furthermore, much of the literature is anecdotal, purely based on expert opinion, or lacks methodological rigour. In reality, there are several papers that advocate the use of passive range of movement (PROM) exercises. Crucially, these have demonstrated that, in fact, there is no significant difference between groups that are mobilized and those that are not in terms of HO formation. Furthermore, those patients with demonstrated HO do not show a worsening or increase in formation if subjected to a passive mobilization regime (Casavant & Hastings 2006; Issak & Egol 2006). Consequently, patients at risk of developing post-traumatic stiffness should have appropriate physiotherapy intervention incorporating relevant mobilization techniques. However, more work is required to identify the optimal strategies for mobilization in this patient group.

Reduction in shoulder external rotation range of movement (ROM) has been reported in patients with LE. Abbot (2001) showed that MWM applied to the elbow results in an increase in the external rotation ROM at the shoulder. The above author suggested that this observation indicates that MWM cause a neurophysiologically mediated decrease in resting muscle tone. This observation further emphasizes the importance of a thorough assessment incorporating the shoulder joint in patients with LE.

Manual therapy to normalize muscle function

The main histopathological feature demonstrated in LE is that of a tendinopathy involving the common wrist extensor origin (Fedorczyk 2006). Microscopic and histology studies have identified angiofibroblastic hyperplasia and a consistent absence of inflammatory cells. These findings are consistent with those demonstrated in achilles and patellar tendinopathies. Manual therapists have long recognized the role of mechanical load in affecting the synthesis and degradation of collagen and influencing tendon remodelling (Mackay et al 2008). Eccentric loading programmes are well described in achilles and patellar tendinopathies (Woodley et al 2007). Despite this, the limited evidence available suggests that eccentric exercise is no better than other standard physiotherapy treatments for chronic lateral epicondylar tendinopathy (or LE) (Croisier et al 2007; Manias & Stasinopoulos 2006; Svernlov & Adolfson 2001). Pathological changes have been demonstrated in both the deep and anterior fibres of the extensor carpi radialis brevis (ECRB) tendon insertion; the ECRB enthesis has extensive attachments to the lateral epicondyle, intramuscular septum, and lateral collateral ligament that are believed to help the dissipation of stress. Tensile, compressive, and shear forces will be specific to the structure and function of this tendon–fibre arrangement, and therefore may necessitate a specific loading approach.

Pain-free grip strength is reduced in LE by an average of 43 to 64% when compared to the unaffected side (Coombes et al 2009). Flexor and extensor deficits have been observed in the wrist and hand of patients with LE when compared to healthy controls (Alizadehkhaiyat et al 2007b). However, metacarpophalangeal extensor strength is not affected. This may reflect a compensation strategy where patients maintain or increase finger extension strength to compensate for the weakness observed in the wrist extensors. As previously discussed there is some limited evidence that a combination of manual therapy directed to the elbow (MWM) and exercise results in short-term improvements in pain-free grip strength.

Electromyographic (EMG) studies have demonstrated a global weakness in the upper limb of patients suffering from LE that affects not only the wrist flexors and extensors, but also the shoulder abductors and external rotators. It is not currently clear whether this is causative or results from the underlying LE. Nevertheless, this does emphasize the importance of addressing global upper limb function in the rehabilitation of patients with LE. Alizadehkhaiyat et al (2009) demonstrated that, even in those patients who reported resolution of symptoms, EMG and strength measurements indicated incomplete functional recovery. The above authors found significant ongoing deficits in global upper limb strength compared to controls. There was no difference between symptomatic LE and those patients with recovered LE. Currently, there is a little evidence regarding the significance of the global upper limb dysfunction and whether it plays a role in recurrence. However, when advising the

therapist to employ evidence-based approach to rehabilitation it is important to consider the relevance of global upper limb strength in optimizing muscle function.

Manual therapy and motor retraining

Investigators have suggested that the greater prevalence of LE in novice tennis players than in expert players may reflect the novice's use of faulty mechanics for certain strokes. Wrist kinematic and EMG data have shown that novice players eccentrically contract their wrist extensor muscles throughout the stroke (Kelley et al 1994). Furthermore, studies have suggested that recreational tennis players transmit more shock impact from their racket to the elbow joint, and use larger wrist flexor and extensor EMG activities during the follow-through phase of the backhand stroke. This is of relevance as follow-through control has been proposed as a critical factor for reduction of shock transmission. Specific differences in ECRB activation levels have been demonstrated in tennis players with LE, compared to asymptomatic players. It is significant that similar abnormal patterns of activation in the common flexor muscles have been observed in golfers with medial epicondylalgia symptoms (Glazebrook et al 1994). Understanding these abnormalities in motor strategies may help us to elucidate predisposing factors for the development of LE and also examine key factors in other at risk populations. To date, however, there is a lack of evidence to demonstrate either how best to address these abnormalities or, crucially, whether addressing them results in symptoms relief. Nevertheless, Alizadehkhaiyat et al (2009) have demonstrated reduced ECRB activity in patients with LE during isometric wrist extension and gripping tasks, which appears to resolve in subjects who have recovered LE. Whether this change in muscle activation results from the resolution of pain or other factors has not been elucidated in this patient group.

Bisset et al (2006b) described the presence of bilateral sensorimotor deficits in patients with LE compared to healthy controls. These deficits remained relatively unchanged despite treatment intervention (Bisset et al 2009). The treatment strategies employed in this later study did not specifically address sensorimotor deficits; however, patients reported improvements in pain-pressure threshold and pain-free grip strength despite the lack of improvement in sensorimotor function. In view of what we understand regarding the influence of sensorimotor deficits on muscle timing, this is commensurate with the alterations observed in motor control in this patient group. However, it is currently not clear what role this plays in the pathophysiology of LE.

Conclusion

It is clear from the literature that there is some limited evidence to support the use of manual therapy combined with exercise to improve pain-free grip strength and pain-pressure threshold in the short term in patients undergoing treatment for LE. Whilst studies have investigated the use of different exercise approaches there is little evidence to support the superiority of one over another. Furthermore, most researchers have failed to investigate the role of therapeutic exercise alone compared to a control or no intervention. However, there is increasing evidence that current strategies may not acknowledge what is understood regarding sensorimotor deficits and global upper limb dysfunction. In an effort to ensure best practice, it is crucial that manual therapists are familiar with the current evidence regarding the pathophysiology of LE and complete a thorough assessment addressing the key areas discussed to facilitate the implementation of appropriate management strategies. The paucity of evidence to guide the management of other elbow pathologies highlights key areas for future research.

5.1   Acupuncture and elbow dysfunction

Jennie Longbottom

The hypothesis that Lateral Epicondylagia (LE) may be the result of a chronic tissue injury with sympathetic involvement is accepted on the basis that healing failed to proceed through the orderly and timely process outlined by Keast and Orsted (1998), failing to produce anatomical integrity and occupational capabilities (Kitchen & Young 2002). In addition, the fourth decade of life predisposes tendon injury through degenerative processes (Hong et al 2004; Khan et al 2002). Occupational strain (Walker-Bone & Cooper 2005) and repetitive upper extremity use are causative factors associated with inadequate tissue healing and chronic states (Pascarelli & Hsu 2001; Waugh et al 2004).

Pain is an inhibitory mechanism, preventing normal function (Chilton 1997; Pomeranz 1996; Trinh et al 2004); therefore, attaining some relief from the primary symptom (pain), secondary improvements in function are plausible. Many physical therapies have been employed both in isolation and in combination in the management of chronic LE including, exercise, manipulation and mobilizations, orthotics and taping, laser, and extracorporeal shock wave therapy. The most recent systematic reviews (Bisset et al 2005; Buchbinder et al 2006) suggest a lack of evidence for the long-term benefit of physical interventions over that of a placebo group.

It has been estimated that there is an average of 12 weeks absenteeism in 30% of those affected by LE (Beller et al 2005). This highlights the importance of selecting the most effective means to manage pain effectively. A review of the current limited available literature and recent trials demonstrates that there is contradictory supporting evidence for the use of acupuncture in the treatment of LE. Brattberg (1983) compared the efficacy of acupuncture versus steroid injections in the treatment of this condition, indicating 62% of patients reported a positive outcome of no pain or much improved pain levels after acupuncture intervention in comparison to 31% who received steroid injections. However, it is unclear from the results how many steroid injections were administered, or what type of steroid was used. Brattberg's (1983) acupuncture group also appeared to have had a longer duration of symptoms prior to treatment, which may well have influenced their response and expectations of treatment.

Molsberger and Hille (1994) studied the immediate analgesic effect of acupuncture with placebo acupuncture for LE in 48 patients. After treatment, 79% of the acupuncture group reported pain relief of at least 50%, but only 25% of the placebo group. This may support the use of acupuncture for an immediate analgesic effect; however, the sample used by the above authors were volunteers, and 50% had expressed a positive expected outcome for acupuncture prior to the study. The main outcome measurement in this study was a subjective measurement of pain; therefore, coupled with the possible influence of bias from treatment expectations, limitations in bias were demonstrated. The acupuncture group were also asked to have carried out elbow movements during treatment, whereas the placebo group were not. It is unclear what these movements were and whether this has an extra influence over the placebo group.

Fink et al (2002a) measured the clinical effectiveness of acupuncture for chronic LE by comparing real acupuncture versus sham. An initial significant reduction in pain was noted for the real acupuncture group and an increase in function over a longer duration was also highlighted in these patients. It is also of interest that both groups had a mixture of subjects with repetitive and non-strenuous occupations, and both subgroups had similar improvements. This provides further limited support for acupuncture again for initial pain relief, but with some longer term functional improvement. It also indicates its effective use in patients, regardless of the daily level of activities of the involved upper limb. The initial pain improvements could be attributed to the nature of the course of the condition or the prolonged sessions of treatment.

Following a systematic review, Trinh et al (2004) concluded that acupuncture has a role in the management of pain but mainly in the short-term relief of lateral elbow pain. However, a Cochrane review by Green et al (2002) stated that acupuncture was limited in its effects with no relief lasting longer than 24 hours after treatment. Nevertheless, these findings still indicate acupuncture is effective for initial pain management and as a precursor to rehabilitation.

The lack of consensus regarding the management of this condition presents scope for further investigation into symptomatic relief and functional improvement.

Acupuncture is recognized in the Western world as a useful complementary medicine procedure (NIHCC 1998). Clinically, its uses have been recognized in the relief of acute pain following surgery (Suzuki et al 2002; Taguchi 2008), as well as for long-term relief from chronic pain following carpal tunnel syndrome (Napadow et al 2007), knee osteoarthritis (Selfe & Taylor 2008), shoulder pain (Filshie 2005), and chronic low back pain (Haake et al 2007). Research has indicated that acupuncture intervention for the relief of pain (Chilton 1997; Tsui & Leung 2002) and management of dysfunction (Fink et al 2002a) may be beneficial in the treatment of LE, provided that attention to the predominant pain presentation and tissue-healing time scales are taken into consideration.

Case Study 1

Lawrence Mayhew

Introduction

A 45-year-old male presented with a 6-month complaint of left lateral elbow pain. The subject had recently started a new job that involved repetitive gripping of an industrial power washer. The discomfort was initially mild, but symptoms and function had become significantly worse, causing further disablement. The severity of the symptoms resulted in three weeks sick leave; anti-inflammatory medication gave little relief of symptoms.

Assessment

On examination, the subject presented with the following symptoms:

- Pain on resisted contractions of the extensor muscles of the forearm;
- A reduced pain-pressure threshold over the lateral humeral epicondyle, which is symptomatic of LE (Bisset et al 2006b; Skinner & Curwin 2006). Pressure-pain threshold refers to the pain elicited on direct palpation of the lateral epicondyle and is quantified through the direct measurement of the amount of pressure required to elicit pain using an algometer;
- Increased sensitivity to touch, a possible indication of sympathetic involvement; and
- Pain and reduced grip during occupational tasks, which were identified as the patient's foremost problems.

The term LE was the nomenclature chosen to classify this patient's condition, since the suffix 'algia' denotes pain and hyperalgesia; both of which were the patient's predominant symptoms and those of chronic LE (Vicenzino & Wright 1996; Waugh 2005). Furthermore, there exists a growing body of knowledge that challenges the original theories about its pathophysiology (Benjamin et al 2006). Mounting evidence suggests that chronic LE does not involve an inflammatory response but is characterized by structural changes within the tendon, neovascularization, disorganized and immature collagen, and mucoid degeneration (Ashe et al 2004; Khan et al 2002).

The term LE encapsulates the many potential pathophysiological mechanisms and underlying causes of LE pain without assuming underlying pathology and appropriately reflects the complexity of the condition (Waugh 2005).

Acupuncture point rationale

The following acupuncture points were selected to treat the subject based on a current clinical reasoning paradigm (Bradnam 2003), in conjunction with up-to-date evidence-based research into chronic pain relief. Table 5.1 lists the acupuncture rationale treatment plan, and outcome measures used. Needles were left in situ for 20 minutes, with stimulation every 5 minutes by manual rotation in order to achieve a constant aching sensation that is identified as being common best practice in musculoskeletal acupuncture treatment (Chilton 1997; Filshie 2005; Haake et al 2007; Selfe & Taylor 2008; Trinh et al 2004; Tsui & Leung 2002).

Physiological reasoning for Acupuncture selection

The physiological mechanisms of acupuncture still remain debatable (Streitberger et al 2008). Point selection was therefore clinically reasoned on the basis of the subject's presentation of:

- Long-term persistent pain;
- The chronic state of the underlying tissues; and
- The most up-to-date research into pain mechanisms and acupuncture analgesia.

The patient presented with localized elbow pain, so local needling to Large Intestine (LI) points LI10 and LI11 was employed to stimulate A-delta (Aδ) and C fibres in order to encourage the release of calcitonin gene-related peptides (CGRP), substance P (SP), and neurokinin. This causes a flare reaction, vasodilation, reddening of the skin, and the release of local endorphins (Carlsson 2002; Delay-Goyet et al 1992). This is clinically significant since patients with chronic pain appear to demonstrate low levels of endorphins and SP (Terenius 1981). Inducing a small inflammatory reaction around affected tissues has also been proven to offer pain relief for up to 2 to 3 days (Besson 1999) and therefore local needling was

(Continued)

Case Study 1 (Continued)

Table 5.1 Physiological reasoning for acupoint selection

Acupoint	Needle size/depth	Treatment plan	Assessment scale	Outcome measures
LI4	0.25 × 25 mm 0.5 cun	2 sessions per week for 3 weeks	VAS before each session	MYMOP Grip dynamometer
LI10	0.25 × 40 mm 1.5 cun	1 session per week for 3 weeks		
LI11	0.25 × 40 mm 1.5 cun			
LI14	0.25 × 40 mm 1 cun			
TE5	0.25 × 40 mm 0.5 cun			

Notes: LI, Large Intestine; MYMOP, Measure Yourself Medical Outcome Profile; TE, Triple Energizer; VAS, Visual Analogue Scale.

used to induce such effects through the surrounding tissues.

Other acupuncture mechanisms associated with relief from chronic pain were targeted using evidence-based needling. Terenius (1981) described the root cause of chronic pain as a result of inadequate afferent influx and the inability to activate endogenous pain modulatory systems. The LI11, LI14, and Triple Energizer (TE) TE5 points were selected to provide attenuation of dermatomal receptive input in the dorsal horn of the spinal cord (Carlsson 2002; Bradnam 2003). Segmental needling has gained wider acceptance for alleviating LE pain within case trials and systematic reviews (Chilton 1997; Trinh et al 2004; Tsui & Leung 2002).

Chronic pain is a prolonged sensitization of the spinal cord and regions within the sensory cortex after the original injury has healed (Bradnam 2003). This leads to over-activation of the sympathetic nervous system contributing to the slow healing of musculoskeletal conditions, and often invisible trophic changes in target tissues (Bekkering & Van Bussel 1998). Needle manipulation at LI4 has been seen to activate descending pain pathways, namely the diffuse noxious inhibitory controls (DNIC) (Dhond et al 2007a; Yan et al 2005). Supraspinal mechanisms via simulation of LI4 have found to deactivate multiple limbic areas that participate in pain processing from the arcuate nucleus in the hypothalamus, precentral gyrus, and superior temporal gyrus (Kong & Randy 2002).

It has been postulated recently that acupuncture affects the cardiovascular system via the autonomic nervous system (Agelink et al 2003; Haker et al 2000). Therefore, it may enhance vagal and suppress sympathetic nerve activity (Wang et al 2002). Needling at LI4 and LI11 has been found to have similar results in heart rate variability (Haker et al 2000), supporting its use within the present case study.

Further empirical evidence indicates the usefulness of using Triple Energizer (TE) on chronic diseases. Haker et al (2000), Agelink et al (2003), Sakai et al (2007), and Streitberger et al (2008) found changes in heart rate variability to be associated with parasympathetic stimulation. In light of these findings, it has been speculated that parasympathetic stimulation by acupuncture also modulates certain functions of the immune system (Mori et al 2008). This speculation arises from the fact that the immune system is modulated by the autonomic nervous system (Kawamura et al 1999; Minagawa et al 1999). Mori et al (2002) demonstrated that acupuncture induced parasympathetic nerve stimulation, resulting in a decrease in the heart rate and a tendency for the leukocyte pattern to normalize. This offers further evidence of parasympathetic responses to acupuncture. Most recently, Mori et al (2008) found pupillary constriction and decreases in pulse wave amplitude during stimulation of TE5. Parasympathetic activation causes pupillary constriction through contraction of the sphincter muscle and relaxation of the dilator muscle (Ohsawa et al 1997). This provides experimental evidence that TE5 modulates central processes via parasympathetic activation and also has segmental effects via the posterior interosseous nerve (Bradnam 2003).

Outcome measures and results

In line with the Standards for Reporting Interventions in Controlled Trials of Acupuncture (STRICTA) Guidelines (MacPherson et al 2002; Prady et al 2008), the outcome measures utilized were both reproducible and validated to assess the usefulness of acupuncture and the measurement of function, whilst being suitably pragmatic to reflect the holistic nature of physiotherapy. The Measure Yourself Medical Outcome Profile (MYMOP)

(Continued)

Case Study 1 (Continued)

is a patient-generated, patient-centred instrument (Paterson 1996) designed to be used as a single method of assessment and thus it complements a case study design (White 2005) in order to evaluate clinical outcomes associated with a course of acupuncture treatment (Paterson & Britten 2003), and is sensitive to clinical change over a 2-month period (Hull et al 2006).

The hand-grip dynamometer is a relatively inexpensive measure of hand strength (Vicenzino & Wright 1996). It is a recognized clinical tool for assessing treatment effectiveness in LE (Bisset et al 2006b) and is easily reproducible. In addition, a VAS was taken at each treatment session as a general measure of pain and symptom severity.

Treatment was initially biweekly for a period of 21 days and became weekly for a further 21 days. This protocol was clinically reasoned on the basis of clinic resources, but previously published protocols for acupuncture treatment of LE were taken into account (Chilton 1997; Fink et al 2002a; Trinh et al 2004; Tsui & Leung 2002; Webster-Harrison et al 2002).

The subject's VAS reduced from 90/100 to 50/100 in a 3-week period. Re-measurement of grip strength at this point found a 17% increase (pre-treatment, 6 kg; at 3 weeks, 8.7 kg). Through weeks 5 and 6 the VAS dropped to a consistent 40/100. As pain became controlled, grip strength measured a 63% rise from pre-test to 10.1 kg at 6 weeks. The MYMOP was re-measured within a 2-month period to assess clinical change (Hull et al 2006). In 6 weeks, a drop of 1.7 (from 5.3 to 3.6) indicated an increase in function and reduction in symptoms.

Discussion

The present case study reports credible evidence that acupuncture provided symptomatic relief and functional improvements in a subject with a 6-month history of lateral elbow pain. A Cochrane review found insufficient evidence to either support or refute the use of acupuncture in the treatment of lateral elbow pain (Green et al 2002); however, its biomedical approach to analysis excluded investigations other than randomized controlled trials (RCT). This exclusion fails to represent the pragmatic nature of physiotherapy and investigations that take a holistic approach. The patient group in the above study was also heterogeneous and therefore a meta-analysis might not have been the most appropriate method of synthesizing the evidence (Trinh et al 2004).

Acupuncture trials have been criticized for providing a lack of standardization, inadequate clinical rationale, and poor quality in reporting details specific to acupuncture interventions (Prady et al 2008), especially the case in reports for elbow pain. Studies such as Chilton (1997), Fink et al (2002a), Trinh et al (2004), Tsui and Leung (2002), and Webster-Harrison et al (2002) used acupuncture as the primary intervention, but differences in dosages, the total number of treatments, the frequency and duration of treatments, number of needles being used, and the type of acupuncture (classical versus anatomical) mean that it is difficult to make effective comparisons.

The present study provides some limited evidence of symptomatic pain relief and an increase in function after an acupuncture intervention that adhered to an evidence-based model incorporating acupuncture research and sound clinical reasoning. The study also refers to STRICTA guidelines (MacPherson et al 2002; Prady et al 2008) to maximize transparency, interpretation, and replication of findings. This is something that many previous investigations have been criticized for failing to do. The limitations of the present study include the lack of information about longer lasting effects of acupuncture, the lack of control, and generalization and limitations of a single study.

Case Study 2

Katy Williams

Introduction

This case study presents a female, 41-year-old police officer, with a keen interest in table tennis; she had developed a progressive onset of right-sided LE some 5 months prior to attending physiotherapy. Treatment initially consisted of manual intervention to address the presenting pain mechanism and mobility issues. Traditional acupuncture, periosteal pecking, and trigger point acupuncture were then used and at times combined, working both systemically and locally to address the local underlying pathologies.

The subject presented to physiotherapy with a diagnosis of right-sided LE following general practitioner advice on regular rest, ice, and a prescription of non-steroidal anti-inflammatory medication (NSAIDS), which had had minimal beneficial effects. Her expectations of progress with physiotherapy were poor, particularly as she was aware that her condition was now chronic, having left it 5 months before requesting a medical review. The subject had joined the police force 6 months earlier and been undertaking basic training in which

(Continued)

Case Study 2 (Continued)

one of the training elements involved self-defence manoeuvres. During a class of repetitive arm-locks she noticed a progressive onset of lateral elbow and forearm pain, increasing as the intensity of the training progressed. She was unwilling to make her medical team aware through fear of failing the training and the condition being documented on her medical records as a source of weakness; she thus struggled to complete her training.

Her condition was further hampered by her hobby, table tennis, in which she regularly trained twice a week and occasionally competed at weekends. This had progressively heightened both the intensity and frequency of her lateral elbow and forearm pain, causing an additional onset of antecubital fossa and dorsal thumb pain.

Assessments

Subjective assessment

The paramount symptom (Fig. 5.4) was pain aggravated by movement and table tennis and eased by ice, rest and deep massage. Pain 1 was worse in the morning with joint stiffness and suffered intermittent flare-ups of increased pain with activity; pain 2 was only present on activities.

Objective assessment

See Table 5.2.

Diagnostic hypothesis

Following analysis of the subjective and objective findings and a thorough review of the literature discussed below, the subsequent hypotheses were reasoned as likely possibilities:

- LE with extensor carpi radialis brevis (ECRB) tendo-periosteal involvement, demonstrating a chronic, nociceptive and mechanic pain presentation;
- Inflammatory pain mechanisms present, with the potential to progress to central sensitization;
- Active supinator trigger point, demonstrating a chronic, nociceptive and mechanical ischaemic involvement of the tissues; and
- Nociceptive pain presentation.

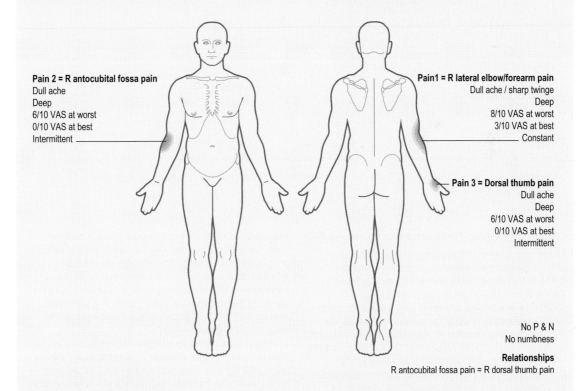

Pain 2 = R antocubital fossa pain
Dull ache
Deep
6/10 VAS at worst
0/10 VAS at best
Intermittent

Pain1 = R lateral elbow/forearm pain
Dull ache / sharp twinge
Deep
8/10 VAS at worst
3/10 VAS at best
Constant

Pain 3 = Dorsal thumb pain
Dull ache
Deep
6/10 VAS at worst
0/10 VAS at best
Intermittent

No P & N
No numbness

Relationships
R antocubital fossa pain = R dorsal thumb pain

Figure 5.4 • Pain presentation.
P&N, pins and needles; R, right; VAS; visual analogue scale; Pain 1, catching elbow/unscrewing jars/pruning shrubs; Pain 2/3, repetitive forehand shots in table tennis >5 minutes play.

(Continued)

Case Study 2 (Continued)

Table 5.2 Objective Assessment

Objective assessment	Findings
Cervical spine	No reproduction of symptoms
Observation	Mild atrophy of wrist/finger extensor muscle bulk
AROM	20° of elbow extension and supination
PROM	10° of elbow extension and supination. Reproduction of pain 1
MS	Isometric power of wrist extensors = 4 Elbow supinator = 4
Neurodynamics ULTT2	No adverse neurodynamics
Special tests	Mill's Test and ECRB Bias Test positive for pain 1
Palpation:	Thickening/tenderness over the tendo-periosteal junction of the common extensor tendon. Reproduction of pain 1
	Active supinator trigger point causing reproduction of pains 1, 2, and 3

Notes: AROM, active range of movement; ECRB, extensor carpi radialis brevis; MS, muscle strength; PROM, passive range of movement; ULTT2, Upper Limb Tension Test 2.

Clinical reasoning for acupuncture intervention

Lateral epicondylalgia can occur at one of four sites around the common extensor origin, the attachment of the ECRB at the tendo-periosteal junction being the most common (Hertling and Kessler 1996; Norris 2001). The tendon has a greater susceptibility to injury, partly explained by overuse or misuse, as well as the mechanical predisposition of the fulcrum effect created by the underlying radial head which greatly contributes to the tensile forces transmitted (Khan et al 2000; Viola 1998). Trigger points (TrPts) of myofascial origin, particularly in the supinator muscle belly, frequently develop as a secondary response, causing pain of a nociceptive and ischaemic nature (Edwards & Knowles 2003; Hecker et al 2008). TrPts radiating from the supinator muscle often refer locally to the lateral humeral epicondyle and into the antecubital fossa, with more distal symptoms referring into the dorsal aspect of the web-base of the thumb (Norris 2001). Occasionally, this can contribute to contracture formation of the anterolateral elbow capsule, through guarding patterns developing in the muscle (Viola 1998). The signs and symptoms demonstrated by this subject were further supported by these findings.

As LE is classified as a degenerative disorder, rather than an inflammatory disorder (Khan et al 2000), based upon findings obtained from recent histopathological investigations of biopsied materials (Khan & Cook 2000; Vicenzino 2003), the tendon responds, under conditions of significantly increased stress, by laying down more tissue through the process of fibroplastic proliferation

(Continued)

Case Study 2 (Continued)

Table 5.3 Acupuncture point protocol

Treatment	Acupuncture	Rationale
1	Local Points: LI11, LI10, LU5 Distal Points: TE5, LI4 (L&R) (endogenous opioid pain modulation point and calming point)	Meridian acupuncture to directly target pain 1/pain 2 and indirectly target pain 3
2	As above Periosteal pecking at tendo-periosteal junction of ECRB	Periosteal pecking to directly target pain 1 at the ECRB origin and to indirectly increase elbow AROM/PROM
3	As above	
4	As above	
5	Treatment as above + TrPt to supinator	TrPt to directly target pain 2 and 3 at the supinator TrPt and to indirectly increase elbow AROM and PROM
6	As above	
7	As above	
8	Local Points: LI1, LI10, LU5	Distal points removed to localize pain inhibitory effects and remove calming effects

Notes: LI, Large Intestine; LU, Lung; TE, Triple Energizer.

(Hertling & Kessler 1996). The resultant effect is tissue hypertrophy, which causes the ECRB tendon to gain in strength at the expense of extensibility (Kochar & Dogra 2002), leading to deformation and microfracturing, causing a low-grade inflammatory response that initiates the viscous cycle of fibroplastic proliferation (Vicenzino 2003).

The mechanism of pain production in LE, particularly chronic pain, has also been under close scrutiny. Several theories that attempt to explain the source exist, including conventional mechanical theories incriminating the local soft tissues and joints, neuropathic and cervicogenic theories, and central nervous system maladaptive process theories (Vicenzino & Wright 1995; Vicenzino 2003; Waugh et al 2004). Findings from recent studies report that LE can progress to developing pain in the form of secondary hyperalgesia, whereby there is a reduction in the pain threshold to noxious stimuli, outside the immediate site of injury (Bisset et al 2005; Fink et al 2002b; Vicenzino 2003). It has been suggested that the underlying mechanism for this is central sensitization, in which there is an increased excitability of and/or a reduction in inhibitory influences on neurones within the central nervous system, rather than a peripheral sensitization of $A\delta$ and C-fibre nociceptors via inflammatory neurotransmitters such as substance P and histamine (Abbot 2001). If this process continues to persist then it is likely to become irreversible (Kochar & Dogra 2002).

For the acupuncture point protocol, see Table 5.3.

Physiological reasoning

Prior to receiving acupuncture as a treatment intervention, the subject received the following interventions:

- MWM to inhibit nociception through dynamic sensory gating; as proposed by Vicenzino et al (2001). This resulted in mild improvements in AROM and PROM, but contact pressure could not be tolerated.
- Friction massage to breakdown scar tissue formation, immediately followed by ultrasound to assist with tissue repair; as proposed by Hertling and Kessler (1996). Again mild improvements in AROM and PROM occurred, but the intensity and frequency of pain heightened.
- The hypothesis of a supinator TrPt as being partly responsible was tested against manual acupressure as a means of reducing hyperactivity of the muscle spindle and unnecessary muscle contraction, as proposed by Norris (2001). Mild improvements in AROM/PROM occurred, but manual deactivation of the TrPt could not be tolerated.

The responses to these treatments helped confirm the original diagnostic hypotheses, though the irritability of the pain mechanisms had been underestimated. On this basis, acupuncture was performed during the fourth treatment session, using the 'layering method' to reason clinically the technique selection and progression (Bradnam 2007). Traditional meridian acupuncture with

(Continued)

Case Study 2 (Continued)

Table 5.4 Outcome measurements

Outcome measurements	First treatment session	Last treatment session
AROM	20° of elbow extension/supination	Neutral zero starting position/full range of elbow extension and supination
MS	4 isometric power of wrist extensors and elbow supinator	5 isometric power of wrist extensors and elbow supinator
Special tests	ECRB Bias Test Positive for pain 1	ECRB Bias Test Negative for pain 1
Palpation	Palpation of tendo-periosteal junction of ECRB positive for pain 1 Activation of supinator TrPt positive for pain 1, 2, and 3	Palpation of tendo-periosteal junction of ECRB negative for pain 1 Activation of supinator TrPt negative for pain 1, 2, and 3
Functional tasks	Unscrewing jar lids: Pain 1 8/10 VAS 5 minutes of repetitive forehand shots in table tennis: Pain 2 and 3 60/100 VAS	Unscrewing jar lids: Pain 1 and 2 0/100 VAS 5 minutes of repetitive forehand shots in table tennis: Pain 2 and 3 0/100 VAS

De Qi activation and frequent re-enforcement was used over a 30-minute duration. A combination of local and distal points was selected to influence nociceptive pain mechanisms. Research suggests that local point needling induces segmental pain-ascending inhibitory effects, through the spinal gate-control mechanism (Carlsson 2002; Moffet 2006), stimulating Aδ fibres, which transmit pain signals to the dorsal horn of the spinal cord (Norris 2001). This in turn mediates inhibition of pain signals carried in C-fibres, by stimulating the release of opioids from enkephalinergic inhibitory interneurones in the dorsal horn (Andersson & Lundeberg 1995). Distal points were selected to induce strong supraspinal pain-descending inhibitory effects (Carlsson 2002) to the periaqueductal grey matter, hypothalamus, and pituitary gland (Bowsher 1998). This in turn mediates further inhibition of pain signals by releasing serotonin, norepinephrine, and adrenocorticotrophic hormone (Moffet 2006).

Periosteal pecking (PP) in a peppering pattern, at a rate of 4 strikes per second over a 60-second duration, was introduced on the fifth session with traditional acupuncture. This technique is thought to encourage scar tissue breakdown whilst encouraging tissue healing and local pain relief (Hansson et al 2007; Mann 1992). Research suggests that this may occur via axon reflexes, causing the release of neuropeptides with resulting trophic effects (Carlsson 2002; Bradnam 2007).

Direct TrPt needling through fanlike manipulation with needle grasp and twitch response was simultaneously introduced on the eighth session, along with traditional acupuncture; followed by static and dynamic muscle stretching. Trigger point needling is thought to activate

the pain inhibitory pathways discussed previously. Research suggests that this reduces ischaemia and increases adenosine-triphosphate concentration, improving control of the calcium pump (Edwards & Knowles 2003); reducing hyperactivity of the muscle spindle and therefore the stretch reflex (Baldry 2002); decreasing acetylcholine release; and reducing unnecessary muscle contraction (Norris 2001).

Systematic reviews of traditional acupuncture for LE suggest that there is insufficient evidence to either support or refute its use as a treatment long term (Bisset et al 2005; Green et al 2002; Trinh et al 2004). It has been proven to be of short-term benefit with respect to pain, based predominantly on the results of two randomized controlled trials conducted by Haker and Lundeberg (1990) and Molsberger and Hille (1994). Findings suggest it relieves pain for significantly longer than placebo, and is likely to result in more than 50% reduction in pain after one session, with an overall lasting improvement following more than 10 sessions. However, no significant differences were found in the long-term (more than 3 months). To date, the majority of studies conducted have used successfully the meridian points selected in this case study (Davidson et al 2001; Fink et al 2002b; Haker & Lundeberg 1990). No studies to date have combined meridian acupuncture, PP, and TrPt acupuncture, indicating that more research is needed in these areas.

Outcome measurements

The objective outcome measures of AROM and isometric muscle strength (MS) were measured, using

(Continued)

Case Study 2 (Continued)

a goniometer and Oxford scale respectively. The subjective outcome measures of the ECRB Bias Test and palpation were recorded as positive or negative for pain, based on the patient's pain response. The subject had the responsibility of undertaking the functional tasks of unscrewing jar lids and playing 5 minutes of repetitive forehand shots in table tennis, prior to attending the sessions, after which she was asked to use the pain VAS to record her pain response between 0 and 100 (Table 5.4).

Conclusion

In conclusion, the subject made significant improvements in all outcome measures, enabling her to resume her full-time post as a police officer and her hobby of table tennis, with no further flare-ups. Her only remaining complaint was the isometric power of her wrist extensors and elbow supinators, with a VAS of 20/100 when unscrewing jar lids; this was overcome through the participation in a home strengthening exercise programme.

The manual techniques undertaken during the first three sessions helped with the confirmation of diagnostic hypotheses, irritability of pain mechanisms, and in assisting with acupuncture technique selection and progression. Most improvements were made following traditional acupuncture intervention and the subsequent introduction of PP combined with TrPt deactivation, enabling individual pathological mechanisms to be worked on locally, whilst providing systemic analgesia.

On reflection, limitations included the validity and reliability of the use of subjective outcome measures of pain response to determine treatment selection and progression, particularly the use of functional tasks that the patient had to undertake and record prior to attending the sessions. Furthermore, no studies have simultaneously combined meridian acupuncture, PP, and TrPt needling, making the results questionable. Findings should therefore be interpreted with caution before making generalizations to clinical practice.

Discussion

This case study has attempted to demonstrate the challenges facing practitioners managing patients with LE, as well as the scope for possible improvement when complementing practice with acupuncture. LE is a prevalent neuromusculoskeletal condition (Abbott 2001; Fink et al 2002b); recent epidemiological studies report that it has an incidence rate of 3% in the general population aged between 40 and 50 years and 15% in high-risk groups, e.g. persons undertaking occupational and/or sporting activities involving repetitive forearm and hand actions (Trinh et al 2004; Waugh et al 2004). Two pathologies were diagnosed with this subject, these being ECRB tendo-periosteal involvement and an active supinator TrPt. The former was diagnosed as the primary pathology based on the mechanism of injury, with treatment being directed in this order. Significant improvements were made in all outcome measures through using a combination of interventions, as advocated in other studies of LE (Davidson et al 2001; Viola 1998). The most efficacious intervention in this case study was the introduction of meridian acupuncture combined with PP and TrPt needling. However, the early intervention of manual therapy facilitated the acupuncture intervention, confirming the hypotheses and status of tissue irritability that reinforced the pain mechanisms. Improvements made with the assistance of acupuncture were related to analgesic effects on the chronic, nociceptive, mechanical, and inflammatory pain mechanisms, through activation of segmental and supraspinal inhibitory pathways with local and distal points respectively (Carlsson 2002; Moffet 2006), supported by the research evidence (Davidson et al, 2001; Fink et al 2002b; Haker & Lundeberg 1990). The use of PP and TrPt needling proved particularly advantageous, providing additional analgesia through the pain-inhibitory pathways, as well as directly breaking down scar tissue formation at the ECRB tendo-periosteal junction (Mann 1992) and thus facilitating recovery and return to function.

References

Abbott, J.H., 2001. Mobilisation with movement applied to the elbow affects shoulder range of movement in subjects with lateral epicondylalgia. Man Ther. 6 (3), 170–177.

Abbott, J.H., Patla, C.E., Jensen, R.H., 2001. The initial effects of an elbow mobilisation with movement technique on grip strength in subjects with lateral epicondylalgia. Man Ther. 6 (3), 163–169.

Agelink, M.W., Sanner, D., Eich, H., 2003. Does acupuncture influence the cardiac autonomic nervous system in patients with minor depression or anxiety disorders? Fortschr Neurol Psychiatr 71 (3), 141–149 [In German].

Alfredson, H., Ljung, B.O., Thorsen, K., et al., 2000. In vivo investigation of ECRB tendons with microdialysis techniques- no signs of inflammation

but high amounts of glutamate in tennis elbow. Acta Orthopaedia Scandinavia 71 (5), 475–479.

Alizadehkhaiyat, O., Fisher, A.C., Kemp, G.J., et al., 2007a. Pain, functional disability and psychological status in tennis elbow. Clin. J. Pain 23 (6), 482–489.

Alizadehkhaiyat, O., Fisher, A.C., Kemp, G.J., et al., 2007b. Upper limb muscle imbalance in tennis elbow: a functional and Electromyographic assessment. J. Orthop. Res. 25 (12), 1651–1657.

Alizadehkhaiyat, O., Fisher, A.C., Kemp, G.J., et al., 2009. Assessment of functional recovery in tennis elbow. J. Electromyogr. Kinesiol 19 (4), 631–638.

Andersson, S., Lundeberg, T., 1995. Acupuncture — from empiricism to science: Functional background to acupuncture effects in pain and disease. Med. Hypotheses 45 (3), 271–281.

Ashe, M.C., McCauley, T., Khan, K.M., 2004. Tendinopathies in the upper extremity: a paradigm shift. J. Hand Ther. 17, 329–334.

Baldry, P., 2002. Superficial versus deep dry needling. Acupunct. Med. 20, 78–81.

Beller, E., Bisset, L., Paungmali, A., et al., 2005. A systematic review and meta-analysis of clinical trials on the physical interventions for LE. Brit. J. Sports Med. 39, 411–422.

Bekkering, R., van Bussel, R., 1998. Segmental Acupuncture. In: Filshie, J., White, A. (Eds.) Medical acupuncture: a Western scientific approach. Churchill Livingstone, Edinburgh.

Benjamin, M., Toumi, H., Ralphs, J.R. et al., 2006. Where tendons and ligaments meet bone: attachment sites ('entheses') in relation to exercise and/or mechanical load. J. Anatomy 208, 471–490.

Berglund, K.M., Persson, B.H., Denison, E., 2008. Prevalence of pain and dysfunction in the cervical and thoracic spine in persons with and without lateral elbow pain. Man Ther. 3 (4), 295–299.

Besson, J.M., 1999. The neurobiology of pain. Lancet 353 (9164), 1610–1615.

Bisset, L., Paungmali, A., Vicenzino, B., et al., 2005. A systematic review and meta-analysis of clinical trials on physical interventions for lateral epicondylalgia. Brit. J. Sports Med. 39, 411–422.

Bisset, L., Beller, E., Jull, G., et al., 2006a. Mobilization with movement and exercise, corticosteroid injection or wait and see for tennis elbow: randomised trial. Brit. Med. J. 4333 (7575), 93.

Bisset, L.M., Russell, T., Bradley, S., et al., 2006b. Bilateral sensorimotor abnormalities in unilateral lateral epicondylalgia. Arch. Phy. Med. Rehabilitat. 87 (4), 490–495.

Bisset, L.M., Coppieters, M.W., Vicenzino, B., 2009. Sensorimotor

deficits remain despite resolution of symptoms using conservative treatment in patients with tennis elbow: a randomised controlled trial. Arch. Phy. Med. Rehabilitat. 90 (1), 1–8.

Bowsher, D., 1998. Introduction to the anatomy and physiology of the nervous system, 5th edn. Blackwell, Oxford.

Bradnam, L., 2003. A proposed clinical reasoning model for Western acupuncture. New Zealand J. Physiotherapy 20, 83–94.

Bradnam, L., 2007. A proposed clinical reasoning model for Western acupuncture. J. Acupun. Assoc. Chart. Physiotherapists 12, 21–30.

Brattberg, G., 1983. Acupuncture therapy for tennis elbow. Pain 16, 285–288.

Buchbinder, R., Green, S., Struijs, P., 2006. Musculoskeletal disorders: tennis elbow. Clin. Evid. 15, 1–3.

Carlsson, C., 2002. Acupuncture mechanisms for clinically relevant long-term effects—reconsideration and a hypothesis. Acupunct. Med. 20 (2-3), 82–99.

Casavant, A.M., Hastings, H., 2006. Heterotopic ossification about the elbow: a therapists guide to evaluation and management. J. Hand Therapy 9, 255–266.

Chilton, S.A., 1997. Tennis elbow: A combined approach using acupuncture and local corticosteroid injection. Acupunct. Med. 15 (2), 77–78.

Cleland, J.A., Whitman, J.M., Fritz, J. M., 2004. Effectiveness of manual physical therapy to the cervical spine in the management of lateral epicondylalgia: a retrospective analysis. J. Orthopaedic Sports Phys. Ther. 34 (11), 713–722.

Coombes, B.K., Bisset, L., Vicenzino, B., 2009. A new integrative model of lateral epicondylalgia. Brit. J. Sports Med. 43 (4), 252–258.

Croisier, J.L., Foidart-Dessalle, M., Tinant, F., et al., 2007. An isokinetic eccentric programme for the management of chronic lateral epicondylar tendinopathy. Brit. J. Sports Med. 41 (4), 269–275.

Cyriax, J., 1945. Deep massage and manipulation, 3rd edn. Hamish Hamilton Medical Books, London.

Davidson, J., Vandervoort, A., Lessard, L., et al., 2001. The effect of acupuncture versus ultrasound on pain level, grip strength, and disability in individuals with lateral epicondylitis: A pilot study. Physiotherapy Canada 1, 195–211.

Delay-Goyet, P., Satoh, H., Lundberg, J.M., 1992. Relative involvement of

substance P and CGRP mechanisms in antidromic vasodilation in the rat skin. Acta Physiologica Scandinavica 146 (4), 537–538.

Dhond, R.P., Kettner, N., Napadow, V., 2007a. Do the neural correlates of acupuncture and placebo effects differ? Pain 128 (1-2), 8–12.

Edwards, J., Knowles, N., 2003. Superficial dry needling and active stretching in the treatment of myofascial pain - A randomised controlled trial. Acupunct. Med. 21, 80–86.

Fedorczyk, J.M., 2006. Tennis elbow: blending basic science with clinical practice. J. Hand Ther. 19 (2), 146–153.

Fernández-Carnero, J., Fernández-de-las-Peñas, C., de la Llave-Rincón, A.I., et al., 2008a. Bilateral myofascial trigger points in the forearm muscles in patients with chronic unilateral lateral epicondylalgia: a blinded, controlled study. Clin. J. Pain 24 (9), 802–807.

Fernández-Carnero, J., Fernández-de-las-Peñas, C., Cleland, J.A., 2008b. Immediate hypoalgesic and motor effects after a single cervical spine manipulation in subjects with lateral epicondylalgia. J. Manip. Physiol. Ther. 31 (9), 675–681.

Filshie, J., 2005. Acupuncture improves short term and long-term pain and disability in patients with shoulder pain compared with a non-penetrating sham treatment. Focus on Alternative and Complementary Therapies 10 (2), 124–125.

Fink, M., Wolkenstein, E., Luennemann, M., et al., 2002a. Chronic epicondylitis: effects of real and sham acupuncture treatment: a randomised controlled patient and examiner, blinded long term trial. Forschende Komplementarmedizin und Klassische Naturheilkunde 9 (4), 210–215.

Fink, M., Wolkenstein, E., Karst, M., et al., 2002b. Acupuncture in chronic epicondylitis: a randomised controlled trial. Brit. J. Rheumatol. 41, 205–209.

Glazebrook, M.A., Curwin, S., Islam, M.N. et al., 1994. Medial epicondylitis. An electromyographic analysis and an investigation of intervention strategies. Am. J. Sports Med. 22 (5), 674–679.

Green, S., Buchbinder, R., Barnsley, L., et al., 2002. Acupuncture for lateral elbow pain (review). Cochrane Database of Systematic Rev. CD003527.

Gummesson, C., Astroshi, I., Ekdah, L.C., 2003. The disabilities of arm, shoulder and hand (DASH) Outcome questionnaire: longitudinal construct validity self related health changes after surgery. Brit. Med. Council Musculoskeletal Disorders 4, 11.

Haake, M., Muller, H.H., Schade-Brittinger, C., et al., 2007. German Acupuncture Trials (GERAC) for chronic low back pain. Arch. Internal Med. 167 (17), 1892–1898.

Haker, E., Lundeberg, T., 1990. Acupuncture treatment in epicondylalgia: a comparative study of two acupuncture techniques. Clin. J. Pain 6, 221–226.

Haker, E., Egekvist, H., Bjerring, P., 2000. Effect of sensory stimulation (acupuncture) on sympathetic and parasympathetic activities in healthy subjects. J. Autonomic Nervous System 79 (14), 52–59.

Hansson, Y., Carlsson, C., Olsson, E., 2007. Intramuscular and periosteal acupuncture for anxiety and sleep quality in patients with chronic musculoskeletal pain—an evaluator blind, controlled study. Acupunct. Med. 25, 148–157.

Harbour, R., Miller, J., 2001. A new system for grading recommendations in evidence-based guidelines. Brit. Med. J. 323, 334–336.

Hecker, H-U., Steveling, A., Peuker, E., et al., 2008. Colour atlas of acupuncture: body points—ear points—trigger points, 2nd edn. Thieme, Stuttgart.

Hertling, D., Kessler, R., 1996. Management of common musculoskeletal disorders: physical therapy principles and methods, 3rd edn. Lippincott Williams and Wilkins, Philadelphia.

Hong, Q.N., Durand, M.J., Loisel, P., 2004. Treatment of LE: where is the evidence? Joint Bone Spine 71, 369–373.

Hull, S.K., Page, C.P., Skinner, B.D., et al., 2006. Exploring outcomes associated with acupuncture. J. Altern. Compl. Med. 12 (3), 247–254.

Issak, P.S., Egol, K.A., 2006. Posttraumatic contracture of the elbow: current management issues. Bull. Hospital Joint Disorders 63 (3), 129–136.

Kawamura, H., Kawamura, T., Kokai, Y., et al., 1999. Expansion of extrathymic T cells as well as granulocytes in the liver and other organs of granulocytecolony stimulating factor transgenic mice: why they lost the ability of hybrid resistance. J. Immunol. 162 (10), 5957–5964.

Keast, D.H., Orsted, H., 1998. The basic principles of wound care. Ostomy Wound Manage 44 (8), 24–31.

Kelley, J.D., Lombardo, S.J., Pink, M., et al., 1994. Electromyographic and cinematographic analysis of elbow function in tennis players with LE. Am. J. Sports Med. 22 (3), 359–363.

Khan, K., Cook, J., 2000. Overuse tendon injuries: where does the pain come from? Sports Med. Arthroscopy Rev. 8, 17–31.

Khan, K., Cook, J., Maffull, N., et al., 2000. Where is the pain coming from in tendinopathy? It may be biochemical, not only structural in origin. Brit. J. Sports Med. 34, 81–83.

Khan, K.M., Cook, J.L., Kannus, P., et al., 2002. Time to abandon the tendinitis myth. Brit. Med. J. 324, 626–627.

Kitchen, S., Young, S., 2002. Tissue repair. In: Kitchen, S. (Ed.), Electrotherapy Evidence Based Practice. Churchill Livingstone, London.

Kochar, M., Dora, A., 2002. Effectiveness of a specific physiotherapy regimen on patients with tennis elbow. Physiotherapy 88, 333–341.

Kong, J., Ma, L., Randy, L., 2002. A pilot study of functional magnetic resonance imaging of the brain during manual and electroacupuncture stimulation of acupuncture points (LI 4, Hegu) in normal subjects reveals differential brain activation between methods. J. Alternat. Complem. Med. 8 (4), 411–419.

Korthals-de Bos, I.B., Smidt, N., van Tulder, M.W., et al., 2004. Cost effectiveness of interventions for LE: results from a randomised controlled trial in primary care. Pharmoeconomics 22 (3), 185–195.

Labelle, H., Guibert, R., Joncas, J., et al., 1992. Lack of scientific evidence for the treatment of lateral epicondylitis of the elbow. J. Bone Joint Surg. 74, 646–651.

Mackay, A.L., Heinemeier, K.M., Anneli Koskinen, S.O., et al., 2008. Dynamic adaptation of tendon and muscle connective tissue to mechanical loading. Connective Tissue Res. 49 (3), 165–168.

MacPherson, H., White, A., Cummings, M., et al., 2002. Standards for reporting interventions in controlled trials of acupuncture. Acupunct. Med. 20 (1), 22–25.

Manias, P., Stasinopoulos, D.A., 2006. A controlled clinical pilot trial to study the effectiveness of ice as a supplement to the exercise programme for the management of lateral elbow tendinopathy. Brit. J. Sports Med. 40, 81–85.

Mann, F., 1992. Reinventing acupuncture: a new concept of ancient medicine, 1st edn.. Butterworth Heinemann, Oxford.

Minagawa, M., Narita, J., Tada, T., et al., 1999. Mechanisms underlying immunologic states during pregnancy: possible association of the sympathetic nervous system. Cell Immunol. 196 (1), 1–13.

Moffet, H., 2006. How might acupuncture work? A systematic review of physiologic rationales from clinical trials. Brit. Med. Council Complementary and Alternative Med. 6, 1–8.

Molsberger, A., Hille, E., 1994. The analgesic effect of acupuncture in chronic tennis elbow pain. Brit. J. Rheumatol. 33 (12), 1162–1165.

Mori, H., Nishijo, K., Kawamura, H., 2002. Unique immuno-modulation by electroacupuncture in humans possible via stimulation of the autonomic nervous system. Neurosci. Lett. 320 (1-2), 21–24.

Mori, H., Ueda, S., Kuge, H., et al., 2008. Pupillary response induced by acupuncture stimulation—an experimental study. Acupunct. Med. 26 (2), 79–85.

Napadow, V., Kettner, N., Liu, J., et al., 2007. Hypothalamus and amygdale response to acupuncture stimuli in carpal tunnel syndrome. Pain 130 (2), 254–266.

NIH Consensus Conference, 1998. Acupuncture. J. Am. Med. Assoc. 280, 1518–1524.

Norris, C., 2001. Acupuncture: treatment of musculoskeletal conditions, 1st edn. Butterworth Heinemann, Oxford.

Ohsawa, H., Yamaguchi, S., Ishimaru, H., 1997. Neural mechanism of pupillary dilation elicited by electroacupuncture stimulation in anesthetized rats. J. Autonom. Nervous Sys. 64 (2-3), 101–106.

Paterson, C., 1996. Measuring outcome in primary care: a patient-generated measure, MYMOP compared to the SF-36 health survey. Brit. Med. J. 312, 1016–1020.

Paterson, P., Britten, N., 2003. Acupuncture for people with chronic Illness: combining qualitative and quantitative outcome assessment. J Altern Complement Med. 9 (5), 671–681.

Pascarelli, E.F., Hsu, Y.P., 2001. Understanding worked related upper extremity disorders. J. Occupation. Rehabilitat. 11 (1), 1–21.

Paungmali, A., O'Leary, S., Souvlis, T., et al., 2003. Hypoalgesic and sympathoexcitatory effects of mobilization with movement for lateral epicondylalgia. Phys. Ther. 83 (4), 374–383.

Pienimaki, T., Tarvainen, T., Siira, P., et al., 2002. Associations between pain, grip strength and manual tests in the treatment evaluation of chronic tennis elbow. Clin. J. Pain 18 (3), 164–170.

Pomeranz, B., 1996. Scientific research in to acupuncture for the relief of pain. J Altern Complement Med. 2 (1), 53–60.

Prady, S.L., Richmond, S,J., Morton, V.M., et al., 2008 A systematic evaluation of the impact of STRICTA and CONSORT recommendations on the quality of reporting for acupuncture trials. [Online]. Available at URL: http://www. plosone.org/article/info%3Adoi%2F1 0.1371%2Fjournal.pone.0001577

Sakai, S., Hori, E., Umeno, K., et al., 2007. Specific acupuncture sensation correlates with EEG's and autonomic changes in human subjects. Autonomic Neurosci. 133 (2), 158–169.

Selfe, T.K., Taylor, A.G., 2008. Acupuncture and osteoarthritis of the knee: a review of randomized controlled trials. Family Community Health 31 (3), 247–254.

Skinner, D.K., Curwin, S.L., 2006. Assessment of fine motor control in patients with occupational-related LE. Man Ther. 12 (3), 249–255.

Smidt, N., van der Windt, D. A., Assendelft, W.J., et al., 2002. Corticosteroid injections, physiotherapy, or a wait and see policy for LE: a randomised controlled trial. Lancet 359 (9307), 657–662.

Smidt, N., Assendelft, W.J., Arola, H., et al., 2003. Effectiveness of physiotherapy for LE: a systematic review. Annals Med. 35 (1), 51–62.

Streitberger, K., Steppan, J., Maier, C., et al., 2008. Effects of verum acupuncture compared to placebo acupuncture on quantitative EEG and heart rate variability in healthy volunteers. J Altern Complement Med. 14 (5), 505–513.

Suzuki, M., Egawa, M., Yano, T., et al., 2002. Post-operative pain which showed resistance in medicine afar lung cancer excision: a case report. J. Jap. Acupun. Moxibust. 689, 29–34.

Svernlov, B., Adolfson, L., 2001. Non-operative treatment regime including eccentric training for lateral humeral epicondylalgia. Scand. J. Med. Sci. Sports 11, 328–334.

Taguchi, R., 2008. Acupuncture anaesthesia and Algesia for clinical acute pain in Japan. Evid Based Complement Alternat. Med. 5 (2), 153–158.

Terenius, L., 1981. Biochemical mediators in pain. Triangle 20 (1–2), 19–26.

Trinh, K., Phillips, S., Ho, E., et al., 2004. Acupuncture for the alleviation of lateral epicondyle pain: a systematic review. Brit. J. Rheumatol. 43, 1085–1090.

Tsui, P., Leung, M.C., 2002. Comparison of the effectiveness of between manual acupuncture and electro-acupuncture on patients with tennis elbow. Acupun. Electrotherapeutics Res. 27 (2), 107–117.

Verhaar, J.A., Walenkamp, G.H., van Mameren, H., et al., 1995. Local steroid injection versus Cyriax type physiotherapy for tennis elbow. J. Bone Joint Surg. 77 (B), 128–132.

Vicenzino, B., 2003. Lateral epicondylalgia: a musculoskeletal physiotherapy perspective. Man. Ther. 8 (2), 66–79.

Vicenzino, B., 2007. Physiotherapy for tennis elbow. Evidence Based Med. 12 (2), 37–38.

Vicenzino, B., Wright, A., 1995. Effects of a novel manipulative physiotherapy technique on tennis elbow: a single case study. Man Ther. 1, 30–35.

Vicenzino, B., Wright, A., 1996. Lateral epicondylalgia I: epidemiology, pathophysiology, aetiology and natural history. Phys. Ther. Rev. 1 (1), 23–34.

Vicenzino, B., Collins, D., Wright, A., 1996. The initial effects of a cervical spine manipulative physiotherapy treatment on the pain and dysfunction of lateral epicondylalgia. Pain 68 (1), 69–74.

Vicenzino, B., Paungmali, A., Buratowski, S., et al., 2001. Specific manipulative therapy treatment for chronic lateral epicondylalgia produces uniquely characteristic hypoalgesia. Man Ther. 6 (4), 205–212.

Vicenzino, B., Cleland, J.A., Bisset, L., 2007. Joint manipulation in the management of lateral epicondylalgia: a clinical commentary. J. Manip. Ther. 15 (1), 50–56.

Viola, L., 1998. A critical review of the current conservative therapies for tennis elbow (lateral epicondylitis).

Australas Chiropr Osteopathy 7, 53–67.

Walker-Bone, K., Cooper, C., 2005. Hard work never hurt anyone: or did it? A review of occupational association with soft tissue musculoskeletal disorders of the neck and upper limb. Ann. Rheum. Dis. 64 (10), 1391–1396.

Walker-Bone, K., Palmer, K.T., Reading, I., et al., 2004. Prevalence and impact of musculoskeletal disorders of the upper limb in the general population. Arthritis. Rheum. 51 (4), 642–651.

Wang, J.D., Kuo, T.B.J., Yang, C.C.H., 2002. An alternative method to enhance vagal activities and suppress sympathetic activities in humans. Auton Neurosci: Basic Clin. 100 (1-2), 90–95.

Waugh, E.J., 2005. Lateral epicondylalgia or epicondylitis: what's in a name? J. Orthopaedic Sports Phys. Ther. 35 (4), 200–202.

Waugh, E., Jaglal, S., Davis, A., et al., 2004. Factors associated with prognosis of lateral epicondylitis after 8 weeks of physical therapy. Arch. Phys. Med. Rehabilitat. 85, 308–317.

Webster-Harrison, P., White, A., Rae, A., 2002. Acupuncture for tennis elbow: an email consensus study to define a standardised treatment in a GP's surgery. Acupunct. Med. 20 (4), 181–185.

White, A., 2005. Conducting and reporting case series and audits: author guidelines for acupuncture in medicine. Acupunct. Med. 23 (4), 181–187.

Woodley, B.L., Newsham-West, R.J., Baxter, G.D., 2007. Chronic tendinopathy: effectiveness of eccentric exercise. Brit. J. Sports Med. 41 (4), 188–198.

Wright, A., Thurnwald, P., O'Callaghan, J., et al., 1994. Hyperalgesia in tennis elbow patients. J. Musculoskeletal Pain 2, 83–97.

Wright, A., Thurnwald, P., Smith, J., 1992. An evaluation of mechanical and thermal hyperalgesia in patients with lateral epicondylalgia. Pain Clinics 5, 221–227.

Yan, B., Li, K., Xu, J., et al., 2005. Acupoint-specific fMRI patterns in human brain. Neurosci. Lett. 383, 236–240.

Zhang, W., Jin, Z., Luo, F., et al., 2004. Evidence from brain imaging with fMRI supporting functional specificity of acupoints in humans. Neurosci. Lett. 354, 50–53.

The thoracic spine

Jennie Longbottom

Introduction

The spinal column forms the keel of the human body, and is exposed to a variety of metabolic, mechanical, and circulatory stresses that contribute to pain. The thoracic spine (T-spine) receives relatively little attention compared with its cervical and lumbar neighbours; this may be attributed to difficulties associated with movement analysis or the belief is that it is less commonly implicated in clinical pain syndromes (Edmonson & Singer 1997). However, within clinical practice the T-spine is frequently found to be a source of musculoskeletal dysfunction. The clinical syndrome of whiplash injury includes neck and upper thoracic pain, as well as cervicogenic headaches (Hong & Simonds 1993), together with more subtle presentations of chest, viscerosomatic, and somatovisceral pain patterns. However, much of the clinical theory, particularly in relation to the influences on spinal posture and movement, is untested (Edmonson & Singer 1997), and equally no consensus on interventions has been established. In comparison to the cervical or lumbar spine, there have been few studies on the effect of manipulation and mobilization techniques for the upper body (Atchinson 2000). An understanding of skeletal, facial, and muscular innervation of the T-spine is essential for effective management of pain and dysfunction.

Most musculoskeletal pain and dysfunction is the result of a failure of adaptation, where self-regulating compensation mechanisms reach a point of exhaustion and decompensation mechanisms become established. The ideal role of the manual therapist is to assist in the restoration of the body to its optimum state, i.e. restoration of homeostatic function. Encouraging self-regulatory mechanisms to function by means of the least-invasive therapeutic interventions, and offering a catalyst for healing and repair, should be the primary aim of the physiotherapist.

Skeletal structures

T1 to T8

The T1 toT8 vertebrae are classified as typical vertebrae, the compressive load on T1 being about 9%

of body weight increasing to 33% at T8 and 47% at T12 (White 1969). The vertebrae articulate with corresponding ribs and costovertebral joints, the upper three to four nerve roots supplying the medial arm and axilla via the brachial plexus. The T2 vertebra ascends to the mid-dorsal level and acromion; it may well influence shoulder pain and dysfunction (Hoppenfield 1977). The costovertebral synovial joints are rich in proprioceptive innervation and are often a source of costovertebral dysfunction with presentation of pain. The T5 to T8 vertebrae are relatively immobile, providing greater stability, together with the thoracic cage, against anterior flexion, facilitating rotation at approximately 10° between T5 and T8. Posterior extension is limited by the shape of the zygapophysial facets and spinous processes (Mootz & Talmage 1999) (Table 6.1).

T9 to T12

The T12 vertebra innervates the iliac crest and lateral cutaneous region of the buttocks, thigh, and pubic region, and may well present with a diagnosis of thoracolumbar syndrome, which is unresponsive to lumbar and sacroiliac mobilization techniques. Here it is essential to examine the thoracolumbar fascia and associated paraspinal muscles for further sources of dysfunction; this is discussed below.

The extent to which features of spinal degeneration and pathoanatomy are related to symptoms remains unclear, and the influence of motion segmental degeneration on the mobility of the thoracic spine has not been established (Edmonson & Singer 1997). Thoracic disc herniations are uncommon lesions that are asymptomatic in most patients (Sheikh et al 2008), and unless affected by Scheurmann's disease, any increased kyphosis in adolescent individuals may be attributed to poor habitual posture rather than structural changes or reduced joint mobility. As the thoracic kyphosis increases with age the associated anatomical changes and decreased mobility will only be ameliorated by compensatory changes in the lumbar and cervical regions and the shoulder girdle (Edmonson & Singer 1997).

Careful observation during active movement testing is required, and thus, any upper thoracic symptoms should include an assessment of the cervical and cervicothoracic junction. Mechanical provocation should include resisted, assisted, active, and passive movements, as well as ischaemic compression (Mootz & Talmage 1999). The sensitivity and specificity of many physical examination processes for recording thoracic range of motion (ROM) are limited (Deyo et al 1992), and these should be contextualized within the overarching results of careful questioning and examination of all structures. Palpation for tenderness is a crucial part of manual therapy assessment for musculoskeletal dysfunction. Mid-thoracic tenderness is not a normal finding in asymptomatic subjects, and as such, it should be viewed as a possible source of pain-presenting structures (Keating et al 2001).

Joint movement assessment

Palpation helps determine the range and quality of motion of individual joints but pure passive movement is difficult to determine at the T-spine (Mootz & Talmage 1999). There are four essential categories of joint play (Maitland 1986):

- Central vertebral (posteroanterior (PA));
- Unilateral vertebral (PA);
- Transverse vertebral; and
- Rib springing.

Reliability studies on motion palpation and joint play have shown much variability (Haas et al 1995), as have discussions about the direct application of manual forces to affect the underlying thoracic joint and restore function (Bereznick et al 2002; Hertzog et al 1993). Generally, direct manipulation techniques are employed in the presence of somatic impairment when tissue reactivity is low, tissue stiffness is dominant, and minimum pain at the end of available range is demonstrated

Table 6.1 Thoracic range of movement guideline

Movement	Measurement	Vertebral level
Flexion	23°	T1 to T12
Extension	10°	C7 to T12
Lateral flexion	20° to 40°	C7 to T12
Rotation	20°	T1 to T12
Costovertebral expansion excursion	Inhalation: 6.5 mm	T8 to T10
	Exhalation: 13 mm	

Adapted from Evans (1994).

(Maitland 1986). In contrast, indirect or positional release techniques are applied to soft tissues and joints in the presence of somatic impairment when this is associated with high levels of tissue reactivity with associated nociceptive hypertonicity (Chaitow et al 2002).

'A time to hold and a time to scold.' (Makofsky 2003)

Pain arising from the thoracolumbar joints may be referred (via the terminal branches of the dorsal rami) into the lower lumbar spine, buttocks, and inguinal area (Dreyfuss et al 1994; Grieve 1988). Careful spinal mobilization and manipulative techniques may be implicated in this area, but only with evidence of the absence of any underlying pathology or neurological involvement. Sustained neural apophyseal glides (SNAGs) (Mulligan 1995) are important in the context of painful movement dysfunction associated with degenerative change (Edmonson & Singer 1997), providing normal physiological load-bearing, and combining elements of active and passive physiological movement with accessory glides along the zygapophysial joint plane (Edmonson & Singer 1997; Mulligan 1995). The Mulligan (1995) concept encompasses a number of mobilizing treatment techniques that can be applied to the spine, including natural apophyseal glides (NAGs), SNAGs, and spinal mobilizations with limb movements (SMWLMs).

Thoracolumbar fascia

The thoracolumbar fascia (TLF) is a critical structure in transferring load from the trunk to the lower extremities (Vleeming et al 1995). The anatomy of the TLF is complex, providing attachment for numerous paraspinal and abdominal muscles, as well as stability to the pelvic girdle when movement of the upper and lower extremities is undertaken. Muscle control in posture and locomotion is reliant on multifactorial integrated systems, the quality of muscle function depending directly on central nervous system (CNS) activity (Janda 1986). Functional stability is dependent on integrated local and global muscle function. Mechanical stability results from segmental (articular) and multisegmental (myofascial) function. Any dysfunction presents as a combination of restriction of normal motion and associated compensations (i.e. give) to maintain function (Comerford & Mottram 2001).

Strategies to manage mechanical stability dysfunction require:

- Specific mobilization of articular and connective tissue restrictions;
- Regaining myofascial extensibility;
- Retraining global stability muscle control of myofascial compensations; and
- Local stability muscle recruitment to control segmental motion (Comerford & Mottram 2001).

Stability re-training targets both the local and global stability systems; the strategy is to:

- Train low-load recruitment to control;
- Limit motion at the site of pathology;
- Actively move the adjacent restriction;
- Regain through range control of motion with the global stability muscles; and
- Regain sufficient extensibility in the global mobility muscles to allow normal function (Comerford & Mottram 2001).

Biopsychosocial influences

Emotional states have a huge impact on basic muscle tone and patterning, influencing muscle and visceral tone both locally and globally (Holstege et al 1996). Even more pertinent to physical intervention is the existence of the sympathetic chain, which is routed along the length of the T-spine and has ganglia in close proximity to the head of each rib. The result is that abdominal and visceral pain may refer to various thoracic levels, and these need to be assessed together with joint structures.

Autonomic nervous system

Sympathetic fibres leave the spinal nerve from levels T1 to L2 to join the sympathetic chain via the white rami communicantes. They travel for up to six T-spinal segments before synapsing with between 4 and 20 postganglionic neurons. The postganglionic neurons exit via the grey rami communicantes to rejoin a peripheral nerve and are distributed to the target tissues (Evans 1997). These nerves supply vasoconstrictor fibres to arterioles, secretory fibres to sweat glands, and pilomotor fibres to the skin (Craven 2008). The head and neck are supplied by levels T1 to T4 and the upper trunk and upper limb by T1 to T9 (Bogduk 2002).

The paired sympathetic trunk consists of ganglia and nerve fibres, and extends along the prevertebral fascia from the base of the skull to the coccyx (Craven 2008). There are two complementary parts of the autonomic nervous system (ANS); the sympathetic nervous system (SNS), which controls excitatory fight or flight reflexes, and the parasympathetic nervous system (PNS), which controls inhibitory rest and repose reactions. These two complementary, but contrasting and contradictory, systems leave the CNS at different sites, and have opposing effects through adrenergic or cholinergic endings.

Visceral fibres pass to the thoracic viscera by postganglionic fibres to:

- The cardiac plexus;
- The oesophageal plexus;
- The pulmonary plexus;
- Abdominal viscera by preganglionic splanchnic nerves;
- The adrenal medulla by the preganglionic greater splanchnic nerve; and
- Cranial and facial structures that accompany the:
  ○ Carotid vessels;
  ○ Larynx; and
  ○ Pharynx.

The greater splanchnic nerve (T5 to T10) ends in the coeliac plexus, while the lesser one (T9 to T10/T11) ends in the aortic and renal plexus. The lumbar sympathetic trunk (L1 to L5) supplies the pelvic viscera, rectum, bladder, and genitalia via the hypogastric nerves, whilst the inferior plexus (S2 to S4) receives parasympathetic branches from the nervi erigentes (Craven 2008).

The parasympathetic nervous system

The PNS is comprised of cranial and sacral components that cause constriction of the pupils, decreases in heart rate and volume, bronchoconstriction, increase in peristalsis, sphincter relaxation, and glandular secretion, whilst the pelvic component inhibits the detrusor muscle of the bladder (Craven 2008).

The cranial outflow is conveyed to the oculomotor nerve (III), facial nerve (VII), glossopharyngeal nerve (1X), and vagal nerves (X). Knowledge of the neural innervation and response of the PNS and SNS is essential for any proposed manual intervention. The insidious nature of thoracic pain and the associated postural dysfunction and stress (DeFranca & Levine 1995) may predispose the ganglion to mechanical pressure (Bogduk 1986), ischaemia (Conroy & Schneiders 2005), and somatic dysfunction via the CNS (Shaclock 1999).

Central pain mechanisms are deeply embodied in the psychophysical problem of pain, and are becoming increasingly recognized as playing a major role in the generation and maintenance of pain and disability associated with neuromusculoskeletal problems. Central mechanisms participate in all pain states, both acute and chronic. They are universally influenced by psychological and physical factors, whether or not a specific pathology can be identified. Common misconceptions that arise are that manual therapy operates on peripheral mechanisms without influencing the central ones and that, when a central problem exists, psychological management is preferable. In reality, as key players in the healing process, central mechanisms are profoundly affected by manual therapy even when it is directed at a peripheral problem. Treatment of peripheral mechanisms can be performed through central techniques because both peripheral and central mechanisms are always part of the same clinical problem. Consequently, manual therapy must integrate central mechanisms into clinical practice as a means of improving therapeutic efficacy and to prevent the descent of acute pain into chronic pain. Hendler (2002) suggested that 25–75% of cases of misdiagnosed complex regional pain syndrome type I (CRPS1) are actually upper extremity nerve entrapment affected more often by the scalenes and pectoralis minor muscles. Given the mounting evidence that chronic muscle pain syndromes may be sympathetically driven or maintained, it may be pertinent that chronic thoracic pain should be approached from the hypothetical perspective of muscle spindles under constant sympathetic excitation, meaning that the term 'sympathetic intrafusal tension syndrome' should replace myofascial pain syndrome as the appropriate description (Berkoff 2005) (Table 6.2).

Uncovering stressful condition-stimuli and evaluating their potential clinical relevance is vital. Relaxation, breathing, biofeedback, and cognitive behaviour therapy techniques are all useful in the management of increased sympathetic sensitivity. Here, the management of physical measures to alleviate pain and discomfort must be integrated in a multidisciplinary manual and biopsychosocial

Table 6.2 Common features and associated disorders of sympathetic intrafusal tension syndrome (SITS)

Presenting symptoms[a]	Associated symptoms[a]
Constant stiffness/discomfort at C7 area	Sleep disturbance
Constant stretching, rubbing, or pressure of pain area	Bruxism and temporo-mandibular joint pain
Active TrPts in scapular muscles reproduce pain pattern	Pain increased with stress
Gradual chronic pain fluctuations with no acute attacks	Worse on waking and end of day

Adapted from Berkoff (2005).
[a] Clinical diagnosis of SITS may be made on the presence of:
- 3 symptoms + 1 associated feature; or
- 2 symptoms + 3 associated features.

approach; a purely biomedical approach to physical therapy is too reductionist. Therapy needs to shift from symptomatic treatment to an emphasis on education, rehabilitation, facilitation of ownership, personal responsibility, and continuing management (CSAG 1994), in order to achieve longer lasting results and restoration of function.

The onset of acute chest pain, which may be very distressing for patient and family, is a major health problem in the Western world, and the most common reason for hospital admissions (McCaig & Nawar 2004). In over 50% of cases, the aetiology appears to be non-cardiac (Chambers et al 1999; Eslick et al 2001) and often no definitive diagnosis can be made (Panju et al 1996). Many thoracic dysfunctions have a mechanical cause originating from the T-spine, and referring to the upper extremities, chest, and cervical and lumbar spine, together with reverse referral patterns (Lee 2003; Proctor et al 1985; Wickes 1980).

The heart, pleura, and oesophagus are all potential generators of visceral pain in the T-spine. Sensory fibres from cardiac and pulmonary structures are routed through T1 to T4 and T5. Irritable bowel syndrome (IBS) is accompanied by altered visceral perception and back pain (Accarino et al 1995; Zighelboim et al 1995), and patients often demonstrate visceral and cutaneous hyperalgesia via viscerosomatic neurons (Tattersal et al 2008). The overlap between fibromyalgia syndrome (FMS) and IBS is considerable, with 70% of patients with FMS

reporting chronic visceral pain and 65% of those with IBS having primary FMS (Veale et al 1991).

Chronic visceral pain syndromes are more common in women than men and manifest such conditions as abdominal pain, migraine, and FMS (Table 6.3), reflecting the influence of hormonal factors on the algesic response both peripherally and centrally. The direct effect of oestrogen, progesterone, and testosterone on organ function, and psychological and social factors cannot be underestimated within the assessment process (Giamberardino 2000; Heitkemper & Jarrett 2001).

Recent findings have indicated that spinal manual therapy produces concurrent hypoalgesia and sympathoexcitatory effects (Sterling et al 2001). Therefore it is pertinent that, with regard to patients exhibiting sympathetically maintained pain or increased hypersensitivity of the SNS, manual mobilization may indeed add to both hypersensitivity and pain pattern. Thus great care should be taken in both the examination of and intervention in any hypersensitive thoracic states.

Myofascial component

Myofascial interscapular pain can confuse clinicians because it can be composite pain referred from as many as 10 different muscles (Whyte-Ferguson & Gerwin 2005) (Fig. 6.1).

One of the commonly overlooked causes of interscapular pain, one responsible for more than 80% of reported cases, is the scalene muscle complex which refers pain into three distinct areas (Spanos 2005):

- The upper two-thirds of the vertebral border and scapula;
- The lateral aspect of upper arm into triceps muscle;
- The whole hand, especially the thumb and the index finger; and
- Under the clavicle into the pectoral area.

The term T4 syndrome represents a clinical pattern involving upper extremity paraesthesia, and pain with or without symptoms into the neck and/or head (Maitland 1986). Even today the syndrome is poorly defined and agreed upon (Grieve 1994). Equally, it appears to be a catch-all phrase used by clinicians for patients whose varied problems seem to be derived from the upper T-spine and are not at all confined to T4 segmental vertebrae. It is not an uncommon

Table 6.3 Myofascial and visceral pain syndromes: viscerosomatic pain presentation

Pain referral pattern	Visceral involvement	Physiological processing
Pectoralis major Pectoralis minor Scapula Forearm	Myocardial infarction	Afferent interactions Increased sympathetic reflexes Increased fluid extravasation Oedema Sympathetic hypersensitivity
Lumbar Groin Thigh Right upper abdominal quadrant Abdominal oblique Rectus abdominus	Urethral colic Biliary colic	
Lower quadrant muscle Pelvic pain and tenderness Low back Abdominal muscle wall Iliopsoas Adductors Piriformis Pelvic floor Right shoulder Rotator cuff C5 and C6	Ovarian/uterine pain Urethral colic Dysmenorrhoea Cystitis Chlamydia Bladder and bowel dysfunction Sexual dysfunction Vulvodynia Liver and gall bladder Phrenic nerve irritation	Increased hypersensitivity and visceral tone of bladder
Mediastinal Pleura Impingement syndrome Frozen shoulder	Diaphragmatic irritation Gall bladder dysfunction	

Adapted from Gerwin (2002).

presentation in clinical practice. Pain may be caused by a variety of structures (Evans 1997):

- Entrapment of segmental spinal nerves carrying afferent fibres from the sympathetic nerves;
- Entrapment or ischaemia of sympathetic nerves over ribs or osteophytes;
- Referred cardiac or oesophageal pain;
- Pain referred from posterior spinal structures; and
- Pain referred from anterior spinal structures.

The sympathetic nerves supply forms a path for expression of T4 syndrome with pain referral occurring in the somatic nerves, referring from a proximal structure supplied at one level to a peripheral structure supplied at the same level (Evans 1997). Evans (1997) suggested that it might not only be the joint that is involved but also the arteriole. Sustained or extreme postures can lead to relative ischaemia, a repetitive strain injury with sympathetic symptoms, and repeated injury and repair, often seen in the more demanding upper quadrant sports such as rowing, gymnastics, and javelin, and prolonged poor posture in the workplace.

Recent findings demonstrating that cervical spinal manipulation produces concurrent hypoalgesia and sympathoexcitatory effects have led to the proposal that spinal manipulation may exert its initial effects by activating descending inhibitory pathways from the dorsal periaqueductal grey area of the midbrain, producing increased pressure-pain thresholds on the side receiving the treatment. Visual analogue scale (VAS) scores decreased along with superficial neck flexor muscle activity (Sterling et al 2001). Manual therapy may include both mobilization (low-velocity oscillatory techniques) and manipulation (high-velocity thrust techniques). Often little difference is found in reported conclusions about the effectiveness of manual therapy in using these techniques (Hurley et al 2005). Thoracic spine manipulation is applied only if extension restriction of T1 to T4 has been identified based upon palpatory examination and gliding motion of the upper thoracic dorsal vertebrae (Fernández de las Peñas et al 2004). Thoracolumbar joint manipulation should be applied in all patients with the aim of restoring free movement at T12 to L1 because the biomechanical analysis of whiplash injury implies a compression spine dysfunction at this level (Panjabi et al 1998; Yoganandan et al 2002). Inconsistencies in manual force application during spinal mobilizations in existing studies suggest that further studies are needed to improve clinical standardization of manual force application (Snodgrass et al 2006).

Determining the source of propagating pain structures is imperative and often complex for the successful resolution of thoracic pain. Manual examination of muscles, joints, fascia, and spinal

Right Scapular = pain	Location of pain	Muscle	Distinguishing characteristics that may be present	% Encountered by Author
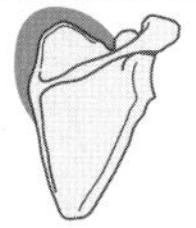	Upper 1/4 of vertebral border	Levator scapula	Pain also at angle of neck, limits rotation to opposite side (often accompanied by 1st rib dysfunction that limits rotation to same side)	30%
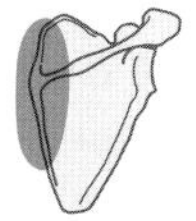	Upper 2/3 of vertebral border	Scalene	Pain in lateral as pect of upper arm; thumb and index finger, 2 finger-like projections over pectoral region almost to nipple level	80%
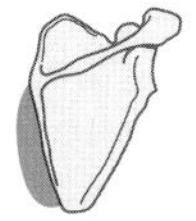	Middle 1/2 of vertebral border	Infraspinatus	Deep pain in front of shoulder and down front of upper arm (biceps)	20%
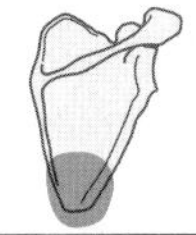	Lower 1/3 of vertebral border (inferior angle) of scapula, fist size	Latissimus dorsi	Light pain in ring and little fingers, triceps	30%
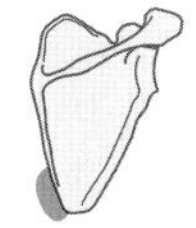	Lower 1/3 of vertebral border, inferior angle of scapula, 2 thumb digits size	Serratus anterior	Pain anterolaterally at mid-chest level. Sense of air hunger with short panting respiration	20%
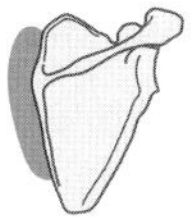	Lower 4/5 of vertebral border, narrow in width	Lower trapezius	Slight burning pain, not severe	10%
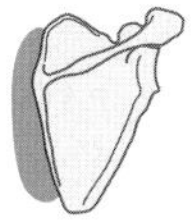	Medial pain inferior end of scapula and lighter in pain along vertebral border	Iliocostalis thoracis	Pain along inferior medial border of scapula, less intense pain along vertebral border	10%
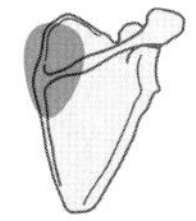	Upper 1/2 of vertebral border and deep pain under scapula	Serratus posterior superior	Pain in entire little finger. Deep pain cannot be reached by patient	5%
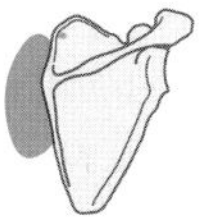	Middle 1/2 of vertebral border and toward spine	Multifidi thoracis	Most pain toward the spine	10%
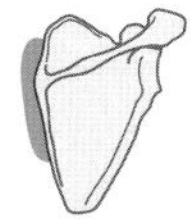	Middle 1/2 of vertebral border between the scapula and paraspinal	Rhomboid	Complaint is of superficial aching pain at rest, not influenced by ordinary movement	5%

Figure 6.1 • Interscapular pain table. Reproduced with kind permission from Lucy Whyte Ferguson & Robert Gerwin (2005), Clinical Mastery in the Treatment of Myofascial Pain, Lippincott Williams and Wilkins.

dysfunction has been the subject of much criticism because of poor reproducibility and validity (Stochkendahl et al 2006). What is paramount is a clear clinical reasoning pathway in order to eliminate, select, and treat appropriate presenting pain structures for effective management and rehabilitation, to prevent the development of chronic pain syndromes.

6.1   Acupuncture interventions with thoracic spine dysfunction

Jennie Longbottom

Stressors are physiological or psychological perturbations that throw the body out of homeostatic balance; the stress response is the set of neural and endocrine adaptations that help us re-establish homeostasis. In traditional Chinese medicine (TCM) a balance between Yin and Yang (homeostasis) ensures both physical and mental health and well being, Acupuncture is believed to aid the restoration of homeostasis. With prolonged stress, increased corticotropin releasing factor is secreted from the hypothalamus into the hypophysial–pituitary circulation, along with a pituitary release of adrenocorticotropic hormone, which rapidly releases glucocorticoids. Glucocorticoids are central to the stress response, targeting energy storage, increasing cardiovascular tone, and inhibiting anabolic processes such as growth, reproduction, healing, inflammation, and immunity (Sapolsky 1992). The stress response now becomes as damaging as the stressor itself. Stressors disrupt physiological regulatory mechanisms, leading to diseased states and altered responses of the psychoneuroimmune system.

It has been estimated that 80% of all illness is stress-induced (Friedman et al 2003; Sapolsky 1992; Walling 2006). One purpose of any healthcare system is to diagnose and treat dysfunctions of the homeostatic mechanisms of any individual in order to maintain the higher level of health and to prevent disease. However, increasingly within the Western world, interventions are directed towards the symptoms of failure of that homeostatic system. The integrated use of acupuncture within a physiotherapeutic toolbox may offer the clinician the ability to directly affect homeostatic stability as a means of restoring health or preventing further disease. The science of neuroimmunology, when combined with the art of TCM acupuncture, may enable the endocrine and immune system to regulate a cascade of cellular processes and changes, through the stimulation of neuropeptides, via needle insertion at selected points in order to maintain, rebalance, and restore health and well being. When Yin and Yang systems are balanced, the neuropeptides are free flowing (Qi) and a sense of well being pervades (Shen). Stress prevents the free flow (Qi stagnation) of peptide-signalling molecules (Pert

1997), creating blockages (Qi excess or stagnation) and weakness (Qi deficiency) that may lead to disease. Reduced output of endorphins and norepinephrine may lead to anxiety and depression (Shen disturbance) (Pert 1997).

A continuous interaction via action potentials within the nerve fibres, which may in fact be acupuncture meridians, exists between the autonomic, central, and endocrine systems. Action potentials are generated in response to a stimulus, whether physical or emotional, positive or negative, and thus, pathological over- or underactivity of neurotransmitters may cause neurological or psychiatric disease (Pert 1997; Sapolsky 1992; Walling 2006). Stress can trigger a cascade of physiological responses, including increased levels of cytokines, interleukin-6, inflammatory chemicals linked to obesity, diabetes, osteoporosis, arthritis (Sapolsky 1992; Pert 1997; Walling 2006), and, at its worst, Alzheimer disease (Sapolsky 1992). During sleep, recalibration and resetting of the CNS takes place in order to restore homeostasis (Kandel et al 1995; Sapolsky 1992). During excess stress, sleep is elusive, and this adds to the imbalance and strain placed upon the system. Acupuncture is known to have an inhibitory effect on cytokine production (Jong et al 2006; Kandel et al 1995; Shah 2008), neuroimmune anti-inflammatory responses (Kavoussi & Evan-Ross 2007), and anxiety and depression (Hansson et al 2007). This is especially so with anxiety and depression in people with dementia, who often demonstrate an improvement in cognitive function, which is thought to be a result of enhanced oxygen content and perfusion in the brain (Lombardo et al 2001). Luo (1987) demonstrated beneficial effects from acupuncture that were similar to those resulting from amitriptylin, but without the associated side effects. Chen (1992) suggested that electroacupuncture (EA) increases serotonin and cerebral blood flow, and the production of hypothalamic and pituitary neuropeptide-releasing factors, oxytocin, vasopressin, and endorphins, many of which have anti-depressant properties. Dudaeva (1990) reported neurophysiological changes using electroencephalography (EEG) during acupuncture treatment for depression, and Hui et al (2000) demonstrated that study participants experiencing de Qi had prominent decreases of functional magnetic resonance imaging (fMRI) signals in the limbic and subcortical regions of the amygdala, hippocampus, caudate, putamen, and anterior cingulate nucleus, which could well contribute to acupuncture efficacy for the treatment of diverse affective and psychosomatic disorders. Acupuncture may be a safe, feasible, and effective method for reducing symptoms of anxiety, sympathetic hypersensitivity, depression, and cognitive impairment before the application of manual interventions for managing pain and dysfunction, i.e. a means of preparing the system and promoting homeostasis to facilitate recovery.

The feeling of well being often reported by subjects receiving acupuncture may enable the ANS to regain some measure of homeostasis via releasing immune-enhancing neuropeptides (Fisher 1988), and suppressing the production and release of inflammatory cytokines (Jeong et al 2003). However, these techniques are adjuncts to the essential premise of changing the amount of stressors to which the individual is subjected. Enabling and supporting autonomic homeostasis will enhance well being, enhancing effective coping strategies, and should always be used within a multidisciplinary approach combining psychological therapies, such as cognitive behaviour therapy, pacing strategies, and counselling in order to offer best available practice.

The limbic structures are implicated in the reward system, and play a key role in most disease and illness responses, including chronic pain and depression, by regulating mood and neuromodulatory responses. For patients, reduction of unpleasantness and restoration of well being and the individual sense of self may be of greater importance than an actual reduction in pain intensity (Lundeberg et al 2007). When patients are asked how an acupuncture treatment makes them feel (self-relevant tasks), there is a shift to one's self as the referent, resulting in activation of the ventral and dorsal medial prefrontal cortex, dorsorostral and posterior cingulate. Treatments that convey general information about well being are related to activation in the ventral medial prefrontal cortex, and anterior cingulate, nucleus accumbens and insula, triggering a cascade of subcortical processing orientating the subject to an increased response potential (Lundeberg et al 2007). If pain is the presenting factor, pain may be alleviated; if sleep is the paramount problem, sleep may be induced by acupuncture; thus acupuncture activates this reward system (Pariente et al 2005).

Dudley et al (2003) demonstrated that EA increases the serotonin and dopamine content of the nuclei accumbens, caudate putamen, and lateral hypothalamus, whereas a decrease in these monoamines is seen in the dorsal raphe nucleus and amygdala. These results demonstrate that acupuncture techniques, as well as non-penetrating placebo controls, activate the patient's expectation and belief regarding a potentially beneficial treatment, thus modulating activity and the reward system (Dhond et al 2007; Lu et al 1998) (Fig. 6.2).

Auricular acupuncture (AA) has been used for various disorders in clinical practice. It has been theorized that different auricular areas have a distinct influence on autonomic function (Gao et al 2008). The selection of AA points for pain relief (Usichenko et al 2005a, b), anxiety and sleep disorders (Chen et al 2007), hypertension (Huang & Laing 1992), gastrointestinal disorders (Takahashi 2006), urinary tract symptoms (Capodice et al 2007), and postoperative vomiting (Kim & Kim 2003) is well documented, although the specificity of AA points is still a matter of conjecture (Gao et al 2008).

The human ear receives innervations from cervical and cranial nerves including the auricular branch of the vagal nerve, great auricular nerve, and auriculotemporal nerve (Peuker & Filler 2002). Gao et al (2008) found that stimulation of the auricle with either manual acupuncture (MA) or EA (100 Hz at 1 mA) can evoke a characteristic pattern of response, including a reduction in blood pressure, bradycardia, and gastric contraction, which may be attributed to an increase in vagal output, mediated by auricular–vagal reflexes. The inferior concha produced the

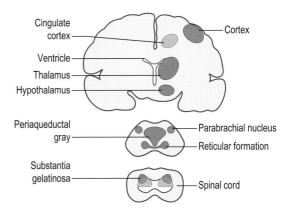

Figure 6.2 • Diagram of limbic structures.
Reproduced with kind permission of Purdue Pharma
LP's *Pain—an illustrated resource*, http://www.purduepharma.com

biggest depressor effect during MA (Gao et al 2008). Stimulation of the outer auditory canal produced enhancement of well being coupled with deactivation of limbic and temporal structures (Kraus et al 2007). These anatomical studies suggest an overlapping distribution of somatic and cranial nerves, which does not support the concept of a specific functional map of the ear, but rather, a general pattern of autonomic changes in response to AA of variable intensity, depending on the level of stimulation, and the use of MA or EA. Gao et al (2008) define the most powerful site for regulation of autonomic functions as the inferior concha, which may further enhance homeostasis as a preparation for manual interventions at the T-spine.

The correlation between chronic pain, chronic thoracic pain, and sympathetic overactivation cannot be underestimated. Abnormality in autonomic functions has been implicated in FMS and acupuncture is frequently applied in managing the symptoms in chronic pain management. It has been demonstrated that acupuncture significantly reduces heart rate, elevated systolic pressure (Furlan et al 2005), complex regional pain syndrome (Baron et al 1999), and whiplash-associated disorders (Passatore & Roatta 2006). Acupuncture may be used to restore balance between the inhibition of the SNS and excitation of the PNS (Nishijo et al 1997).

A study by Jang et al (2003) looking at the effect on neural pathways on using acupuncture points Heart (HT) 7 and Pericardium (PC) 6 showed that signals from EA at these two points could converge to the dorsal horn neurons at T2 to T3. Liu et al (1996) investigated the receptive fields on the body surface and the physiological types of 18 neurons, reporting that information from PC6 and Stomach (ST) 36 can converge to the neurons at T2 to T3 dorsal horn and influence sympathetic inhibitory activity at this level (Liu et al 1996).

Kavoussi and Evan-Ross (2007) found that sympathetic nerves were inhibited and parasympathetic nerves excited after stimulation of ST36, supporting the Chinese therapeutic principle of adjusting and harmonizing the internal environment to achieve stability (Unchald 2008). This model parallels the modern notion of re-establishing homeostasis by regulating the interactions between the ANS, innate immunity, and the body as a whole. The cholinergic anti-inflammatory pathway provides simple, cohesive, and integrative biomedical evidence for the systemic immunoregulatory actions of acupuncture at selected points, and for AA as an integrated tool within manual medicine for the treatment of a number of cytokine-mediated diseases; these are plausible, evidence-based interventions (Kavoussi & Evan-Ross 2007; Tracey 2005, 2007).

Caution should be exercised when directly needling the Bladder, Huatuojiaji, and Governor Vessel points over the sympathetic chain in patients who demonstrate increased sympathetic excitability, for fear of increasing sympathetic hypoexcitability and potentially aggravating the patient and the SNS system. Preference for AA and specific distal points such as PC6, ST36, and HT7, together with specific parasympathetic points such as BL10, Gall Bladder (GB) 20, and BL28 (Longbottom 2006) may provide a gentler, more effective way of promoting balance and homeostasis in the ANS.

 ## Case Study 1

Kenny Cross

Introduction

A 63-year-old female accountant had experienced an insidious onset of upper abdominal pain, which she described as a deep ache of one year in duration prior to her physiotherapy consultation. Her right upper abdominal pain was worse than the left. The subject reported a 20-year history of chronic low back pain (CLBP) related to a diagnosis of lower lumbar disc herniation and had experienced intermittent symptoms since its onset. Within the past year she had experienced right shoulder, neck, and scapula symptoms that had alleviated over time. Her LBP was asymptomatic at the time of assessment.

Following a medical diagnosis of gall bladder lesion, the subject underwent a series of abdominal investigations (i.e. blood analysis, computed axial tomography scan, and endoscopy). All findings were negative. An electrocardiogram investigation was normal. She had received osteopathic treatment over a 2-month period prior to physiotherapy. This was focused on her T-spine, and appeared to aggravate her pain.

The subject reported symptoms as constant intense ache in the upper abdominal area rating it as 60/100 on the VAS. Aggravating factors included supine lying, and prolonged activity, e.g. walking, gardening, or housework for more than 10 minutes, which increased her symptoms

(Continued)

Case Study 1 (Continued)

to 90/100 on the VAS. There were no abnormal symptoms relating to loss of appetite, fever, or altered bowel or bladder function. Symptoms within the upper and lower extremities were also normal. The subject described a feeling of exhaustion throughout the day relating to sleep deprivation caused by her constant pain and she had limited her self-employed accountancy work to less than 8 hours per week because of pain and fatigue.

Objective findings

Postural dysfunction was present in the form of slight chin poke, rounded shoulders, and a small increase in thoracic kyphotic curvature. Lower abdominal muscles laxity was present. Active arm elevation increased the abdominal discomfort (right greater than left) and the client was unable to sustain this position due to her symptoms.

Cervical and thoracic rotation mobility was approximately 70%, but it was limited by tightness, not pain. Lumbar mobility was 80% without pain provocation. The subject demonstrated a predominantly apical breathing pattern, which was confirmed with tape measure diaphragm expansion. At rest it was 787\ mm, and 800 mm on full inhalation (measured immediately inferior to the xiphoid process). She was unaware of the lack of diaphragmatic and lateral costal expansion with relaxed and full inhalation.

Palpation revealed an asymmetrical breathing pattern, with reduced mobility of the right lateral costal inhalation expansion, reduced thoracic cage mobility, and a positive diaphragmatic expansion restriction. A significant painful tightness to palpation was found inferior to both rib cages. Spinal assessment revealed general articular hypomobility throughout the T- and lumbar spines, but without symptom provocation. Palpation of the thoracic and lumbar multifidi muscles failed to elicit active trigger points (TrPts) or reproduce symptoms. However, there was a degree of hypertonus within the multifidus, latissimus dorsi, and quadratus lumborum muscles. On palpation of the external abdominus oblique (EAO) muscle a taut band and twitch response reproduced the subject's pain. The right EAO was significantly more provocative than the left and more provocative than the rectus abdominus (RA) palpation. There was poor recruitment ability in the deep lumbar multifidi and transversus abdominus (TA) muscles and reduced deep neck flexor recruitment.

This subject was experiencing chronic anterior abdominal myofascial dysfunction. The active EAO and RA myofascial trigger points (MTrPts) created a diaphragmatic constriction. The overall findings suggested a long-standing relationship with muscle imbalance, and respiratory and postural dysfunction, possibly associated with her history of chronic LBP and thoracic kyphosis. Family stress and guarding pain adaptations result in a cycle of pain, and heightened emotional and SNS responses had exacerbated her symptoms. On the initial assessment, the subject had poor pain tolerance to light palpation of the EAO or diaphragm fascia.

Management plan

The overall management of this patient was significantly assisted by previous medical interventions that had ruled out underlying pathologies. Acupuncture was the initial modality of choice because of the sensitivity of the MTrPts, and the subject's anxiety and heightened SNS responses (Table 6.4).

Table 6.4 Point Selection

Point	Rationale
ST36	Enhance general energy and Qi metabolism. Regulation of overall function. Strong He-Sea point regulating distal meridian to inner body. Calms the spirit. Acupuncture point of the stomach meridian with a vital role in digestion and healthy well being preventing stagnation. Component of stomach meridian covering anterior thorax.
CV12	Associated with the anterior aspect of the trunk. Regulates the Yin energy and acts as a reservoir when energy is in short supply. Reduces abdominal pain and discomfort. Influential in respiratory stagnation and has a close relationship with the lungs. Influential point of the Fu organs. Anterior-Mu point of the stomach.
GV20	Scalp acupuncture point. General tonification and reduction of sympathetic excitability. General well being and PNS stimulation.
External oblique MTrPt	Alleviate MTrPt localized to the upper abdominal region, and refers pain into adjacent areas and across the midline. Stretch shortened muscle tissue and restore normal motor end-plate function. Release of diaphragmatic constriction.
Rectus abdominus MTrPt	Alleviate MTrPt localized to the central anterior abdominal region and refers pain into adjacent areas. Stretch shortened muscle tissue and restore normal motor end-plate function. Assist in the release of diaphragmatic constriction.

Notes: ST, Stomach; CV, Conception Vessel; GV, Governing Vessel; MTrPt, myofascial trigger point; and PNS, parasympathetic nervous system.

(Continued)

Case Study 1 (Continued)

Table 6.5 Treatment regime

Treatment	Points	Manual intervention	Outcome
1	GV20 ST36 CV12	Basal and diaphragmatic breathing exercises TA recruitment	Constant 6/10 Unable to sleep Reduced diaphragmatic expansion (860 mm) Unable to recruit TA
2	CV12 ST36	R and L EAO MTrP release TA recruitment Education Pacing Walking 10 min daily	Constant 2/10 Sleeping intermittent Increased respiratory expansion by 20 mm Active shoulder elevation to 80% pain free
3	No change	R and L EAO trigger points TA recruitment in crook lying	Intermittent 1/10 Normal sleep patterns Increased thoracic rotation to >85°
4	No change	R and L EAO MF TrPt release RA MTrP release MET to soft tissue at T-spine Manual mobilizations at T-spine TA recruitment Lateral costal breathing exercises	Intermittent 1/10 Sleeping well Expansion increased by 25 mm. Full TA recruitment Full pain-free shoulder movement
6	No change	ISQ	Pain free Functional pain-free mobility achieved Sleeping normally Unrestricted full inhalation achieved. Expansion increased by 45 mm. Independent TA to moderate to advanced level Returning to work

Notes: GV, Governor Vessel; ST, Stomach; CV, Conception Vessel; MTrPt, myofascial trigger point; TA, transversus abdominus; EAO, external abdominal oblique; RA, rectus abdominus.

The initial short-term aims were to:
- Reduce sympathetic excitability;
- Improve well being;
- Improve energy levels;
- Relax the diaphragmatic constriction;
- Provide a window of opportunity to improve overall respiratory function; and
- Enhance patient relaxation.

The long-term aims of the intervention were to:
- Improve movement and the muscle recruitment patterns of the upper quadrant;
- Improve the patient's function;
- Restore good sleep patterns;
- Restore diaphragmatic and lateral costal breathing patterns by 80%;
- Achieve improved core muscle recruitment especially, activation of TA;
- Reduce the global muscle activity of EAO and RA by at least 50%; and
- Restore coping mechanisms by empowerment of the patient.

Outcome measurements and results

The subject demonstrated a consistent improvement, achieving 95% pa in relief with acupuncture, manual soft-tissue release, and a home programme. Diaphragmatic basal and lateral costal expansion improved by more than 80% without her reporting any tension or limitation on full inhalation. She increased her diaphragmatic expansion by 45 mm (Table 6.5). The subject achieved independence in a home programme for muscle recruitment patterns. She also progressed to moderate, but not advanced levels, and had potential for further improvement. Full recovery of arm movements was achieved, along with a 90% return of full cervical,

(Continued)

Case Study 1 (Continued)

thoracic, and lumbar spine mobility. The subject returned to unrestricted work and walking activities. Gardening and housework tasks were pain free.

At 3 and 6 months' telephone follow-up, she continued to report a significant improvement, although she reported experiencing short episodes of abdominal discomfort associated with challenging family emotional situations. Breathing exercises and relaxation techniques helped to resolve these episodes. No exacerbations of LBP were reported and this patient continued to progress in functional mobility with regard to gardening and unlimited walking exercise.

Clinical reasoning for acupuncture

Since this patient's upper abdominal connective tissue and T-spine were sensitive to direct pressure, acupuncture provided a treatment modality that eased symptoms in a way that was tolerable for the patient. Acupuncture was applied to the Governor Vessel (GV) 20 to produce PSN stimulation, relaxation, and well being, and Conception Vessel (CV) 12 to facilitate a localized physiological response to the abdominal area. The CV12 and RA MTrPts are similar in location and could elicit a localized response for pain relief and circulation, relaxing the upper abdominal area and diaphragm via the pain-gate mechanism (Melzack et al 1977).

Acupuncture MTrP release reduced the diaphragmatic constriction by inhibiting EAO and RA overactivity. The subject's subsequent enhanced ability to stretch the previously tight and dysfunctional upper abdominal and diaphragmatic tissues enabled the restoration of improved diaphragmatic basal and lateral costal mobility, and overall respiratory function. The increase in respiratory volume increased her

cardiorespiratory functions such as walking and stair activity, and contributed to further functional restoration.

In his classification of fatigue patterns, Seem (2000) describes diaphragmatic constriction as a ventral pain associated with an overactive SNS. The main suggested muscles involved are the RA, upper abdominal oblique, and pectoralis muscles. Abdominal problems such as IBS, chronic bloating, constipation, and diarrhoea have been associated with this type of constriction. The point ST36 is suggested to elicit a strong sympathetic inhibitory response, coupled with further positive outcomes such as improved energy levels, pain relief, muscle and mood relaxation, and improved respiratory function.

Another treatment modality, transcutaneous electrical nerve stimulation (TENS), might have been of benefit to modulate chronic pain symptoms for this subject, at bilateral points BL10 and BL28. Using high-intensity, low-frequency TENS (2 Hz) for 30 to 40 minutes has been proven to provide supraspinal pain modulation. The release of oxytocin and beta-endorphins (Uvnas-Moberg et al 1993) is thought to aid in the reduction of anxiety, inhibition of pain memory, improvement of sleep, and enhancement of analgesia. This would have been a useful self-management tool preventing any patient reliance on manual intervention, but since this subject progressed well and returned to normal function, it was not necessary.

This present case study has demonstrated the use of an eclectic treatment approach that integrated manual therapy techniques to release tightness in the myofascial pain presentation, and exercises and manual therapy to improve muscle balance, respiratory dysfunction, and lifestyle, providing optimum outcome and independence of care to the patient.

Case Study 2

Helen Sankey

Introduction

This case study involves a 25-year-old female patient who presented with insidious onset right-sided cervical, thoracic, and right arm pain. This correlated with an increase in her anxiety and insomnia symptoms. The clinical impression was that of T4 syndrome and postural dysfunction. The treatment combined acupuncture, exercise, postural correction, and manual therapy. After six sessions of physiotherapy pain was reduced by 50%, while sleep duration and quality was improved subjectively. This case study discusses clinical reasoning, the pain-relieving mechanisms of acupuncture, and the current available research surrounding acupuncture and cervical pain, thoracic pain, anxiety disorders, and insomnia.

A 25-year-old female presented with a 6-month history of insidious onset right-sided cervical, thoracic, and right arm pain (Fig. 6.3). There had been no change in activity associated with the onset of the pain, but she had noted an increase in panic attacks a few weeks before the onset of pain. The cause of her worsening panic attacks was unknown. No previous history of the presenting symptoms was noted, apart from stiffness since an injury at age 7 which had been treated with a neck brace for 6 weeks.

Subjective assessment

The subject had had a history of panic attacks and intermittent insomnia since the death of her father 7 years earlier; she was placed on Paracetamol and

(Continued)

Case Study 2 (Continued)

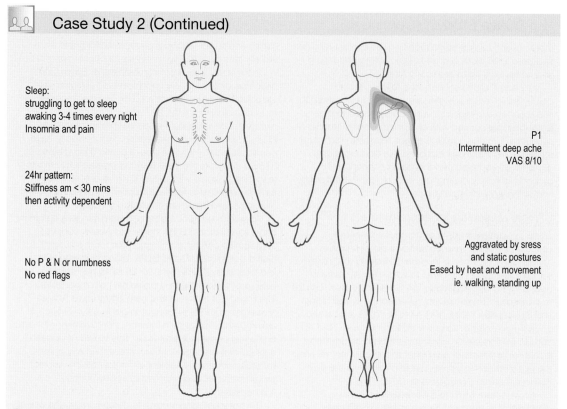

Sleep:
struggling to get to sleep
awaking 3-4 times every night
Insomnia and pain

24hr pattern:
Stiffness am < 30 mins
then activity dependent

No P & N or numbness
No red flags

P1
Intermittent deep ache
VAS 8/10

Aggravated by sress
and static postures
Eased by heat and movement
ie. walking, standing up

Figure 6.3 ● Presenting condition.

Citalopram for the management of anxiety. She worked in an office and was mostly desk-based, but had found increasing difficulty sitting for more than 30 minutes without increase in P1.

Objective assessment

On observation she had a forward head posture with increased thoracic kyphosis and anterior inferior positioning of her glenoid bilaterally, with associated medial rotation of the scapula on the right. On being asked to put herself into what she considered to be a good posture she corrected her lower thoracic and lumbar position, but retracted her shoulder girdle.

- Active range of movement (AROM) of her cervical spine was limited in:
  ○ Left side flexion 4/5 range tightness;
  ○ Retraction 4/5 range tightness; and
  ○ All other movements had full pain-free range.
- The AROM of her thoracic spine was reduced in all directions:
  ○ Flexion 3/4 range P1;
  ○ Right rotation 3/4 range P1;
  ○ Left rotation 3/4 range P1;
  ○ Right side flexion 1/2 range P1;

  ○ Left side flexion 3/4 range P1;
  ○ Extension 1/3 range P1.
- Passive ROM was equal to AROM.
- Palpation of levator scapulae and upper and middle fibres of trapezius were extremely tender, with resulting reproduction of P1 into neck. Passive accessory intervertebral movements (PAIVMs) and central posterior-anterior intervertebral movements were checked from C3 to T6:
  ○ C3 to C6: full pain-free range; and
  ○ C6 to T6: pain immediately and resistance early in range, pain limited glide at all levels.
- There was full reproduction of P1 on palpation of T2 and T3.

Impression and clinical reasoning

From the distribution of pain it could be hypothesized that the origin of the pain is from the C5 or C6 nerve root, as it lies in a C5 to C6 dermatome pattern, and/or pain from the anterior disc at C5 referring into the thoracic spine, Cloward's area (Cloward 1959). However, P1 could not be reproduced from cervical spine movements or PAIVMs at these levels. Pain at P1 could be reproduced from PAIVMs at T2 and T3 and

(Continued)

Case Study 2 (Continued)

thoracic spine movements were significantly reduced, consistent with a mechanical dysfunction of the thoracic spine. The conclusion was that the origin of the pain was T4 syndrome involving T2 and T3. The syndrome is characterized by paraesthesia, numbness, or upper extremity pains associated with or without headaches and upper back stiffness. Upper thoracic joint dysfunction, especially in the region of the T4 segment, appeared to be the major cause of the upper extremity symptoms and non-traumatic onset is common (DeFranca & Levine 1995).

There was tenderness on palpation of Levator scapulae and upper and middle fibres of trapezius with some reproduction of P1. The pain was eased by heat, consistent with myofascial pain from these muscles, combined with poor posture and poor activation of stability muscles around the shoulder girdle; coupled with the insidious onset of pain and aggravation of symptoms in static positions, this indicates a postural strain on the soft tissues.

It was therefore concluded that the mechanism of pain was peripheral mechanical nociceptive pain.

The increased anxiety, panic attacks, and insomnia were associated with the mechanism of her pain, as symptoms were exacerbated and improved simultaneously. It is known that pain is strongly associated with anxiety and depressive disorders. Indeed primary care patients who present with symptoms of muscle pain, headache, or stomach pain are approximately 2.5 times more likely to screen positively for panic disorder, generalized anxiety disorder, or major depressive disorder (Means-Christensen et al 2008). It is also found that certain psychological symptoms (low energy, disturbed sleep, worry) are prominent among pain patients, and that for these patients psychological distress amplifies dysphoric physical sensations, including pain (Von Korff & Simon 1996). Depression and anxiety can adversely affect the course of chronic physical illnesses. Biological mechanisms include increased inflammatory response and disruption of the hypothalamic–pituitary–adrenal axis (HPA) (Sobel & Markov 2005). It has been hypothesized that anxiety disorders are related to a deficiency in the endogenous opioid system (Sher 1998), coupled with the result that stressful life events and psychological dysfunction were statistically higher in a group of chronic regional pain syndrome (CRPS) patients versus a control group. Interestingly insomnia also correlated with the experience of a stressful life event (Geertzen et al 1998). The subject's anxiety and panic disorder was triggered by a stressful life event; it could therefore be hypothesized that this pain presentation may have similar presentations to that of CRPS mechanism. Leriche (1918) proposed that CRPS could involve overactivity of the SNS as surgical sympathectomy produced some relief of symptoms. However, it has

been found that SNS metabolites are not raised in the affected limb as would be expected, and plasma levels of adrenaline and noradrenalin were found to be lower in the affected side, leading to the theory that CRPS is caused by hypersensitivity to SNS neurotransmitters (Drummond et al 1991).

Another theory is abnormal opioid modulation; under normal conditions, opioids are released in large numbers from regional sympathetic ganglia after injury, which prevents excessive autonomic activity in the injured limb. If no opioids are released, dystrophic changes, similar to those observed in the early stages of CRPS, can occur, possibly caused by the complications of disuse (Hannington-Kiff 1991). It has also been proposed that CRPS is a neuropsychiatric disorder, an exaggerated inflammatory response or an abnormal immune response (Muir & Vernon 2000) or caused by a viral infection (Muneshige et al 2003). With the current level of research it is impossible to say what the exact mechanism of pain would be for this case study patient. The pain-relieving mechanisms of acupuncture will be discussed later in this paper.

Presenting pain mechanisms

Listed below are the subjective and objective markers that the treatment was designed to affect:

- Sleep latency and awakening 3–4 times per night;
- Improve posture;
- Reduce pain from the presenting VAS of 80/100; and
- Improve AROM of thoracic extension 1/3 P1 and right rotation 1/2 P1.

Treatment rationale

AROM exercises were taught for the thoracic spine to regain the ROM; the subject was advised to take a brisk walk for 30 minutes to increase heart rate, in order to reduce anxiety. It must be noted that training programs must exceed 10 weeks for significant changes in trait anxiety to occur (Petruzzello et al 1991). Using a mirror and facilitation, the subject was educated on the effects of poor posture and taught posture correction to reduce the strain on the soft tissues. Scapula setting was added to correct the position of the scapula, activate serratus anterior and lower fibres of trapezius, and reduce the increased activity in levator scapulae and upper/mid-trapezius (Mottram 1997). The thoracic spine was mobilized using grade II central posterior–anterior glides progressing to grade III mobilizations to treat T4 syndrome (DeFranca & Levine 1995).

Acupuncture intervention

Acupuncture was used to reduce the severity of her pain, and to address her anxiety and insomnia to help the patient cope better with her pain. Points were chosen (Table 6.6), following the Western model of acupuncture outlined by Bradnam (2007). Points are selected

(Continued)

Case Study 2 (Continued)

Table 6.6 Treatment rationale

Session	Points used	Treatment length (mins)	Outcome measures	Adverse effects	Other treatment
1	LI 4[B] HT7[B] LI11[B]	20	VAS 80/100 Sleep latency 7/7 Awake 3–4 treatments	None	Active ROM exercises Brisk walk \30 minutes Posture correction
2	LI4[B] HT7[B]	25	VAS 80/100 Sleep latency improved 2/7	None	Active and active assisted ROM exercises
3	LI4[B]	25	VAS 70/100	None	Scapula setting
4	LI4[B]	25	VAS 50/100	None	Mobilizations to the thoracic spine
5	LI4[B]	25	VAS 50/100	None	Mobilizations to the thoracic spine

Notes: B, bilateral; LI, Large Intestine; HT, Heart; ROM, range of movement.

depending on the type of pain mechanism and the state of the tissues. In this case the primary pain mechanism was peripheral nociceptive with possible centrally evoked pain. This model proposes a layering mechanism in order to facilitate local, spinal, sympathetic, central, or immune effects. As the patient's condition was chronic (a 6-month history of symptoms), treatment was aimed at stimulating local tissue by utilizing local points. In this case the patient declined acupuncture to the painful area due to fear and hypersensitivity.

Large intestine 11 (LI11) was chosen as it lies along the painful segment to give a spinal effect; LI 4 was chosen as it produces central effects and stimulates the T1 myotome, which can affect sympathetic outflow at this level (Bradnam 2007) and is a well-researched pain-relieving point (Mayer et al 1977). Heart 7 (HT7) and Pericardium 6 (PC6) are extrasegmental and were chosen to effect supraspinal mechanisms. These points are commonly used to treat anxiety and insomnia symptoms (Cheuk et al 2007; Pilkington et al 2007; Sok et al 2003).

Acupoints Bladder 10 (BL10) and Gall Bladder 20 (GB20) were added to stimulate the PNS. They lie between the spinous processes of C1 and C2 and between the occiput and C1, respectively, and are therefore innervated by the PSN (Krassioukov & Weaver 1996).

Outcomes at the final session

Sleep latency was still present due to rumination, but there were subjective improvements in sleep quality and duration and the subject was no longer waking during the night. She was able to demonstrate good posture, but struggled to keep it at work. She had improved function and reported sitting at work for approximately one and a quarter hours before symptoms increased. The pain score was now 40/100 VAS and AROM of

thoracic extension presented with 2/3 stiffness and right rotation 3/4 stiffness.

Research

A review of the literature surrounding treatment searches was conducted on AMED, CINAHL, and MEDLINE. Searches were conducted using keywords: *acupuncture* and *neck pain, cervical pain, thoracic pain, sleep, insomnia* and *anxiety disorders*. No studies were found on thoracic pain, so it was decided to evaluate studies that looked at cervical pain since the area of the patient's pain was lower cervical, upper thoracic and could be classified as neck pain if a full assessment was not completed. A Cochrane review in 2006 looked at the evidence surrounding acupuncture and neck disorders and concluded that there is moderate evidence that acupuncture relieves pain when compared to some sham treatments, measured at the end of the treatment, and that those who received acupuncture reported less pain at short-term follow-up than those on a waiting list. There is also moderate evidence that acupuncture is more effective than inactive treatments for relieving pain post-treatment and this is maintained at short-term follow-up (Trinh et al 2006).

A recent Cochrane review (Cheuk et al 2007) evaluated the effects of acupuncture on insomnia and concluded that based on individual trials, acupuncture and acupressure may help to improve sleep quality scores when compared to placebo, but that current evidence is not sufficient or extensive enough to support its use. From this study, the commonly used acupuncture points for insomnia were H7 (5 studies), ear Shenmen (3 studies), GV20 (3 studies), and PC6 (3 studies). Looking at another review article PC7, Triple Heater 5 (TH5), Shenmen auricular point, LI20, Kidney 17 (KID17), and extra Huatuojiaji points were also used widely to treat insomnia (Sok et al 2003).

(Continued)

Case Study 2 (Continued)

A study by Spence et al (2004) looked at the effects of acupuncture in 18 subsyndromal anxious adult subjects. The study's limitations were a small sample size, the absence of a control group, and inadequate description of the acupuncture given. It was only stated that a traditional Chinese method of acupuncture was used and that the session lasted for an hour; it did not state the length of time the needles were in or whether they were stimulated. The trial did, however, use a range of valid outcome measures. The study found that 10 sessions of acupuncture treatment over 5 weeks was associated with a significant increase in endogenous melatonin secretion (measured in urine samples), polysomnographic measures of sleep onset latency, arousal index, total sleep time, sleep efficiency, and a reduction in anxiety scores.

A recent systematic review (Pilkington et al 2007) examined the research on acupuncture for anxiety disorders. It concluded that positive findings are reported, but there is insufficient evidence for firm conclusions to be drawn. Their search identified four randomized control trials (RCTs) and two non-RCTs in patients with generalized anxiety disorder; the other trials included in the study were related to situational anxiety. Only one of the RCTs was well designed, but had a small sample size. It compared acupuncture at GV20, HT7, PC6, BL62, and Sishencong or EX HN1 to sham acupuncture in patients with generalized anxiety disorder or minor depression. They found significant improvements in clinical global impression in the acupuncture group after 10 sessions, but notably not after five (Eich et al 2000).

Limitations and recommendations

This study has limited application, as it is a single case study design. To improve treatment outcomes, local points such as BL13, or the Huatuojiaji points in the upper thoracic spine could have been used; however, the patient declined in this case. To affect the myofascial

element of pain, GB21 could have been used, as it is located in the trapezius muscle.

From the research, GV20 or auricular points could be included for both insomnia and anxiety symptoms, or BL62 or EX HN1 for anxiety. Acupuncture would be increased to 10 sessions, if funding permitted, as this is the number of treatments required to achieve a significant difference in outcomes. Among the trials reviewed it was noted that insufficient or inappropriate outcome measures were used to measure the effect of acupuncture treatment. To measure the effect of treatment in this study a validated anxiety scale and a validated sleep scale were needed. Thoracic spine ROM should be measured at every session to measure the treatment effect over time.

Conclusion

This case study has endeavoured to present the clinical reasoning behind an integrated acupuncture treatment approach, to explore the mechanisms surrounding the effects of this treatment, and to evaluate and discuss the relevant research related to that treatment. In this case study the combination of acupuncture with exercise, postural correction, and manual therapy was beneficial in improving posture and muscle control around the shoulder girdle and improving function (sitting), reducing pain VAS scores, and subjectively improving sleep quality and duration. The evidence for the pain-relieving mechanisms of acupuncture is strong, but trials which show its effectiveness for treating specific types or areas of pain are poor in quality, but do show moderate effectiveness in neck disorders. Evidence to support the use of acupuncture to treat symptoms of anxiety or insomnia is poor; there is some evidence that acupuncture causes a significant increase in endogenous melatonin secretion and this case study does support this by showing an improvement in sleep quality and duration. There is a need for good quality research within all the areas of acupuncture that this study reviewed.

References

Accarino, A., Azpiroz, F., Malagelda, J., et al., 1995. Selective dysfunction of mechanosensitive intestinal afferents in the irritable bowel syndrome. Gastroenterology 108 (636), 643.

Atchinson, J., 2000. Manipulation efficacy: upper body. J. Back Musculoskeletal Rehabil. 15, 3–15.

Baldry, P., 2002. Superficial versus deep dry needling. Acupunct. Med. 20 (2–3), 78–81.

Baron, R., Levine, J., Fields, H., 1999. Causalgia and reflex sympathetic dystrophy: does the sympathetic nervous system contribute to the generation of pain? Muscle Nerve 22, 678–695.

Bereznick, D., Ross, K., McGill, S., 2002. The frictional properties at the thoracic skin-fascia interface; implications in spinal manipulation. Clin. Biomech. 17 (4), 297–303.

Berkoff, G., 2005. Upper back pain. In: Whyte-Ferguson, L., Gerwin, R. (Eds.) The Clinical Mastery in the Treatment of Myofascial Pain. Lippincott Williams and Wilkins, Philadelphia, pp. 187–211.

Bogduk, N., 1986. Research design or what is T4 syndrome? Define exactly what the phenomenon of interest is. NZ J. Physiother. 14 (3), 9–11.

Bogduk, N., 2002. Innervation and pain patterns of the thoracic spine. In: Grant, R. (Ed.), Physical Therapy in the Cervical and Thoracic Spines, third ed. Churchill Livingstone, Edinburgh.

Bradnam, L., 2007. A proposed clinical reasoning model for Western acupuncture. J. Acupunct. Assoc. Chart. Physiotherap. (Jan.), 21–30.

Cabyoglu, M.T., Ergene, N., Tan, U., 2006. The mechanism of acupuncture and clinical applications. Int. J. Neurosci. 116 (2), 115–125.

Capodice, J., Jin, Z., Bemis, D.L., et al., 2007. A pilot study for acupuncture for lower urinary tract symptoms related to chronic prostatitis/chronic pelvic pain. Chin. Med. 2, 1.

Chaitow, L., Wilson, E., Morrisey, D., 2002. Positional Release Techniques. Elsevier Science, London.

Chambers, J., Bass, C., Mayou, R., 1999. Non-cardiac chest pain: assessment and management. Heart 82, 656–657.

Chen, H., Chen, Y., Shi, C., et al., 2007. Auricular acupuncture treatment for insomnia: a systematic review. J. Altern. Complement. Med. 13, 669–676.

Chen, X.H., Han, J.S., 1992. All 3 typical types of opiod receptors in the spinal cord are important for 2/15 Hz electroacupuncture analgesia. Eur. J. Clin. Pharmacol. 211 (2), 203–210.

Cheng, R.S.S., Pomeranz, B., 1980. Electroacupuncture analgesia is mediated by sterospecific opiate receptors and is reversed by antagonists of type I receptors. Life Sc. 26, 631–638.

Cheuk, D.K.L., Yeung, W.F., Chung, K.F., et al., 2007. Acupuncture for insomnia. Cochrane Database Syst. Rev. 3, CD005472.

Chu, J., Schwartz, I., 2002. The muscle twitch in myofascial pain relief: effects of acupuncture and other needling methods. Electroencephalogr. Clin. Neurophysiol. 42 (5), 307–311.

Chu, J., Zhonghua, Y.X.Z.Z., 2002. The local mechanisms of acupuncture. Chin. Med. J. 65 (7), 299–302.

Cloward, R.B., 1959. Cervical discography. A contribution to the aetiology and mechanism of neck, shoulder and arm pain. Annuals Surg. 150, 1052–1064.

Comerford, M., Mottram, S., 2001. Functional stability re-training: principles and strategies for managing mechanical dysfunction. Man. Ther. 6 (1), 3–14.

Conroy, J., Schneiders, A., 2005. The T4 syndrome. Man. Ther. 10 (4), 292–296.

Craven, J., 2008. The autonomic nervous system, sympathetic chain and stellate ganglion. Anaesth. Intensive Care Med. 9 (2), 39–41.

CSAG, , 1994. Report of Clinical Standards Advisory Group committee on back pain. HMSO, London.

DeFranca, C., Levine, L., 1995. The T4 syndrome. J. Manipulative. Physiol. Ther. 18 (1), 34–37.

Deyo, R., Raineville, J., Daniel, K., 1992. What can the history and physical examination tell us about low back pain?. JAMA 268, 760–765.

Dhond, R., Kettner, N., Napadow, V., 2007. Do the neural correlates of acupuncture and placebo effects differ?. Pain 128 (1–2), 8–12.

Drewes, A.M., Jennum, P., 1995. Epidemiology of myofascial pain, low back pain, morning stiffness and sleep related complaints in the general population. J. Musculoskelet. Pain 3 (Supp 1), 68.

Dreyfuss, P., Tibiletti, C., Dreyer, S., 1994. Thoracic zygaphophyseal joint pain patterns: a study in normal volunteers. Spine 19 (7), 807–811.

Drummond, P.D., Finch, P.M., Smythe, G.A., 1991. Reflex sympathetic dystrophy: the significance of differing plasma catecholamine concentrations in affected and unaffected limbs. Brain 1 (114), 2025–2036.

Edmonson, S., Singer, K., 1997. Thoracic spine: anatomical and biomechanical considerations for manual therapy. Man. Ther. 2 (3), 132–143.

Edwards, J., Knowles, N., 2003. Superficial dry needling and active stretching in the treatment of myofascial pain-a randomised control trial. Acupunct. Med. 21 (3), 80–83.

Eich, H., Agelink, M.W., Lehmann, E., et al., 2000. [Acupuncture in patients with minor depression or generalised anxiety disorders—results of an experimental study.]. Fortschritte der Neurologie-Psychiatrie 68 (3), 137–144 [In German.].

Eslick, G., Jones, M., Talley, N., 2001. Acute chest pain and health care seeking behaviour; role of reflux symptomology. J. Gastroenterol. Hepatol. 16, A106.

Evans, R., 1994. Illustrated Essentials in Orthopaedic Physical Assessment. Mosby, St Louis.

Evans, P., 1997. T4 syndrome: some basic science. Physiotherapy 83 (4), 186–189.

Fernández de las Peñas, C., Fernández Carnero, J., Plaza Fernández, A., et al., 2004. Dorsal manipulation in whiplash injury treatment: a randomised controlled trial. J. Whiplash Relat. Disord. 3 (2), 55–72.

Fink, M., Wolkenstein, E., Luennemann, M., 2002. Chronic epicondylitis: effects of real and sham acupuncture treatment: a random controlled patient and examiner blind long-term trial. Forschende Komplementärmendizin und Klassische Naturheilkunde 9 (4), 210–215.

Fisher, E., 1988. Opioid peptides modulate immune function: a review. Immunopharmacology 10, 265–326.

Forst, R., Ingenhorst, A., 2005. Myofascial pain syndrome. Internist 46 (11), 1207–1217.

Friedman, M., Bowden, V., Jones, E., 2003. Family Nursing: Research, Theory and Practice, fifth ed. Prentice Hall, Upper Saddle River, NJ.

Furlan, R., Furlan, S., Colombo, F., et al., 2005. Abnormalities of cardiovascular neural control and reduced orthostatic tolerance in patients with primary fibromyalgia. J. Rheumatol. 32, 1787–1793.

Gao, X., Zhang, S., Zhu, B., et al., 2008. Investigation of specificity of auricular acupuncture in regulation of autonomic function in anaesthetised rats. Auton. Neurosci. 138 (1–2), 50–56.

Geertzen, J.H., de Bruijn-Kofman, A.T., de Bruijn, H.P., et al., 1998. Stressful life events and psychological dysfunction in Complex Regional Pain Syndrome type I. Clin. J. Pain. 14 (2), 143–147.

Giamberardino, M., 2000. Sex-related and hormonal modulation of visceral pain. In: Fillingim, R. (Ed.), Sex, Gender and Pain. International Association for the Study of Pain (IASP), Seattle.

Grieve, G., 1988. Common Vertebral Joint Problems, second ed. Churchill Livingstone, Edinburgh.

Grieve, G., 1994. Grieve's Modern Manual Therapy, second ed. Churchill Livingstone, Edinburgh.

Haas, M., Panzer, D., Peterson, D., et al., 1995. Short term responsiveness on manual thoracic end-play assessment to spinal manipulation; a randomised controlled trial of construct validity. J. Manipulative Physiol. Ther. 18 (9), 582–589.

Hannington-Kiff, J.G., 1991. Does failed natural opioid modulation in regional sympathetic ganglia cause reflex sympathetic dystrophy?. Lancet 338, 1125–1127.

Hansson, Y., Carlsson, C., Olsson, E., 2007. Intramuscular and periosteal acupuncture for anxiety and sleep quality in patients with chronic musculoskeletal pain-an evaluator blind, controlled study. Acupunct. Med. 25 (4), 148–157.

Heitkemper, M., Jarrett, M., 2001. Gender differences and hormonal modulation in visceral pain. Curr. Pain Headache Rep. 5, 35–43.

Hertzog, W., Conway, P., Kawchuk, Y., et al., 1993. Forces exerted during spinal manipulative therapy. Spine 18, 1206–1212.

Holstege, G., Bandler, R., Saper, C., 1996. The Emotional Motor System. Elsevier Science, Amsterdam.

Hong, C., Simonds, D., 1993. Response to treatment for pectoralis minor. Myofascial Pain Syndrome after whiplash. J. Musculoskelet. Pain 1 (1), 89–131.

Hong, C.Z., Simons, D.G., 1998. Pathophysiological and electrophysiological mechanisms of myofascial trigger points. Arch. Phys. Med. Rehabil. 79 (7), 863–872.

Hoppenfield, S., 1977. Orthopaedic Neurology: A Diagnostic Guide to Neurological Levels. JB Lippincott, Philadelphia.

Huang, H., Laing, S., 1992. Acupuncture at otoacupoint heart treatment for vascular hypertension. J. Tradit. Chin. Med. 12, 133–136.

Hubbard, D.R., Berkoff, G.M., 1993. Myofascial trigger points show spontaneous needle EMG activity. Spine 18, 1803–1807.

Hui, K.K.K., Lui, J., Makris, N., et al., 2000. Acupuncture modulates the limbic system and subcortical gray structures of the human brain: evidence from fMRI studies in normal subjects. Hum. Brain Mapp. 9 (1), 13–25.

Hurley, D., McDonough, S., Baxter, G., et al., 2005. A descriptive study of the usage of spinal manipulative therapy techniques within a randomised clinical trial in acute low back pain. Man. Ther. 10, 61–67.

Janda, V., 1986. Muscle weakness and inhibition (pseudoparesis) in back pain syndromes. In: Grieve, G. (Ed.), Modern Manual Therapy of the Vertebral Column. Churchill Livingstone, Edinburgh.

Jang, I., Cho, K., Moon, S., et al., 2003. A study on the central neural pathway of the heart, Nei-Kuan (EH-6) and Shen-Men (He-7) with neural tracer in rats. Am. J. Chin. Med. 31 (4), 591–609.

Jeong, H., Hong, S., Nam, Y., et al., 2003. The effect of acupuncture on proinflammatory cytokine production in patients with chronic headache: a preliminary report. Am. J. Chin. Med. 31 (6), 945–954.

Jong, M., Hwang, S., Chen, F., 2006. Effects of electro-acupuncture on serum cytokine level and peripheral blood lymphocyte subpopulation at immune-related and non-immune-related points. Acupunct. Electrother. Res. 31 (1–2), 45–59.

Kandel, E., Schwartz, J., Jessell, T., 1995. Essentials of Neural Science and Behaviour. McGraw-Hill, New York.

Kavoussi, B., Evan-Ross, B., 2007. The neuroimmune basis of anti-inflammatory acupuncture. Integr. Cancer Ther. 6, 251–257.

Keating, L., Lubke, V., Powell, T., et al., 2001. Mid thoracic tenderness: a comparison of pressure pain threshold between spinal regions, in asymptomatic subjects. Man. Ther. 6 (1), 34–39.

Kim, C., Kim, K., 2003. Clinical observations on postoperative vomiting treated by auricular acupuncture. Am. J. Chin. Med. 31, 475–480.

Krassioukov, A.V., Weaver, L.C., 1996. Anatomy of the autonomic nervous system. Phys. Med. Rehabil. 10 (1), 1–14.

Kraus, T., Kraus, K., Hosl, O., et al., 2007. BOLD fMRI deactivation of limbic and temporal brain structures and mood enhancing effect by transcutaneous vagal nerve stimulation. J. Neural Transm. 114 (11), 1485–1493.

Lee, D., 2003. The Thorax: An Integrated Approach. D Lee Physiotherapist Corporation, Surrey, Canada.

Leriche, R., 1916. De la causalgia envisage comme une nevrite due sympathique et de son traitment par la denudation et l'excision des plexus nerveux peri-arteriels. Presse Med. 24, 178–180.

Liu, J., Chen, S., Cao, Q., et al., 1996. Influence of neuronal excitation and inhibition of rostral ventrolateral medulla on the effect of electroacupuncture of Nei-Kuan acupoint. Zhen Ci Yan Jui 21, 34–38.

Lombardo, N., Dresser, M., Malivert, M., et al., 2001. Acupuncture as treatment for anxiety and depression in persons with dementia; results of a feasibility and effectiveness study. Alzheimer's Care Q. 2 (4), 28–41.

Longbottom, J., 2006. Not so simple pain: the complexity of chronic pain management. J. Acupunct. Assoc. Chart. Physiotherap. 2, 16–24.

Lu, X., Hikosaka, O., Miyachi, S., 1998. Role of monkey cerebella nuclei in skill for sequential movement. J. Neurophysiol. 79 (5), 2245–2254.

Lundeberg, T., Lund, I., Naslund, J., 2007. Acupuncture-self appraisal and the reward system. Acupunct. Med. 25 (3), 87–99.

Maitland, G., 1986. Vertebral Manipulation, fifth ed. Butterworth Heinemann, Oxford.

Makofsky, H., 2003. Position-assisted combination technique (PACT) in the management of type II impairment in the thoracic and lumbar spine. J. Man. Manip. Ther. 11 (4), 213–222.

Mayer, D.J., Price, D.D., Raffi, A., 1977. Antagonism of acupuncture analgesia in man by the narcotic antagonist naloxone. Brain Res. 121, 368–372.

McCaig, L., Nawar, E., 2004. National hospital ambulatory medical care survey.

Means-Christensen, A.J., Roy-Byrne, P. P., Sherbourne, C.D., et al., 2008. Relationships among pain, anxiety, and depression in primary care. Depress. Anxiety 25 (7), 593–600.

Melzack, R., Stillwell, D.M., Fox, E.J., 1977. Trigger points and acupuncture points for pain: correlations and implications. Pain 3, 3–23.

Mootz, R., Talmage, D., 1999. Clinical assessment strategies for the thoracic area. Top. Clin. Chiropr. 6 (3), 1–19.

Mottram, S., 1997. Dynamic stability of the scapula. Man. Ther. 2 (3), 123–131.

Muir, J.M., Vernon, H., 2000. Review of the literature. Complex regional pain syndrome and chiropractic. J. Manipulative Physiol. Ther. 23 (7), 490–497.

Mulligan, B., 1995. Manual Therapy NAGS, SNAGS, MWM's, third ed. Plane View Services, Wellington.

Muneshige, H., Toda, K., Kimura, H., et al., 2003. Does a viral infection cause complex regional pain syndrome. Electrother. Res. 28 (3), 183–192.

Nishijo, K., Nishijo, H., Mor, H., et al., 1997. Decreased heart rate by acupuncture stimulation in humans via facilitation of cardiac vagal activity and suppression of cardiac sympathetic nerve. Neurosci. Lett. 227, 165–168.

Panjabi, M., Nibu, K., Cholewicki, J., 1998. Whiplash injuries and the potential for mechanical instability. Eur. Spine J. 7, 484–492.

Panju, A., Farkouth, M., Sackett, D., et al., 1996. Outcome of coronary care unit with a diagnosis of chest pain not yet diagnosed. Can. Med. Assoc. 155, 541–546.

Pariente, J., White, P., Frackowiak, R., et al., 2005. Expectancy and belief modulate the neuronal substrates of pain treated by acupuncture. Neuroimage 25 (4), 1161–1167.

Passatore, M., Roatta, S., 2006. Influence of sympathetic nervous system on sensorimotor function: whiplash associated disorders (WAD) as a model. Eur. J. Appl. Physiol. 98, 423–449.

Pert, C., 1997. Molecules of Emotion. Simon and Schuster, Sydney.

Petruzzello, S.J., Landers, D.M., Hatfield, B.D., et al., 1991. A meta-analysis on the anxiety-reducing effects of acute and chronic exercise. Outcomes and mechanisms. Sports Med. 11 (3), 143–182.

Peuker, E., Filler, T., 2002. The nerve supply of the human auricle. Clin. Anat. 15, 35–37.

Pilkington, K., Kirkwood, G., Rampes, H., et al., 2007. Acupuncture for anxiety and anxiety disorders—a systematic literature review. Acupunct. Med. 25 (1–2), 1–10.

Pomeranz, B., Chui, D., 1976. Naloxone blocks acupuncture analgesia and causes hyperalgesia: endorphin is implicated. Life Sci. 19, 1757–1762.

Proctor, D., Dupius, P., Cassidy, J., 1985. Thoracolumbar syndrome as a cause of back pain: a report of two cases. Can. Chiropr. Assoc. 29 (2), 71–73.

Sapolsky, R., 1992. Stress, the Aging Brain and the Mechanisms of Neuron Death. MIT Press, Cambridge, MA.

Seem, M., 2000. Acupuncture Physical Medicine, fifth ed. Blue Poppy Press, Boulder, CO.

Shaclock, M., 1999. Central pain mechanisms: a new horizon in manual therapy. Aust. J. Physiother. 45, 83–92.

Shah, P., 2008. Uncovering the biochemical milieu of myofascial trigger points using in vivo microdialysis. International MYOPAIN Society. J. Musculoskelet. Pain 16 (1–2), 17–20.

Sheikh, H., Samartzis, D., Perez-Cruet, M., 2008. Techniques for the operative management of thoracic disc herniation: minimally invasive thoracic microdiscectomy. Orthop. Clin. N. Am. 38 (3), 351–361.

Sher, L., 1998. The role of the endogenous opioid system in the pathogenesis of anxiety disorders. Med. Hypotheses 50 (6), 473–474.

Snodgrass, S., Rivett, D., Robertson, V., 2006. Manual forces applied during posterior-to-anterior spinal mobilization: a review of the evidence. J. Manip. Physiol. Ther. 29, 316–329.

Sobel, R.M., Markov, D., 2005. The impact of anxiety and mood disorders on physical disease: the worried not-so-well. Curr. Psychiatry. Rep. 7 (3), 206–212.

Sok, S.R., Erlen, J.A., Kim, K.B., 2003. Effects of acupuncture therapy on insomnia. J. Adv. Nurs. 44 (4), 375–384.

Spanos, T., 2005. Interscapular pain: a myofascial composite syndrome. In: Whyte-Ferguson, L., Gerwin, R. (Eds.) Clinical Mastery in the Treatment of Myofascial Pain, first ed. Lippincott, Williams & Wilkins, Philadelphia, pp. 213–226.

Spence, D.W., Kayumov, L., Chen, A., et al., 2004. Acupuncture increases nocturnal melatonin secretion and reduces insomnia and anxiety: a preliminary report. J. Neuropsychiatry Clin. Neurosci. 16 (1), 19–28.

Sterling, M., Jull, G., Wright, A., 2001. Cervical mobilisation: concurrent effects on pain, sympathetic nervous system activity and motor activity. Man. Ther. 6 (2), 72–81.

Stochkendahl, M., Christensen, H., Hartvigsen, J., et al., 2006. Manual examination: critical literature review of reproducibility. J. Manip. Physiol. Ther. 29, 475–485.

Takahashi, T., 2006. Acupuncture for functional gastrointestinal disorders. J. Gastroenterol. 41, 408–417.

Tattersal, J., Cervero, F., Lumb, B., 2008. Effects of reversible spinalisation on the visceral input to viscerosomatic neurons in the lower thoracic spinal cord of the cat. J. Neurophysiol. 56, 785–796.

Thomas, K.P., MacPherson, H., Ratcliff, J., et al., 2005. Long-term clinical and economic benefits of offering acupuncture care to patients with chronic low back pain. Health Technol. Assess. 9 (32), 1–109.

Tracey, K., 2005. Fat meets the cholinergic anti-inflammatory pathway. J. Explor. Med. 202 (8), 1017–1021.

Tracey, K., 2007. Physiology and immunology of the cholinergic anti-inflammatory pathway. J. Clin. Invest. 117 (2), 289–296.

Trinh, K., Graham, N., Gross, A., et al., 2006. Cervical overview group. Acupuncture for neck disorders. Cochrane Database Syst. Rev. 3, CD004870.

Unchald, P., 2008. Traditional Chinese medicine: some historical and epistemological reflections. Soc. Sci. Med. 24, 1023–1029.

Usichenko, M., Dinse, M., Mermsen, T., et al., 2005a. Auricular acupuncture for pain relief Latter total hip arthroplasty-a randomized controlled trial. Pain 114, 320–327.

Usichenko, M., Hermsen, T., Witsstruck, A., et al., 2005b. Auricular acupuncture for pain relief after ambulatory knee arthroscopy; a pilot study. Evid. Based Complement. Alternat. Med. 2, 185–189.

Uvnas-Moberg, K., Bruzelius, G., Alster, P., et al., 1993. The antinociceptive effect of non-noxious sensory stimulation is mediated partly through oxytocinergic mechanisms. Acta Physiol. Scandinavica 149, 199–204.

Veale, D., Kavanagh, G., Fielding, J., et al., 1991. Primary fibromyalgia and the irritable bowel syndrome: different expressions of a common pathogenic process. Br. J. Rheumatol. 30, 220–222.

Vleeming, A., Pool-Goudzwaard, A., Stoeckart, R., et al., 1995. The posterior layer of the thoracolumbar fascia: its function in load transfer from spine to legs. Spine 20, 753.

Von Korff, M., Simon, G., 1996. The relationship between pain and depression. Br. J. Psychiatry Suppl. 30, 101–108.

Walling, A., 2006. Therapeutic modulation of the psychoneuroimmunesystem by medical acupuncture creates feelings of enhanced well-being. J. Am. Acad. Nurse Pract. 18, 135–143.

White, A., 1969. An analysis of the mechanics of the thoracic spine in man. Acta. Orthop. Scand. Suppl. 127, 8–92.

Whyte-Ferguson, L., Gerwin, R., 2005. Hip and groin pain: the disordered hip complex. In: Whyte-Ferguson, L., Gerwin, R. (Eds.) Clinical Mastery of Myofascial Pain. Lippincott Williams and Wilkins, Philadelphia, pp. 271–301.

Wickes, D., 1980. Effects of thoracolumbar manipulation on arterial flow to the lower extremity. J. Manip. Physiol. Ther. 3 (1), 3–7.

Yoganandan, N., Pintar, F., Cusick, J., 2002. Biomechanical analysis of whiplash injuries using an experimental model. Accid. Anal. Prev. 34, 663–671.

Zighelboim, J., Talley, N., Phillips, S., et al., 1995. Visceral perception in irritable bowel syndrome. Dig. Discuss. Sci. 40, 819–825.

The lumbar spine

7

Claire Small

Introduction

The assessment and management of low back pain (LBP) has been shown to be a frustrating and costly challenge for both clinicians and the patients whom they treat (Waddell 1998). Despite the publication of large volumes of research on the subject, evidence regarding the most effective management strategies is limited and often contradictory.

Borkan et al (1998) determined that the greatest difficulties in research into LBP are associated with the individual nature of a patient's presentation. Upon identifying the importance of this individuality, these authors called for future investigations to focus on the subclassification of patients to facilitate the identification of effective management strategies. Consistent with this is the fact that many randomized controlled trials (RCTs), systematic reviews, and the more recent meta-analyses, which do not account for patient-specific presentation, fail to identify effective treatment modalities, since the heterogeneous groupings of patients create a wash out effect in which findings that may have been relevant to a subgroup of patients are not identified.

In the absence of any demonstrable pathology, there has been a growing trend to avoid a specific, patient-centred approach to management and focus instead on a general approach to management, as recommended in the European Guidelines for the management of back pain (Airaksinen et al 2006; Van Tulder et al 2006). The US Joint Clinical Practice Guidelines (Chou et al 2007) identify seven recommendations and categories of LBP that adhere strongly to the European Guidelines.

Recent publications have demonstrated that subclassification leads to both identification of specific dysfunction in certain patient populations (Dankaerts et al 2006) and that treatment based on a classification system improves outcomes (Brennan et al 2006; Cleland et al 2006). Because no one classification system has been shown to encompass all patient presentations, authors have suggested that combinations of systems with weightings on the importance of characteristics between domains for each individual are required (McCarthy et al 2004). This approach reflects the clinical reasoning to assessment and management advocated by many authors (Jones & Rivett 2004), in which consideration is given to determining the presence of any pathoanatomical source of symptoms, the pain mechanisms involved in symptom manifestation, the nature of any movement dysfunction or impairment, and the influence of psychosocial factors. In considering the role of Manual Therapy (MT) in the management of individuals with low back pain, it should be recognized that the manual therapist of today is a different creature to that of 5 to 10 years ago. Manual Therapy now extends beyond the traditional definition, which included manual techniques such as joint mobilization and manipulation to encompass specific exercise therapy, as reflected in the International Federation of Orthopaedic Manual Therapists (IFOMT) definition of Orthopaedic Manual Therapy (www.ifomt.org). Much of this shift in focus occurred following publication of research that identified the role that altered motor control played in the manifestation of many musculoskeletal problems. In a general sense the focus of Manual Therapy is on the treatment of movement dysfunction. In addition to dealing with specific pathoanatomical diagnoses and addressing any relevant psychosocial component to the patient's presentation, the modern manual therapists needs to direct treatment towards four elements when addressing the movement dysfunction present:

- Manual therapy to relieve pain;
- Manual therapy to improve joint movement;
- Manual therapy to normalize muscle function; and
- Exercise therapy and motor retraining.

Manual therapy for the relief of pain

Pain is not just a psychological disincentive to move normally. Several recent studies utilizing an experimental pain model have shown changes in motor control and muscle function in both the deep, local system, i.e. the transversus abdominus and multifidus muscles (Hides et al 1994; Hodges & Richardson 1996; Hodges 2001; Hodges et al 2003), and the more superficial trunk muscles, i.e. erector spinae (Gregory et al 2007; Indahl et al 1997), which are usually more associated with phasic activity and movement. It has been proposed that motor control changes result in tissue damage and pain (Sahrmann 1998) through poor movement patterns that place pathological levels of stress on joints and soft tissue. With the recognition that pain can cause

subtle but significant alterations in motor function, the potential for a vicious cycle is evident (Moseley & Hodges 2005; Panjabi 1992). Thus, therapists must aim to use all techniques at their disposal to modulate pain mechanisms, including mobilisation, manipulation, massage and acupuncture. The use of traditional Manual Therapy techniques, such as joint mobilization, as methods for relieving pain has long underpinned physiotherapy practice, but it is only in recent years that the neurophysiological effects of Manual Therapy have been investigated. Studies by Sterling et al (2001), Skyba et al (2003), Sluka et al (2006), and Moss et al (2007) have all shown a reduction in hyperalgesia in response to treatment with joint mobilization. Clinically, this rationale is supported by several studies that demonstrate the effect of traditional Manual Therapy as a mechanism of pain relief for patients suffering both acute and chronic LBP (Ferreira et al 2007; Koes et al 2006; van Tulder et al 1997).

Abolishing pain will not necessarily restore correct motor function but it may facilitate rehabilitation aimed at the restoration of normal movement patterns. Hides et al (1996) showed that the resolution of LBP did not correspond with a restoration of normal muscle size in all cases of patients presenting with acute first episode LBP, despite a return to normal function. This alteration in muscle size remained present in some cases at 3-year follow-up, and in many cases it was associated with recurrences of LBP (Hides et al 2001). Likewise, Moseley and Hodges (2000) showed altered motor activity in the presence of experimentally induced LBP that did not resolve spontaneously with the resolution of symptoms in all cases. Other studies showed that subjects who lacked this spontaneous return normal motor control were also more likely to have higher fear/avoidance scores on questionnaires that examined beliefs about pain behaviour. The conclusion of these findings is that long-lasting resolution of pain and restoration of function requires normalization of joint function and muscle behaviour.

Manual therapy to improve joint movement

The role of altered joint mobility in the presence of LBP has long been recognized (Twomey & Taylor 2005). Altered mobility can be characterized as general (i.e. mobility of the trunk as a whole) or segmental (i.e. between two consecutive vertebra). The two most commonly used methods to restore segmental joint mobility to the spinal regions are manipulative thrust and mobilization techniques. Two of the more common mobilization techniques include passive accessory intervertebral movements (PAIVM's) and passive physiological intervertebral movements (PPIVM's) as described by Maitland et al (2006).

Studies over several years have questioned the reliability of manual segmental mobilization in both the examination (Seffinger et al 2004) and treatment (Bronfort et al 2004) of patients with spinal pain. In addition, it has been concluded by several authors that manual mobilization is only accurate and reproducible in the presence of pain, and that examination or treatment of altered joint range of motion is flawed (Bogduk 2004).

Recent studies have shown that therapists can reliably detect altered joint stiffness in the absence of pain (Fritz et al 2005; Stochkendahl et al 2006), and that treatment directed at joint restriction/hypomobility can result in improved clinical outcomes (UK BEAM Trial Team 2004). The evidence is strengthened by the use of a subclassification system in which manipulation and mobilization techniques are used only in the management of patients who demonstrate signs and symptoms in their history and physical examination that will respond favourably to this form of treatment, so-called clinical prediction rules (Childs et al 2004; Flynn et al 2002). These criteria included back pain of less than 16 days duration, no symptoms distal to the knee, low fear-avoidance beliefs regarding movement and activity, identification of at least one hypomobile segment of the lumbar spine with posterior–anterior mobilization, and hip internal rotation greater than 35°.

Joint hypomobility is one element of the musculoskeletal system that may be contributing to altered movement within a movement dysfunction paradigm. When managing spinal conditions, it is essential that therapists examine the adjacent joints of the hip, pelvis, and thoracic regions for restrictions of movement. Subgrouping using a movement impairment classification has identified changes in hip function (Van Dillen et al 2007) and pelvic function (Vleeming et al 2008) in certain groups of patients with low back pain. Restoring joint hypomobility in these regions may be important in restoring correct patterns of motion and permitting pain-free function for these individuals.

Manual therapy to normalize muscle activity

In the case of spinal movement dysfunction, evidence of altered motor control abounds in the literature (Hodges & Moseley 2003; Van Dieen et al 2003). Much of the well-publicized literature shows evidence of altered control of the small, deep muscles of the spinal region that have been shown to control shear forces and intra-abdominal pressure during movement (Hides et al 1994; Hodges & Richardson 1996; Pool-Goudzwaard et al 2005; Smith et al 2006). Nevertheless, despite a great deal of research illustrating deficits in this deep, local system in the presence of both actual and experimental pain, there has been no conclusive evidence that treatment regimes aimed at addressing these deficits have a significant effect on LBP or result in improved function.

Critics of spinal stabilizing exercises argue that this lack of evidence suggests that the presence of these motor control deficits are overemphasized in the management of spinal dysfunction and that psychosocial factors are of greater importance. Many of these researchers advocate treatment utilizing pain education and cognitive behavioural therapy in patient management with what has become known as a hands-off approach (Frost et al 2004; Hay et al 2005; Watson 2007). Together, this hands-off approach and the growth of the core stability concept have seen a reduction in the use of traditional Manual Therapy techniques by clinicians. An overemphasis on spinal stability has led to therapists treating all patients suffering from chronic LBP with stabilization exercises and pain education, while failing to recognize the more complex nature of the motor control dysfunctions that exist in patients with LBP (O'Sullivan 2005).

It would seem that motor control training has suffered the same fate as physical interventions in general, in that much of the evidence has failed to account for patient-specific presentations, and instead, investigates the effect of a particular exercise programme on heterogeneous groupings of patients. The use of patient subclassification has begun to highlight altered muscle activity that may previously have been obscured within the data, in which patients who demonstrated a reduction in activity of certain muscles negated the presence of overactivity in other subjects (Dankaerts et al 2006; Hodges et al 2007). Specifically, subgrouping has shown that, in addition to a deficit in the function of the deep, local muscles, subjects with LBP often demonstrate elements of muscular overactivity. The presentation of this muscle overactivity is more variable than the timing delay consistently reported in the transversus abdominis, multifidus, diaphragm, and the pelvic floor muscles. Studies have demonstrated changes in the activity of the erector spinae in specific groups of patients with LBP (Geisser et al 2005; Gregory et al 2007). Similar findings are seen with respect to the flexion relaxation response of the low back muscles, and the hamstrings (Leinonen et al 2000), quadratus lumborum, external oblique, rectus abdominis (Silfies et al 2005), and gluteus medius (Nelson-Wong et al 2008).

A recent study by Hodges et al (2007) highlighted the potential problem of an excessive focus on the timing delay often present in the deep local muscle system. In a group of patients with experimentally induced pain, a net increase in trunk muscle activity was evident, suggesting a need to reduce the activation of some muscles. Together with the work of Reeves et al (2007), the above study suggests that interventions should be aimed at optimizing rather than increasing stability using a combination of both increasing and reducing muscle activation to restore a normal motor control pattern.

The potential for overactivity of these muscles to be a source of pain has been well documented by JG Travell and DG Simons in their work detailing the trigger point (TrPt) referral patterns of various muscles. A myofascial trigger point (MTrPt) is a hyperirritable spot, usually within a taut band of skeletal muscle, that is painful on compression and can give rise to characteristic referred pain, motor dysfunction, and autonomic phenomena (Simons et al 1998). It has been postulated that altered or increased muscle activity may result in pain in the low back and pelvic region because of the development of both active and latent trigger points. Likewise, the presence of definitive lumbopelvic pathology, such as a lumbar disc irritation or hip joint irritation may result in muscular referred pain not specifically related to the initial pathology (Indahl et al 1997).

Support exists for an association between the use of spinal mobilization, manipulation, and improved muscle function (Lehman et al 2001; Sterling et al 2001). Although the exact mechanism is not fully understood, several researchers have demonstrated altered reflex activity following spinal manipulation (Herzog et al 1999; Katavich 1998; Murphy et al 1995). In a review of the neurophysiological effects of spinal manipulation, Pickar (2002) concluded that manipulation evokes paraspinal muscle reflexes and alters motorneuron excitability, but that the effects of spinal manipulation on these somato-somatic reflexes may be quite complex, producing excitatory and inhibitory effects. Studies by Lehman et al (2001) and Lehman and McGill (2001) have shown a reduction in exaggerated muscle activity in the trunk muscles of subjects with LBP in response to manipulation. These studies would suggest that traditional Manual Therapy is capable of both reducing the trunk muscle activity seen in patients with LBP and reducing the pain and overactivity seen in the presence of TrPts.

Other non-invasive methods of treating TrPts that have traditionally been utilized by manual therapists include stretching (Huguenin 2004) and active release techniques (Lee 2004). In recent years, there has been a marked increase in the use of dry needling to manage TrPts. This technique involves the insertion of an acupuncture needle into the region of the TrPts aiming to reproduce the patient's symptoms and stimulate a local muscle twitch response (Shah et al 2006), and it is becoming a common tool in the repertoire of the modern manual therapist. The treatment of TrPts within a movement dysfunction paradigm would suggest that these areas of overactivity are commonly associated with the presence of altered control elsewhere within the system that must be addressed for optimal stability and control.

Exercise therapy and motor retraining

The past 10 years have seen major changes in our understanding of the role that the muscular system plays in the manifestation of back pain. The clinician is no longer focused solely on muscular strength as a management strategy; instead the focus has shifted towards the control of spinal movement. The role of the muscle system in helping the spine function in an optimal fashion is dependant on its ability to match the timing and pattern of muscle recruitment with the constantly changing demands placed upon the system (Hodges 2000). Well-known studies by several authors have shown alterations in the timing and activation of the deep muscle system, including the transversus abdominis (Hodges & Richardson 1996); multifidus (Moseley et al 2004); diaphragm (Hodges et al 2002); and pelvic floor (Smith et al 2007). It is this work that has received overwhelming attention in modern Manual Therapy and has potentially led to an excessive focus in treatment. Studies by Hides et al (1994) and Tsao and Hodges (2007) have shown that addressing these deficits with very specific motor training is capable of normalizing the motor function of these deep muscles; yet clinical trials examining the benefit of stabilization exercises have failed to show any greater benefit than other treatment, including the use of general exercise (Cairns et al 2006; Hayden et al 2005b).

It would seem logical to imagine that improved motor control and function would result from releasing overactive muscle and reducing tone, in addition to normalizing activity of the transversus abdominis and segmental multifidus where functional deficits are commonly seen. To date, much of the research work looking at the use of motor retraining has focused on activation patterns of the transversus abdominis and multifidus muscles, and has not addressed potential overactivity and the presence of TrPts (Ferreira et al 2007; Koumantakis et al 2005; Standaert et al 2008). It may be because of this lack of attention to muscular overactivity that these studies have failed to show a benefit from retraining, despite overwhelming evidence that dysfunction exists in the local muscle system. Likewise, appropriate use of deep muscle retraining exercises in patients who have been subclassified as having a deficit in this element of their motor control pattern results in better outcomes than a general application to any patient experiencing LBP (Hicks et al 2005).

Conclusion

Current evidence would suggest that the manual therapist has a valuable role to play in managing LBP by addressing movement dysfunction. However, because of the variable nature of patients' presentations, detailed assessment of motor control, muscular overactivity, joint hypomobility, pain response, and psychosocial factors are all essential in order to determine the nature of the underlying condition and establish the most effective treatment approaches.

7.1 Acupuncture in low back pain

Jennie Longbottom

Introduction

The detailed model of clinical reasoning described above outlines a means of achieving effective management of LBP and, acupuncture must follow the same model whether the clinician is:

- Using acupuncture as a precursor to Manual Therapy;
- Integrating acupuncture at the same time as Manual Therapy; or
- Using acupuncture as a pain modulation post-Manual Therapy.

'The important questions are when and how?'

Acute back pain

The mechanisms by which acupuncture reduces pain levels have been thoroughly studied (Bowsher 1998; Carlsson 2002; Clement-Jones et al 1980; Ma 2004; Pomeranz 1996); there are thought to be three mechanisms of pain relief that acupuncture seems to trigger (Lundeberg 1998, cited in Bradnam 2007). Primarily, pain relief is initiated at the periphery by axonal reflexes, dichotomizing nerve fibres, local endorphin release, and the release of neuropeptides (i.e. substance P, bradykinin, prostaglandins, histamine) from afferent nerve endings (Carlsson 2002; Kaptchuk 2002). Here, neuropeptides produce local vasodilation and control local immune response, thereby improving tissue healing. Secondarily, according to pain-gate theory (Wall 1978; Wall et al 1984), acupuncture is thought to reduce pain through the spinal mechanisms, by attenuating the nociceptive input in to the dorsal horn of the spinal cord. Needling also alters the sympathetic outflow (Sato et al 1997, cited in Bradnam 2007) and changes motor output (Yu et al 1995, cited in Bradnam 2007). Spinal effects have the potential to produce strong analgesic effects and may occur immediately (Bradnam 2007; Irnich 2002).

Finally, acupuncture provides pain relief through the activation of pathways from the brain, via diffuse noxious inhibitory controls and descending inhibitory pathways from the hypothalamus to the periaqueductal grey matter (PAG) in the brainstem (Takeshige et al 1992), utilizing neurohormonal responses and central control of the autonomic nervous system (ANS) (Bradnam 2007; Carlsson 2002).

Acupuncture may be used as an anti-inflammatory agent, although the potential anti-inflammatory effects of this treatment remain controversial in clinical trials and the underlying mechanisms are still unclear (Kim et al 2006). Systemic opioids can modulate inflammatory reactions in both the central nervous system (CNS) and at peripheral sites (McDougall et al 2004). McDougall et al (2004) demonstrated that both high-frequency electroacupuncture (HFEA) at 80 to 100 Hz, and low-frequency electroacupuncture (LFEA) at 2 to 4 Hz, applied at acupoint Stomach (ST) 36, significantly reduced peripheral leukocyte migration at the peripheral inflammatory site. Their result is consistent with the theory that specific acupuncture point stimulation as opposed to non-acupuncture stimulation is required to efficiently produce an anti-inflammatory effect (Carneiro et al 2005). Both acupuncture and EA have been shown to enhance opioid release under inflammatory conditions, as compared to the normal state (Ceccherelli et al 1999; Sekido et al 2004), provided de Qi is achieved at the acupoint. Both laboratory and clinical evidence have shown that it is the parasympathetic nervous system that plays the leading role in the downregulation of cytokine synthesis and the containment of somatic inflammation (Kavoussi & Ross 2007).

The vagal nerve outflow innervates the major organs and has been found to play a systemic immunoregulatory and homeostatic role known as the cholinergic anti-inflammatory pathway (Tracey 2002). The parasympathetic origin of the non-specific anti-inflammatory actions of acupuncture stimulates the vagal nerve, and inhibits the inflammatory response and suppresses the development of paw swelling and inflammation in mice (de Jong et al 2005).

The cholinergic pathway proposed by Tracey (2002) could offer a plausible mechanism for the anti-inflammatory effects of acupuncture (Andersson 2005), supporting the use of auricular acupuncture where the vagal nerve is easily stimulated and may produce a systemic anti-inflammatory effect (Ulett & Han 2002). Sections of the Stomach and Spleen meridians (Fig. 7.1) known to generate parasympathetic stimuli correspond closely to the

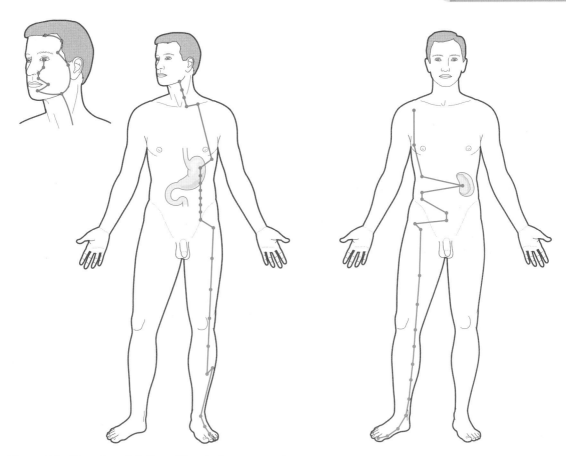

Figure 7.1 • Neural modulation of innate immune system.
Illustration reprinted with kind permission of the publishers from *A manual of acupuncture* by Peter Deadman and Mazin Al-Khafaji, with Kevin Baker. *Journal of Chinese Medicine* Publications, 2007.

path of the vagal nerve and may contribute to the acupuncture action of homeostasis by regulating interactions between the ANS and the CNS, the Yin and Yang of the regulatory action of homeostasis.

> 'The cholinergic anti-inflammatory pathway provides simple, cohesive and integrative biomedical evidence for the systemic immunoregulatory actions of acupuncture and auriculotherapy as an adjunct to manual and conventional medical treatment for a number of cytokine-mediated diseases.'
>
> (Tracey 2007)

Chronic low back pain

Chronic LBP is a common complaint, with up to 80% of the UK population reporting an episode during their lifetime (Dillingham 1995). Despite the prevalence and the increasing cost of LBP there is

much debate and conflicting evidence regarding the most effective management for this condition. Recent Cochrane reviews (Assendelft et al 2004; Furlan et al 2005; Hayden et al 2005a) investigating various forms of management for chronic LBP do not appear to recommend one specific treatment approach. As a consequence more people are turning to complementary therapies, including acupuncture, to help manage their symptoms. There have been many recent RCTs investigating the efficacy of acupuncture for chronic LBP; however, it is difficult to draw conclusions from many of these studies due to methodological flaws. A Cochrane systematic review (Furlan et al 2005) investigated the effects of acupuncture for non-specific LBP and reviewed 24 studies, which specifically focused on chronic LBP. Their findings concluded that when compared with no treatment at all there is evidence for acupuncture providing short-term pain relief and functional improvement in those with chronic LBP. When compared with conventional or alternative therapies acupuncture was found to be no more effective in reducing pain or improving function. However, when acupuncture was used in conjunction with conventional therapies there was greater pain reduction and functional improvement then just therapy alone, suggesting that acupuncture may be a good adjunct to therapies such as physiotherapy for the management of chronic LBP. However, conclusions made from systematic reviews are limited as they are unable to categorize LBP, which may lead to poor results and one treatment being no more effective.

Since then there have been further RCTs investigating this topic. Thomas et al (2006) compared the effects of a short course of traditional acupuncture with 'usual care' for patients with chronic non-specific LBP. A total of 241 patients were randomized into an acupuncture group ($n = 160$) and usual management ($n = 81$). The acupuncture group received acupuncture treatments along with massage and advice on diet and exercises. The usual care group received mixed management, including physiotherapy and medication. The findings concluded that there was only weak evidence for acupuncture over usual care for non-specific LBP at 12 months but stronger evidence at 24 months. However, as the acupuncture group received massage and advice on exercises and the group sizes were unequal, it could be argued that the difference in improvements made cannot be attributed solely to the effects of acupuncture.

Brinkhaus et al (2006) conducted an RCT to investigate the efficacy of acupuncture compared with sham acupuncture and no acupuncture at all in chronic LBP patients. This study comprised 301 patients randomized into the three groups. The study concluded that acupuncture was more effective than no acupuncture at all in chronic LBP. However, there was no significant difference between acupuncture and sham acupuncture long term, suggesting that the location and placement of needles may not be as significant as thought. However, overall this study concludes that acupuncture is a beneficial form of treatment for pain chronic LBP patients.

The German acupuncture trials for chronic LBP (Haake et al 2007) compared the effectiveness of acupuncture, sham acupuncture, and 'conventional treatment' in reducing chronic LBP. This was a multicentre, blinded RCT involving 1162 patients. The conventional therapy group involved patients receiving physiotherapy, massage, heat, electrotherapy, injection, guidance, and referral to back school. This group arguably typifies standard physiotherapy management in this country. This study concluded that acupuncture (verum or sham) was significantly more superior and effective in reducing chronic LBP than conventional therapy. Patients in the acupuncture groups also were noted to have had a significant reduction in pain medication use. These findings contrast with that of the Cochrane review (Furlan et al 2005), which found acupuncture to be no more effective. Interestingly this study also concluded that there was no significant difference between sham and verum acupuncture, which supports the results of Brinkhaus et al (2006) and therefore questions current beliefs about pain modulation from acupuncture (discussed later). Nevertheless this study provides strong evidence due to its size and sound methodology that acupuncture is more effective than conventional therapy in reducing pain in patients with chronic LBP.

Overall it appears that the evidence regarding the effectiveness of acupuncture in reducing chronic LBP is growing. The Cochrane review (Furlan et al 2005) concluded that acupuncture could be a useful adjunct to conventional therapy whereas more recent studies conclude that acupuncture is more effective than conventional therapy, i.e. physiotherapy. After reviewing this recent evidence, acupuncture was selected as an appropriate treatment option for the following case study.

 ## Case Study 1

Siobhan Byrne

Introduction

A 33-year-old female presented with a 15-year history of central lower lumbar pain. The subject had received physiotherapy in the past consisting of manual and exercise therapy with little improvement; this was followed by a lumbar spine X-ray showing mild degenerative changes.

Subjective assessment

The subject reported an aching pain of 9/10 on a numeric pain rated scale (NPRS). The pain was aggravated by bending, lifting, and driving for more than 30 minutes and it was eased by lying supine with heat. She reported disturbed sleep, but no referred pain and no red flags.

(Continued)

Case Study 1 (Continued)

Objective assessment

The assessment findings showed the subject had an increased lumbar lordosis and increased tone in her paraspinal muscles. Lumbar spine flexion was limited to below the subject's knees and reproduced her pain. Extension and side flexion were not comparable. She had a positive slump test that reproduced her pain in addition to cervical spine sensitization, indicating symptoms of a neurogenic origin. PAIVMs in the lower lumbar spine were inconclusive because the subject was allodynic. She had normal movement in her upper and low thoracic spines but was allodynic around her T6 region, and this condition was accompanied with stiffness. The diagnosis was a movement impairment disorder into flexion (O'Sullivan 2005) with central sensitization.

Treatment

Initial management of this subject focused on desensitizing the nervous system through restoring the correct movement pattern of flexion. This approach almost restored full-range movement (ROM) of lumbar spine flexion, but she still complained of disturbed sleep and 6/10 NPRS. Acupuncture was selected as an appropriate treatment for pain relief, whilst the patient continued with her home exercise programme (Table 7.1).

Physiological reasoning for acupuncture selection

It has been documented that identification of the predominant pain mechanisms is key for acupuncture point selection and, therefore, its effectiveness (Lundeberg & Ekholm 2001). The present subject had a combination of pain mechanisms that were driving her symptoms, predominantly centrally evoked pain with secondary maintained nociceptive pain. O'Sullivan (2005) suggested that movement impairment disorders are associated with abnormal, significant muscle guarding, resulting in compressive loading on the joints, excessive stability (rigidity), and tissue strain. These are all sources of ongoing nociceptive (somatic) pain. However, because of the chronicity of the subject's condition and central sensitization, it is likely that ongoing stimulation of the peripheral nociceptors was centrally maintained. For this reason, acupuncture treatment included both local and distal points. Initially the Bladder points (BL) 23 and (BL25) were used bilaterally, which had an effect on the peripheral and spinal mechanisms. As a result of needle introduction into the skin, chemoreceptors and A-delta (Aδ) fibres are stimulated, releasing chemicals including endorphins, which act to cause local vasodilation, facilitate healing, and provide a local analgesic effect, i.e. peripheral mechanism (Bradnam 2007). The needle also stimulates A-beta (Aβ) fibres, which have an effect on the dorsal horn. At the spinal cord level, there is an increase in the production of serotonin and the release of other neurotransmitters, causing inhibition at the dorsal

horn (spinal mechanism). This has a further analgesic effect and increases the feeling of well being and muscle relaxation. Local points BL23 and BL25 were specifically chosen since they are both recognized as important points for reducing LBP (Liangyue et al 1999). These both regulate and remove blockages of Qi and, therefore, are important in chronic conditions (Liangyue et al 1999). After the initial acupuncture treatment showed no adverse effects, additional acupuncture points were gradually added; BL24 and Huatuojiaji points at L3 to L5 were included to further stimulate local acupuncture mechanisms and increase dorsal horn inhibition.

The Large Intestine 4 (LI4) acupoint was also used throughout the treatment as a distal point. Acupuncture is also thought to have an effect on the supraspinal mechanisms or descending nociceptive inhibitory control (DNIC) through stimulation of C fibres. Among the higher centres affected are the pituitary and pineal glands, the hippocampus, the periaqueductal grey matter, and the hypothalamus. These centres are stimulated and collectively increase the production of endorphins, cortisone, serotonin, endogenous opioids, oxytocin, and melatonin. These chemicals have an analgesic effect, and promote healing, well-being relaxation, and sleep. These effects were specifically sought from needle insertion. Oxytocin is a chemical that serves to block pain memory and, therefore, is particularly useful in chronic pain patients. Because this patient was also suffering from disturbed sleep, the increase in the production of melatonin was thought to be desirable since it can help promote good sleep patterns. Bradnam (2007) suggested that these supraspinal mechanisms are best accessed through the hands because of their large representation in the somatosensory cortex. The LI4 point was specifically chosen since it is widely recognized as the most important analgesic point in the body (Liangyue et al 1999).

Overall outcome of treatment

Following two treatments of Manual Therapy and exercises, there was a significant improvement in the subject's lumbar spine flexion and the quality of its movement. Her pain levels also dropped from a 9/10 to 7/10 NPRS; however, sleep was still disturbed by pain. After four acupuncture treatments, the subject reported that pain was 3/10 on average and that her sleep was no longer disturbed. Lumbar spine flexion also improved further, allowing her to place her fingers flat on the floor with no reproduction of pain.

Discussion and limitations

Using O'Sullivan's (2005) proposed classification for chronic LBP a diagnosis of non-specific LBP, movement impairment disorder was made for this subject. Initial management focused on restoring the impaired movement (flexion), as recommended by O'Sullivan (2005). Movement was successfully restored; because of

(Continued)

Case Study 1 (Continued)

Table 7.1 Treatment Choice

Day	Pre-treatment Marker	Treatment	Post treatment marker
1	LS flexion: below knee, P1 NPRS 9/10	TS mobilizations LS flexion PPIVMs in side lying Education re: diagnosis HEP: pelvic tilts, LS flexion with improved pattern	LS flexion: to floor NPRS 7/10
22	LS flexion: to toes NPRS 7/10	TS mobilizations Pelvic tilt in standing, facilitation of LS flexion in standing	LS flexion: to floor improved pattern of movement NPRS 6/10
34	LS flexion: to floor, P1 NPRS 7/10	LI4 (B) BL23 (B) BL25 (B) Prone lying, 20 mins	LS flexion: fingers flat on floor NPRS 4/10
37	LS flexion: fingers flat on floor NPRS 4/10	LI4 (B) BL23 (B) BL24 (B) BL25 (B) Prone lying, 20 mins	NPRS 3/10
41	NPRS 4/10	LI4 (B) BL23 (B) BL24 (B) BL25 (B) HJJ points L3–L5 bilateral Prone lying, 20 mins	NPRS 3/10
49	NPRS 3/10 Reports improved sleep, not waking	LI4 (B) BL23 (B) BL24 (B) BL25 (B) HJJ points L3-L5 bilateral Prone lying, 20 mins	NPRS 3/10

Notes: NPRS, numeric pain rated scale; LS, lumbar spine; TS, thoracic spine; B, bilateral unilateral posterior–anterior mobilizations to T5 toT7; HEP, home exercise programme.

the other pain mechanisms involved (central sensitization) and the chronicity of the condition, her pain levels remained at 7/10 NPRS. With the adjunct of acupuncture combined with the Manual Therapy there was a further reduction in pain levels and an improvement in sleep.

The present case study shows that a combination of both manual and exercise therapy, and acupuncture was of benefit to this subject. However, since multiple treatments were used, it is not possible to specifically attribute the improvements to one particular treatment. Nevertheless, it could be argued that the greatest reduction in pain and the improvements in sleep patterns came after acupuncture treatment commenced. Although the outcomes support current evidence concluding that acupuncture is a beneficial treatment for chronic LBP, it is not possible to generalize the results from any case study because of the minimal sample size ($n = 1$). Another limitation of the present case study is that treatment was incomplete and therefore, the final outcomes and, more importantly, the long-term effects are unknown.

The combination of therapies used to treat the CNS in the present case was appropriate to recovery; exercises were essential as a means of restoration of normal movement patterns; and acupuncture was used to relieve pain through inhibiting the DNIC and releasing endogenous opioids. This non-specific tissue treatment approach for patients with a diagnosis of non-specific LBP is likely to be successful.

(Continued)

Case Study 2

Hannah Edwards

Introduction

A 41-year-old lady presented to physiotherapy complaining of central and right-sided lumbar spine pain (Fig. 7.2). She had initially felt her pain 2 years previously whilst attending a yoga class; she had felt her back 'go' and was left with severe pain in the same distribution as her current pain. The severity of her pain settled, but she was left with a residual dull ache. She had been able to self-manage this problem with simple analgesics, non-steroidal anti-inflammatory agents (NSAIDs) and by attending Pilates classes.

In 2007 the subject was involved in a road traffic accident (RTA), in which she was struck from behind whilst stationary. This caused an increase in the severity of her pain and about 1 week later, whilst flexing forwards, her pain increased severely, causing 10 days of enforced bed rest. She was consequently reviewed by a rheumatologist and underwent a magnetic resonance imaging (MRI), which revealed lumbar 4-5 and L5–S1 disc bulges, L4-5 end-plate oedema and annular tear; she was referred to physiotherapy seeking pain relief.

From the above findings described (Table 7.2), it was concluded that the majority of the subject's pain was a consequence of her disc pathology. Contributory factors included hypomobile motion segments, facet joint irritation, and propagation of pain memory, which was compounded by the presence of a legal claim and yellow flags.

The likelihood of disc degeneration with age is increased by end-plate damage. From 20 to 65 years of age the end-plate thins and cell death occurs in the superficial layers of the cartilage. The vascular changes in the subchondral bone results in decreased permeability of the end-plate to nutrients for the disc, as does ossification of the end-plate, which restricts fluid exchange, causing disc dehydration, and a vulnerability to damage or disc prolapse (Ferguson & Steffen 2003).

The solid matrix of the intervertebral disc (IVD) is organized into a gelatinous nucleus pulposus and a highly organized angle ply lamellae structure, the annulus fibrosus (Iatridis & Gwynn 2004).

Mechanical overloading from hyperflexion, torsion, and fatigue loading is considered to be a potential cause of disc failure. Iatridis and Gwynn (2004) studied the mechanisms for damage within the IVD, concluding that fibre failure and interlaminar shear stresses can cause delamination and the propagation of annular tears from focal disruptions or existing cracks.

Table 7.2 Objective assessment

Aggravating factors	Bending: gives pain with immediate onset. Sitting: 30 mins gives a gradual onset of pain. Breast stroke
Easing factors	Walking Supine lying Heat
24-hour pattern	O/W: Stiff O/R: Eases quickly with movement AM–PM phased return back to work, pain increases + + after 3 hours of sitting. Night—Sleeping pattern initially disturbed but is now improving
Drug history	No steroids No anticoagulants Regularly taking NSAIDs
Past medical history	Fractured wrist Ophthalmic surgery
Investigations	MRI showing L4-5, L5–S1, disc dehydration and bulge with L4–L5 annular tear.
Social history	Works as a tax inspector, involving visiting companies and office-based duties
Hobbies	Swimming Pilates Walking
No red flags and all special questions	

Notes: NSAIDs, Non-steroidal anti-inflammatory drugs; MRI, magnetic resonance imaging.

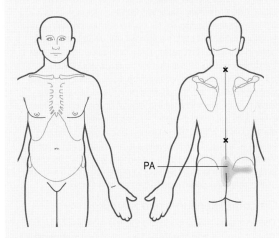

Figure 7.2 • Pain presentation.

PA

(Continued)

Case Study 2 (Continued)

Oliver and Middleditch (1991) introduced the idea of gradual disc prolapse. The injury starts with the annular lamellae, being distorted to form radial fissures. Nuclear pulp then breaks the distorted lamellae, causing a protrusion. This can then progress to the pulp extruding from the outer lamellae. Because of the insidious nature of the events leading to the disc prolapse the final straw is usually a trivial event such as bending to pick up an object from the floor, as in the case of the present subject.

Bogduk (1994) noted that the outer annulus fibrosus of an IVD is supplied by the complex and free nerve endings of the mixed sinuvertebral nerve, and therefore can be a source of somatic pain. Pain provocation studies have confirmed that the posterior annulus is the most frequent tissue of origin in severe chronic LBP (Kuslich et al 1991). Bogduk (1997) stated that pain is aggravated by any movement that stresses the annulus, in particular flexion and rotation in the direction that produced the lesions.

Chemical pain will also be present as a result of irritation of the nociceptive nerve endings by inflammatory exudates, which are produced as a result of trauma. The annulus also contains some unmyelinated and small myelinated fibres that are thought to act as silent nociceptors responding to algesic chemicals, produced during inflammation (Kesson & Atkins 2005).

It should also be noted that acquired disorders of a single component of a motion segment cannot exist without affecting the functions of the components of the segment, i.e. sacroiliac joint (SIJ) hypomobility.

The anatomical changes of disc degeneration or prolapse lead to a loss of fluid pressurization and decreased disc height that contribute directly to the changes in the local stress/strain state within the disc, and indirectly to facet joint degeneration and pain (An et al 2004). This may explain the underlying regular compression pattern during lumbar spine active range of movement (AROM).

The treatment management plan was to:
- Reduce pain;
- Improve range of movement;
- Mobilize motion segments;
- Increase core stability; and
- Restore function.

Physiological reasons for treatment selection

The first six treatments consisted of manual techniques and core stability strengthening. The subject 's poor core stability was addressed with basic transversus abdominis setting combined with gluteal strengthening and motor control of the multifidus. She also continued with Pilates and a graduated return to swimming.

The subject's pain decreased from a deep constant compression pain that she rated as 70/100 on the visual analogue scale (VAS) to an intermittent ache that she rated at 40 to 50/100. Her AROM of lumbar flexion improved, as did her function. However, after six treatments, the improvement in her symptoms plateaued and it was agreed that another form of treatment should be employed; hence acupuncture was utilized.

Synaptic plasticity is fundamental to many neurobiological functions, including memory and pain. Central sensitization refers to the increased synaptic efficacy established in somatosensory neurons in the dorsal horn of the spinal cord following intense peripheral noxious stimuli, tissue injury, or nerve damage. This heightened synaptic transmission leads to a reduction in pain threshold, an amplification of pain responses, and a spread of pain sensitivity to non-injured areas. In the prefrontal cortex (PFC) the amygdala long-term potentiation, a long-lasting, highly localized area of synaptic strength is a synaptic substrate for memory and learning. Hence, by using acupuncture to stimulate the PFC and amygdala, the memory of chronic pain may be inhibited.

Meng et al (2003) attempted to determine whether acupuncture is an effective and safe adjunct to standard therapy in chronic LBP in older people. They compared a standard therapy control group, acupuncture plus standard therapy group, an acupoints supplementary protocol group, and a crossover group. Their results confirmed that acupuncture plus standard therapy does decrease back pain and disability in a clinically and statistically significant manner, when compared to standard therapy alone.

All studies reviewed by the present author used a non-prescriptive or semi-standardized approach to formulating acupuncture treatment. However, some common themes are present. Macpherson et al (2004) (Table 7.3) investigated the patterns of diagnosis and treatment of LBP. They identified that the Bladder and Gall Bladder meridians are most commonly utilized for the treatment of LBP; Brinkhaus et al (2006) (Table 7.4) used a semi-standardized approach to the acupuncture points utilized during their study.

In all sessions de Qi sensation was achieved at all points. A marked parasympathetic reaction was achieved when using BL23, Governor Vessel (GV) 4 and HJJ points at the L2/L3 segment. All treatments were carried out for 20 minutes. Care was taken on the first treatment not to overstimulate local points close to the damaged tissue. However, since no adverse reactions were reported, treatment was progressed to include local points, thus increasing dorsal horn and segmental inhibition. Treatment was also progressed to utilize more distal points within the segment because Lundeberg (1998) reported that this was a good progression for the treatment of chronic pain. Treatment was also progressed away from general analgesia to more specific treatment of the affected segments (L4-5, L5-S1) (Table 7.5).

Outcome measures and results

The outcome measures included the active range of lumbar flexion and the VAS. The initial six treatments

(Continued)

Case Study 2 (Continued)

Table 7.3 Common acupuncture points for low back pain

Point	Dermatome
Local points	
BL23	L4
BL26	L4/5
BL53	S1/S2
BL54	S1/S2
GB30	S2
Huatuojiaji points at Lumbar Spine	
Distal points	
BL40	S1/S2
BL60	S1
BL62	S1
KID3	S2
KID7	S2
GB34	L5
GB41	S1
LIV3	L5
GV14	C6
GV20	C2

Adapted from MacPherson et al (2004).

Table 7.4 Commonly used points for low back pain

Point	Dermatome
Local points	
BL20 to 34	L1 to S2
BL41	
BL50 to 54	S1 to S2
LIV3	L5
GB30	S1
GV3 to GV6	L3 to S1
Huatuojiaji (HJJ) at lumbar spine	
Distal points	
GV4	C6 to C7
GV20	C2
2 distal points selected from below	
SI 3	C5
BL 60/62	S1 to S2
KID 3/KID 7	S2
GB31/GB34/GB41	L5 to S1
GV14/GV20	C6-7 & C2

Adapted from Brinkhaus et al (2006).

were based upon Manual Therapy techniques and exercise. The subject's VAS dropped from 70/100 to 40/100; her SIJ shear test became pain free, and her range of lumbar flexion improved from touching the knees to being able to reach to 51 mm below the pole of the patella, but continued to be restricted by pain. All other lumbar movements were full and pain free. The subject's function had improved, thus allowing her to return to full-time work. After the initial acupuncture session, she cited a reduction of her VAS to 30/100 and a general improvement in function (she was able to swim 750 m with no adverse effects). After the next three sessions her VAS was reported to be at 20/100 and her lumbar flexion improved to being able to reach 178 mm below the distal pole of her patella. She also reported a 75% improvement since treatment had began and was unable to identify any activity of daily living that was restricted. Acupuncture was continued as her symptoms and the level of function continued to improve, and since she continues to report improvements in her symptoms; the final outcome of treatment cannot be reported.

Limitations

Because the subject's main symptom was pain, it was difficult to utilize a reliable and valid objective outcome measure, and the results of this treatment regime are based primarily upon her subjective pain score. It must also be recognized that no recommendations for treatment or efficacy of treatment can be made because this was only a single-patient case study. Finally, the acupuncture regime had not been previously validated because most research encouraged the selection of acupuncture points according to individual symptoms.

Discussion

The present case study describes the physiotherapeutic management of a patient suffering from chronic LBP, including clinical reasoning and a discussion of previous research. The treatment plan was devised by considering the mechanism of injury, the pathophysiology of the injury, the pain mechanisms, the chronicity of the injury, and the subject's reduction in function.

Manual techniques were initially used as the treatment of choice. Derosa and Porterfield (1992) reported that manual techniques give rise to the following physiological responses:

- Manual techniques influence the fluid dynamics of the injured areas: static fluid dynamic causes an alteration in the chemical balance of soft tissues,

(Continued)

Case Study 2 (Continued)

Table 7.5 Point rationale

Treatment 1	Aim: General and Lumbar analgesia avoiding local overstimulation
Points	LIV3[B], LI4[B], BL23[B], BL40[B], BL62[B]
Rationale	LIV3 and LI4: major analgesic points
	BL23: empirical point for back pain, segmental inhibition, dorsal horn inhibition.
	BL62: back pain point (within S1 dermatome and myotome)
	BL40: back pain point (within S1 dermatome and myotome)
Treatment 2	Aim: general and lumbar analgesia emphasizing dorsal horn inhibition
Points	LIV3[B], LI4[B], BL23[B], BL40[B], BL62[B], HJJ[B], GV4.
Rationale	LIV3 & LI4: major analgesic points
	BL23: empirical point for back pain, dorsal horn inhibition.
	BL62: back pain point (within S1 dermatome)
	BL40: back pain point (within S1 dermatome)
	HJJ & GV4: Spinal pain, dorsal horn inhibition, segmental inhibition
Treatment 3	Aim: lumbar analgesia emphasizing dorsal horn inhibition
Points	BL23[B], BL40[B], BL62[B], HJJ[B], GV4
Rationale	BL23: empirical point for back pain, dorsal horn inhibition.
	BL62: back pain point (within S1 dermatome)
	BL40: back pain point (within S1 dermatome)
	HJJ & GV4: spinal pain, dorsal horn inhibition
Treatment 4	Aim: lumbar analgesia emphasizing dorsal horn inhibition
Points	BL23[B], BL40[B], BL62[B], BL2[B], HJJ[B], GV4, GB34[B]
Rationale	BL23: empirical point for back pain, dorsal horn inhibition.
	BL62: back pain point (within S1 dermatome)
	BL40: back pain point (within S1 dermatome)
	BL25: back pain, segmental inhibition L4/L5
	HJJ & GV4: spinal pain, dorsal horn inhibition
	GB34: distal point in L4 segment, He-sea point influential with muscular disorders

Notes: B, bilateral.

thereby stimulating the nociceptive system and impeding healing.

- Manual techniques generate afferent input to the CNS, consequently modulating pain and alterations in the state of muscle contraction.

Kesson and Atkins (2005) documented manipulation-induced hypoalgesia and recognized that restoration of functional movement may itself cause a reduction in pain levels. Exercise is also an integral component of any treatment of LBP. It is thought that muscles act as shock absorbers and that strengthening muscle increases stiffness, thereby optimizing a patient's ability to attenuate forces converging on the lumbar spine. Exercise programmes can prepare individuals to self-manage their low back problem, as well as reducing emotional distress and illness behaviour (Derosa & Porterfield 1992). The necessity for the inclusion of a graded exercise programme was also reinforced by Lindström et al (1992): their graded exercise programme significantly reduced long-term sick leave, and on average, allowed their subjects to return to work 5.1 weeks before the control group.

By combining a Manual Therapy approach and independent exercise, the present subject's pain decreased, functional movement improved, and her general feeling of well being and function were enhanced. However, the gain through manual treatments did plateau, and, therefore, the use of acupuncture was indicated.

Yan et al (2005) demonstrated point-specific patterns using functional magnetic resonance imaging (fMRI) in 37 healthy volunteers while needling LI4 and Liver (LIV) 3, as compared to sham points. Common activation areas for LI4 and LIV3 were in the middle temporal gyrus and cerebellum, along with deactivation areas in the middle frontal gyrus and inferior parietal lobule. Acupuncture at LIV3 evoked specific activation in the post-central gyrus, posterior cingulate, and parahippocampal gyrus, thereby assisting pain modulation.

Liu et al (2004) also noticed a dramatically increased induced activation of the periaqueductal grey matter (PAG) in humans with both LI4 and a non-acupuncture point. However, it appeared that the PAG activation was far greater when utilizing the acupuncture point. Also, as previously mentioned, acupuncture may have had an effect on the present subject's pain memory through effects on the hippocampus and amygdala, thereby combatting her chronic pain.

Despite this evidence, many researchers have compared the effects of acupuncture with that of a placebo and hence, it is difficult to determine the cause of the present subject's reduction in pain. Campbell (2006) reported that acupuncture can produce complex brain changes in areas connected with brain transmission and pain perception, but these effects also occurred in response to placebo treatments. Lewith and Vincent (1996) identified the release of neural substrates during acupuncture for non-painful indications; however, when considering the treatment of pain, a far less specific response emerges involving overlapping neural substrates activated by both placebo and expectation.

(Continued)

Case Study 2 (Continued)

This was further supported by Ezzo et al (2000) who wrote:

We conclude there is limited evidence that acupuncture is more effective than no treatment for chronic pain; and inconclusive evidence that acupuncture is more effective than placebo, sham acupuncture or standard care.

Therefore it is difficult to establish which component of the present subject's treatment was most beneficial; however, a combined approach with a possible contribution from a placebo effect, or her expectations, has greatly improved her symptoms and function.

Conclusions

Using a combined approach to treatment was most beneficial for the present subject. Manual techniques, core stability conditioning, and the individual exercise programme all helped to decrease pain, restore movement patterns, increase strength, decrease fear avoidance behaviour, and promote self-management. Acupuncture caused a general decrease in pain and possibly aided the management of her original chronic pain memory.

References

Airaksinen, O., Brox, J.I., Cedraschi, C., et al., 2006. European guidelines for the management of chronic non-specific low back pain. Eur. Spine J. 15 (Suppl 2), S192–S300.

An, H.S., Howard, S., Anderson, P., et al., 2004. Introduction: disc degeneration. Spine 29 (23), 2677–2678.

Andersson, J.L., 2005. The inflammatory reflex-introduction. J. Intern. Med. 257 (2), 122–125.

Assendelft, W.J.J., Morton, S.C., Yu, E.I., et al., 2004. Spinal manipulative therapy for low back pain. Cochrane Database Syst. Rev., CD000447.

Bogduk, N., 1994. Innervation, pain patterns, and mechanisms of pain production. In: Twomey, L., Taylor, J. (Eds.) Physical therapy of the low back, 2nd edn. Churchill Livingstone, New York, pp. 93–109.

Bogduk, N., 1997. Clinical anatomy of the spine and sacrum. Churchill Livingstone, London.

Bogduk, N., 2004. Management of chronic low back pain. Med. J. Aust. 180, 79–83.

Borkan, J.M., Koes, B., Reis, S., 1998. A report from the Second International Forum for Primary Care Research on Low-back Pain: re-examining priorities. Spine 23, 1992–1996.

Bowsher, D., 1998. Mechanisms of acupuncture Chapter 6. In: Filshie, J., White, A. (Eds.) Medical acupuncture, a Western scientific approach. Churchill Livingstone, Edinburgh.

Bradnam, L., 2007. A proposed clinical reasoning model for

Western acupuncture. Journal of the Acupuncture Association of Chartered Physiotherapists, 21–30.

Brennan, G.P., Fritz, J.M., Hunter, S.J., et al., 2006. Identifying subgroups of patients with acute/subacute 'non specific' low back pain: results of a randomised clinical trial. Spine 31, 623–631.

Brinkhaus, B., Witt, C., Jena, S., et al., 2006. Acupuncture in patients with chronic low back pain. Arch. Intern. Med. 166, 450–457.

Bronfort, G., Haas, M., Evans, R.L., et al., 2004. Efficacy of spinal manipulation and mobilisation for low back and neck pain: a systematic review and best evidence synthesis. Spine 4, 335–356.

Cairns, M.C., Foster, N.E., Wright, C., 2006. Randomised controlled trial of specific stabilisation exercises and conventional physiotherapy for recurrent low back pain. Spine 31 (19), E670–E681.

Campbell, A., 2006. Point specificity of acupuncture in the light of recent clinical and imaging studies. Acupunct. Med. 24 (3), 118–122.

Carlsson, C., 2002. Acupuncture mechanisms for clinically relevant long-term effects reconsideration and a hypothesis. Acupunct. Med. 20 (2–3), 82–99.

Carneiro, E.R., Carneiro, C.R., De Castro, M.A., et al., 2005. Effect of electro-acupuncture on bronchial asthma. J. Altern. Complement Med. 11, 127–134.

Ceccherelli, F., Gagliardi, G., Visentin, R., et al., 1999. The

effects of parachlorophenylalinine and naloxone on acupuncture and electroacupuncture modulation of capsaicin-induced neurogenic oedema in the rat hind paw: a controlled blind study. Clinical Experiments in Rheumatology 17, 655–662.

Cherkin, D., Eisenberg, M.D., Sherman, K., et al., 2001. Randomised control trial comparing traditional Chinese medical acupuncture, therapeutic massage, and self-care education for chronic low back pain. Arch. Int. Med. 161, 1081–1088.

Childs, J.D., Fritz, J.M., Flynn, T.W., et al., 2004. A clinical prediction rule to identify patients with low back pain to benefit from spinal manipulation: a validation study. Ann. Intern. Med. 141, 920–928.

Chou, R., Quaeem, A., Snow, V., et al., 2007. Diagnosis and treatment of low back pain: a joint clinical practice guideline from the American College of Physicians and the American Pain Society. Ann. Intern. Med. 147 (7), 478–491.

Cleland, J.A., Fritz, J.M., Whitman, J.M., et al., 2006. The use of a lumbar spine manipulation technique by physical therapists in patients who satisfy a clinical prediction rule: a case series. J. Orthop. Sports Phys. Ther. 36, 198–199.

Clement-Jones, V., McLoughlin, L., Tomlin, S., et al., 1980. Enkephalin levels in human cerebrospinal fluid after acupuncture for headache. Lancet 2 (8201), 946–949.

Dankaerts, W., O'Sullivan, P., Burnett, A., et al., 2006. Altered patterns of superficial trunk muscle activation during sitting in non-specific chronic low back pain: importance of subclassification. Spine 31, 2017–2037.

de Jong, W.J., van der Zanden, E.P., The, F.O., et al., 2005. Stimulation of vagal nerve attenuates macrophage activation by activating Jak2-STAT3 signalling pathway. National Immunology 6, 8444–8451.

Derosa, C., Porterfield, J., 1992. A physical therapy model for the treatment of low back pain. Phys. Ther. 72 (4), 261–272.

Dillingham, T., 1995. Evaluation and management of low back pain: and overview. State of the Art Reviews 9 (3), 559–574.

Ezzo, J., Berman, B., Hadhazy, V.A., et al., 2000. Is acupuncture an effective treatment for Chronic pain: a systematic review. Pain 86 (3), 217–225.

Ferguson, S.J., Steffen, T., 2003. Biomechanics of the aging spine. Eur. Spine J. 12 (Suppl 2), S97–S103.

Ferreira, M.L., Ferreira, P.H., Latimer, J., 2007. Comparison of general exercise, motor control exercise and spinal manipulative therapy for chronic low back pain: A randomised trial. Pain 13, 31–37.

Flynn, T., Fritz, J., Whitman, J., et al., 2002. A clinical prediction rule for classifying patients with LBP who demonstrate short-term improvement with spinal manipulation. Spine 27, 2835–2843.

Fritz, J.M., Whitman, J.M., Childs, J. D., 2005. Lumbar spine segmental mobility assessment: an examination of the validity for determining intervention strategies in patients with low back pain. Arch. Phys. Med. Rehabil. 86, 1745–1752.

Frost, H., Lamb, S.E., Doll, H.A., et al., 2004. Randomised controlled trial of physiotherapy compared with advice for low back pain. Br. Med. J. 329, 708–714.

Furlan, A.D., Van Tulder, M.W., Cherkin, D.C., et al., 2005. Acupuncture and dry needling for low back pain. Cochrane Database Syst. Rev., CD001351.

Geisser, M.E., Wiggert, E.A., Haig, A.J., et al., 2005. A randomised controlled trial of Man therapy and specific adjuvant exercise for chronic low back pain. Clin. J. Pain 21, 463–470.

Gregory, D.E., Brown, S.H., Callaghan, J.P., 2007. Trunk muscle responses to suddenly applied loads: do individuals who develop discomfort during prolonged standing respond differently? J. Electromyogr. Kinesiol. 18 (3), 495–502.

Haake, M., Muller, H., Schade-Brittinger, C., et al., 2007. German acupunctures trials (GERAC) for chronic low back pain. Arch. Intern. Med. 167 (17), 892–898.

Hay, E.M., Mullis, R., Lewis, M., et al., 2005. Comparison of physical treatments versus a brief pain-management programme for back pain in primary care: a randomised clinical trial in physiotherapy practice. Lancet 365, 2024–2030.

Hayden, J.A., Van Tulder, M.W., Malmivaara, A., et al., 2005a. Exercise therapy for treatment of non-specific low back pain. Cochrane Database Syst. Rev., CD000335.

Hayden, J.A., Van Tulder, M.W., Tomlinson, G., 2005b. Systematic review: Strategies for using exercise therapy to improve outcome in chronic LBP. Ann. Intern. Med. 142, 766–785.

Herzog, W., Scheele, D., Conway, P.J., 1999. Electromyographic responses of back and limb muscles associated with spinal manipulative therapy. Spine 24, 146–153.

Hicks, G.E., Fritz, J.M., Delitto, A., et al., 2005. Preliminary development of a clinical prediction rule for determining which patients with LBP will respond to a stabilisation exercise programme. Arch. Phys. Med. Rehabil. 86, 1753–1762.

Hides, J.A., Stokes, M.J., Saide, M., et al., 1994. Evidence of lumbar multifidus wasting ipsilateral to symptoms in patients with acute/subacute low back pain. Spine 19, 165–172.

Hides, J.A., Richardson, C.A., Jull., G.A., 1996. Multifidus muscle recovery is not automatic after resolution of acute first episode low back pain. Spine 21, 2763–2769.

Hides, J.A., Jull, G.A., Richardson, C.A., 2001. Long-term effects of specific stabilising exercises for first episode low back pain. Spine 26, 243–248.

Hodges, P.W., 2000. The role of the motor system in spinal pain: implications for rehabilitation of the athlete following lower back pain. J. Sci. Med. Sport 3, 243–253.

Hodges, P.W., 2001. Changes in motor planning of feedforward postural responses of the trunk muscles in low back pain. Exp. Brain Res. 141, 261–266.

Hodges, P.W., Moseley, G.L., 2003. Pain and motor control of the lumbopelvic region: effect and possible mechanisms. J. Electromyogr. Kinesiol. 13, 361–370.

Hodges, P.W., Richardson, C.A., 1996. Inefficient muscular stabilisation of the lumbar spine associated with low back pain: a motor control evaluation of transversus abdominis. Spine 21, 2640–2650.

Hodges, P.W., Gurfinkel, V.S., Brugmagne, S., et al., 2002. Coexistence of stability and mobility in postural control: evidence from postural compensation for respiration. Exp. Brain Res. 144, 293–302.

Hodges, P.W., Moseley, G.L., Gabrielsson, A., et al., 2003. Experimental muscle pain changes feedforward postural responses of the trunk muscles. Exp. Brain Res. 151, 262–271.

Hodges PW, Cholewicki J, Coppieters M et al 2007 Trunk muscle control in back pain: how can the variability be explained? *Proceedings of the 11th World Congress of Physical Therapy, Vancouver.*

Huguenin, L.K., 2004. Myofascial trigger points: the current evidence. Phys. Ther. in Sport 5, 2–12.

Iatridis, J., Gwynn, I., 2004. Mechanisms for mechanical damage in the intervertebral disc annulus fibrosus. J. Biomech. 37, 1165–1175.

Indahl, A., Kaigle, A.M., Reikeras, O., et al., 1997. Interaction between the porcine lumbar intervertebral disc, zygapophysial joints and paraspinal muscles. Spine 22, 2834–2840.

Irnich, D., Behrens, N., Gleditsch, J.M., et al., 2002. Immediate effects of dry needling at distant points in chronic neck pain: results of a randomized, double-blind, sham-controlled crossover trial. Pain 99 (1–2), 83–89.

Jones, M., Rivett, D., 2004. Clinical reasoning for manual therapists. Butterworth-Heinemann, Oxford.

Kaptchuk, T.J., 2002. Acupuncture: theory, efficacy, and practice. Ann. Intern. Med. 136, 374–383.

Katavich, L., 1998. Differential effects of spinal manipulative therapy on acute and chronic muscle spasm: a proposal for mechanisms and efficacy. Man. Ther. 3, 132–139.

Kavoussi, B., Ross, E., 2007. The neuroimmune basis of anti-inflammatory acupuncture. Integr. Cancer. Ther. 6 (251), 257.

Kesson, M., Atkins, E., 2005. Orthopaedic medicine: a practical approach. Elsevier, London.

Kim, H.W., Roh, D.H., Yoon, S.Y., et al., 2006. The anti-inflammatory effects of low and high frequency electroacupuncture are mediated by peripheral opioids in a mouse air pouch inflammation model. J. Altern. Complement Med. 12 (1), 39–44.

Koes, B.W., Van Tulder, M.W., Thomas, S., 2006. Diagnosis and treatment of low back pain. Br. Med. J. 332, 1430–1434.

Koumantakis, G.A., Watson, P.J., Oldham, J.A., 2005. Trunk muscle stabilisation plus general exercise versus general exercise only: randomised controlled trial of patients with recurrent low back pain. Phys. Ther. 85, 209–225.

Kuslich, S.D., Ulstrom, C.L., Michael, C.J., 1991. The tissue origin of low back pain and sciatica: a report of pain response to tissue stimulation during operations on the lumbar spine using local anesthesia. Orthop. Clin. North Am. 22 (2), 181–187.

Lee, D.G., 2004. The pelvic girdle, 3rd edn. Elsevier Science, Edinburgh.

Lehman, G.J., McGill, S.M., 2001. Spinal manipulation causes variable spine kinematic and trunk muscle electromyographic responses. Clin. Biomech. 16, 293–299.

Lehman, G.J., Vernon, H., McGill, S.M., 2001. Effects of a mechanical pain stimulus on erector spinae activity before and after a spinal manipulation in patients with back pain: a preliminary investigation. J. Manipulative Physiol. Ther. 24, 402–406.

Leinonen, V., Kankaanpaa, M., Airaksinen, O., et al., 2000. Back and hip extensor activities during trunk flexion/extension: effects of Low Back pain and rehabilitation. Arch. Phys. Med. Rehabil. 81, 32–37.

Lewith, G.T., Vincent, C., 1996. On the evaluation of the clinical effects of acupuncture: a problem reassessed and a framework for future research. J. Altern. Complement Med. 2 (1), 79–90.

Liangyue, D., Yijun, G., Shuhui, H., et al., 1999. Chinese acupuncture and moxibustion. Foreign Languages Press, Beijing, China.

Lindström, I., Ohlund, C., Eek, C., et al., 1992. The effect of graded activity on patients with subacute low back pain: a randomized prospective clinical study with an operant-conditioning behavioral approach. Phys. Ther. 72 (4), 279–290.

Liu, W.C., Feldman, S.C., Cook, D. B., et al., 2004. fMRI study of acupuncture-induced periaqueductal gray activity in humans. Neuroreports 15, 1937–1940.

Lundeberg, T., Ekholm, J., 2001. Pain— from periphery to brain. Journal of the Acupuncture Association of Chartered Physiotherapists, 13–19.

Ma, S.X., 2004. The neurobiology of acupuncture towards CAM. Evid. Based Complement. Alternat. Med. 1 (1), 41–47.

McCarthy, C.J., Arnall, A., Strimpakos, N., et al., 2004. The biopsychosocial classification of non-specific low back pain: a systematic review. Phys. Ther. Reviews 9, 17–30.

McDougall, J.J., Bake, C.L., Hermann, P.M., 2004. Attenuation of knee joint inflammation by peripherally administered endorphin-1. J. Mol. Neurosci. 22, 125–137.

Macpherson, H., Thorpe, L., Thomas, K., et al., 2004. Acupuncture for low back pain: traditional diagnosis and treatment of 148 patients in a clinical trial Complement. Ther. Med. 12, 38–44.

Maitland, G.D., Hengeveld, E., Banks, K., et al., 2006. Maitland's vertebral manipulation, 7th edn. Butterworth-Heinemann, Oxford.

Meng, C.F., Wang, D., Ngeow, J., et al., 2003. Acupuncture for chronic low back pain older patients: a randomised, controlled trial. Rheumatology 42, 508–557.

Moseley GL, Hodges PW 2000 Is variability in postural adjustments a key to normalisation of control after symptoms has resolved? *Proceedings of IFOMT Cape Town*.

Moseley, G.L., Hodges, P.W., 2005. Are the changes in postural control associated with low back pain caused by pain interference? Clin. J. Pain 21, 323–329.

Moseley, G.L., Nicholas, M.K., Hodges, P.W., 2004. Does anticipation of back pain predispose to back trouble? Brain 127, 2339–2347.

Moss, P., Sluka, K., Wright, A., 2007. The initial effects of knee joint mobilization on osteoarthritic hyperalgesia. Man. Ther. 12, 109–118.

Murphy, B.A., Dawson, N.J., Slack, J.R., 1995. Sacroiliac joint manipulation decreases the H-reflex. Electromyogr. Clin. Neurophysiol. 35, 87–94.

Nelson-Wong, E., Gregory, D.E., Winter, D.A., et al., 2008. Gluteus medius muscle activation patterns as a predictor of low back pain. Journal of Clin. Biomech. 23 (5), 545–553.

O'Sullivan, P.B., 2005. Diagnosis and classification of chronic low back pain disorders: maladaptive movement and motor control Impairments as underlying mechanism. Man. Ther. 10, 242–255.

Oliver, J., Middleditch, A., 1991. Functional anatomy of the spine. Churchill Livingstone, London.

Panjabi, M.M., 1992. The stabilising system of the spine. Part II: Neutral zone and instability hypothesis. Journal of Spinal Disorders 5, 390–396.

Pickar, J.G., 2002. Neurophysiological effects of spinal manipulation. Spine 2, 357–371.

Pomeranz, B., 1996. Scientific research into acupuncture for the relief of pain. J. Altern. Complement Med. 2 (1), 53–60.

Pool-Goudzwaard, A.L., Slieker ten Hove, M.C., Vierhout, M.E., 2005. Relations between pregnancy-related low back pain, pelvic floor activity and pelvic floor dysfunction. Int. Urogynecol. J. Pelvic Floor Dysfunct. 16, 468–474.

Reeves, P.N., Narendra, K.S., Cholewicki, J., 2007. Spine stability: the six blind men and the elephant. Clin. Biomech. 22, 266–274.

Sahrmann, S.A., 1998. Diagnosis and treatment of movement impairment syndromes. Elsevier, Edinburgh.

Seffinger, M.A., Najm, W.I., Mishra, S. I., et al., 2004. Reliability of spinal palpation for diagnosis of back and neck pain: a systematic review of the literature. Spine 29, E413–E425.

Sekido, R., Keisou, I., Masakazu, S., 2004. Corticotropin-releasing factor and Interleukin-1 + are involved in the electroacupuncture-induced analgesic effect on inflammatory pain elicited by carrageenan. Am. J. Chin. Med. 32 (2), 269–279.

Shah, J.P., Desai, M., Phillips, T.M., et al., 2006. Local Biochemical Milieu in the upper trapezius muscle with active, latent and absent myofascial trigger points compared to the gastrocnemius muscle with absent myofascial trigger points. Arch. Phys. Med. Rehabil. 87, E25.

Silfies, S.P., Squillante, D., Maurer, P., et al., 2005. Trunk muscle recruitment patterns in specific chronic low back pain populations. Clin. Biomech. 20, 465–473.

Simons, D.G., Travell, J.G., Simons, L.S., 1998. Myofascial pain and dysfunction: the trigger point manual, vol. i: Upper half of body, 2nd edn. Williams and Wilkins, Baltimore.

Skyba, D.A., Radhakrishnan, R., Rohlwing, J.J., et al., 2003. Joint manipulation reduces hyperalgesia by activation of monoamine receptors but not opioid or GABA receptors in the spinal cord. Pain 106, 159–168.

Sluka, K.A., Skyba, D.A., Radhakrishnan, R., et al., 2006. Joint mobilization reduces hyperalgesia associated with chronic muscle and joint inflammation in rats. J. Pain 7, 602–607.

Smith, M.D., Russell, A., Hodges, P.W., 2006. Disorders of breathing and continence has a stronger association with back pain than obesity and physical activity. Aust J Physiother 52, 11–16.

Smith, M.D., Coppieters, M.W., Hodges, P.W., 2007. Postural activity of the pelvic floor muscles is delayed during rapid arm movements in women with stress urinary incontinence. Int. Urogynecol. J. Pelvic Floor Dysfunct. 18, 901–911.

Standaert, C.J., Weinstein, S.M., Rumpeltes, J., 2008. Evidence-informed management of chronic low back pain with lumbar stabilization exercises. Spine 8, 114–120.

Sterling, M., Jull, G., Wright, A., 2001. Cervical mobilization: concurrent effects on pain, sympathetic nervous system activity and motor activity. Man. Ther. 6, 72–81.

Stochkendahl, M.J., Christensen, H. W., Hartvigsen, J., et al., 2006. Manual examination of the spine: a systematic critical literature review of reproducibility. J. Manipulative Physiol. Ther. 29, 475–485.

Takeshige, C., Sato, T., Mera, T., et al., 2002. Descending pain inhibitory system involved in acupuncture analgesia. Brain Res. Bull. 29 (5), 617–634.

Thomas, K., Macpherson, H., Thorpe, L., et al., 2006. Randomised controls trial of a short course of traditional acupuncture compared with usual care for persistent non-specific low back pain. Journal of Acupuncture Association of Chartered Physiotherapists 1 (3), 47–56.

Tracey, I., 2002. The inflammatory reflex. Nature 420, 853–859.

Tracey, K., 2007. Physiology and immunology of the cholinergic anti-inflammatory pathway. J. Clin. Invest. 117 (2), 289–296.

Tsao, H., Hodges, P.W., 2007. Persistence of improvements in postural strategies following motor control training in people with recurrent low back pain. J. Electromyogr. Kinesiol. 18 (4), 559–567.

Twomey, L.T., Taylor, J.R., 2005. Physical Therapy of the low back, 3rd edn. Churchill Livingstone, Edinburgh.

UK BEAM Trial Team, 2004. United Kingdom back pain exercise and manipulation (UK BEAM) randomised trial: effectiveness of physical treatments for back pain in primary care. Br. Med. J. 329, 1377–1385.

Ulett, G.A., Han, S., 2002. The biology of acupuncture. Warren H Green, St Louis, MO.

Van Dieen, J.H., Selen, L.P., Cholewicki, J., 2003. Trunk muscle activation in low-back pain patients, an analysis of the literature. J. Electromyogr. Kinesiol. 13, 333–351.

Van Dillen, S., Gombotto, D., Collins, J., et al., 2007. Symmetry of timing of hip and lumbopelvic rotation motion in 2 different subgroups of people with low back pain. Arch. Phys. Med. Rehabil. 88, 351–360.

Van Tulder, M.W., Koes, B.W., Bouter, L.M., 1997. Conservative treatment of acute and chronic non-specific low back pain. A systematic review of randomized controlled trials of the most common interventions. Spine 22, 2128–2156.

Van Tulder, M.W., Becker, A., Bekkering, T., et al., 2006. European guidelines for the management of acute non-specific low back pain in primary care. Eur. Spine J. 15 (Suppl. 2), 168–184.

Vleeming, A., Albert, H.B., Ostgaard, H.C., et al., 2008. European guidelines for the diagnosis and treatment of pelvic girdle pain. Eur. Spine J. 17, 794–819.

Waddell, G., 1998. The problem, social interactions, treatment: the scientific evidence In: Waddell, G. (Ed.), The back pain revolution. Churchill Livingstone, Edinburgh, pp. 1–8, 204-205, 265-267.

Wall, P.D., 1978. The gait control theory of pain. Brain 101, 1–18.

Wall, P.D., Melzack, R., Bonica, J.J., 1984. Textbook of pain. Churchill Livingstone, Edinburgh.

Watson P 2007 Managing low back pain from a cognitive perspective. In Proceedings of the 6th Interdisciplinary World Congress on Low Back and Pelvic Pain, Barcelona.

Yan, B., Li, K., Xu, J., et al., 2005. Acupoint specific MRI patterns in human brain. Neurosci. Lett. 383, 236–240.

8

The sacroiliac joint and pelvis

Howard Turner

CHAPTER CONTENTS

Introduction

The pelvis has a curious place in the history of manual therapy. Perhaps more than any other joint complex in the body there is a mystique about the relevance of disorders of the sacroiliac joint (SIJ) and pubis, and confusion about their management. However, there is a growing body of evidence to support the notion that disorders of the pelvis form a significant pain subgroup and increasing insight into appropriate approaches to management. The SIJ is a well-documented source of buttock and leg pain in cases of chronic low back pain, pregnancy-related pain, post-partum pain, and chronic groin pain in athletes. Furthermore, there is evidence that SIJ pain and dysfunction are associated with a disruption of normal neuromuscular control of the trunk, the hip, and the knee, and this may be related to the pathogenesis of symptoms in these areas.

Manual therapy to the region aims to restore normal movement and alignment to the pelvis, and improve stability through rehabilitation. The biomechanical literature provides some support for the application of manual therapy, but little work has been published to validate it. However, there is support for rehabilitation incorporating motor learning strategies to improve the activation of the core musculature.

Clinical relevance

The SIJ is a relatively common cause of pain. Fluoroscopically guided anaesthetic injections suggest that 15–25% of chronic low back pain emanates from the SIJ (Maigne et al 1996; Schwarzer et al 1995). The incidence of pelvic-mediated pain is probably higher in the population with pregnancy-related low back and pelvic pain. Half or more of all pregnant women develop low back and pelvic pain (Bjorklund & Bergström 2000; Kristiansson et al 1996; Ostgaard et al 1991), and based on their clinical presentation, it has been estimated that around 50% of these individuals have symptoms emanating from the SIJ and pubis (Ostgaard et al 1991). Anecdotal suggestions that pelvis-related pain accounts for a proportion of groin and proximal lower-limb presentations in the sporting population have been strengthened by a recent study on groin pain by Mens et al (2006). Some 26% of the athletes in this study had a reduction of symptoms on the application of an SIJ stabilization belt when provoked using manually resisted adduction. Adduction force also improved, suggesting that either the pelvis is the source of pain or the mechanism of pain production is related in some other way to SIJ stability (Mens et al 2006).

As well as being clinically relevant because of its capacity to produce pain, dysfunction of movement and control of the pelvis may be clinically relevant to the development or maintenance of symptoms elsewhere. SIJ motion is considered to be important for shock absorbance during weight-bearing activities (Adams et al 2002), and therefore, a disruption to normal movement may mechanically and adversely affect adjacent structures. There also appears to be neuromuscular relationships. Hungerford et al (2003) identified disrupted neuromuscular control of the trunk and hip in a group of subjects with possible SIJ pain, and O'Sullivan et al (2002) identified disrupted respiratory and pelvic floor function in a similar population. Marshall and Murphy (2006) showed that manipulation of the SIJ can reverse timing deficits in the anterolateral abdominals, and Suter et al (1999) showed that it can improve the electromyographic activity of the vastii and extensor strength at the knee in anterior knee pain patients. These are intriguing results that help to support anecdotal evidence of a relationship between pelvic dysfunction and an array of other pain patterns.

The clinical picture

The availability of motion at the SIJ is well established (Jacob & Kissling 1995; Sturesson et al 1989; Vleeming et al 1992a). It is a synovial joint, but it is also surrounded by a strong capsuloligamentous complex so movement is limited. The best estimates of motion come from studies that have radiographically tracked the movement of implanted metalwork. In weight-bearing, these studies identify only small amounts of movement, on average 2° of rotation and 2 mm of translation (Jacob & Kissling 1995; Sturesson et al 1989, 2000; Vleeming et al 1992a). Studies of passive movement in fresh cadavers reveal more movement and a greater variation of movement, i.e. 3° to 17° of rotation (Smidt et al 1997).

Doppler studies have investigated the stiffness of the SIJ by measuring the conduction of vibration across the joint; if the vibration is conducted intact the joint is stiffer than if it attenuates as it crosses the joint (Buyruk et al 1999). The most interesting work has looked at the characteristics of the postpartum pelvic pain population. Contrary to popular conception, the difference between women in pain and those that are not is not that they are more mobile, but that they have asymmetrical stiffness values side to side (Damen et al 2001, 2002).

There are several features of the emerging understanding of the SIJ's stability mechanisms that are relevant to clinical practice. Arguably the most important amongst them is that the joint's stability is under dynamic muscular control. A number of muscles have the capacity to compressively stabilize the joint, from the inner core and pelvic floor to more superficial muscles, such as the gluteus maximus, the long head of biceps femoris, and the latissimus dorsi (Pool-Goudzwaard et al 2004; Richardson et al 2002; Snijders et al 1993a,b, 1998, 2006; van Wingerden et al 2004; Vleeming et al 1990a, 1992b). Deficits in neuromuscular control are implicated strongly in the pathogenesis of pain and dysfunction of this area.

Diagnosis

A clinical protocol for diagnosing pain of SIJ origin has also become clearer in the past few years. Recent injection studies have shown that a clinical examination incorporating provocation testing (Fig. 8.1) of the SIJ can accurately identify individuals with SIJ-mediated pain (Laslett et al 2003, 2005a,b; Petersen et al 2004; Young et al 2003). The clinical picture of SIJ-mediated pain that has arisen from these studies is one of unilateral pain with no referral up into the lumbar spine. Pain is often focused over the involved joint, and the sacral sulcus is often tender. Pain may refer down the lower limb and into the foot (Dreyfuss et al 1996; Fortin et al 1994a,b, Maigne et al 1996; Schwarzer et al 1995; Slipman et al 2000; van der Wurff et al 2006; Young et al 2003). Whilst it is very common for SIJ-mediated pain to be centred over the joint, it is worth noting that both this and tenderness of the sacral sulcus have low specificity to SIJ pain involvement (Dreyfuss et al 1996).

Traditionally, the diagnosis of SIJ dysfunction has been made by a palpation assessment of movement at the joint (Bourdillon et al 1992; DiGiovanna & Schiowitz 1999; Fowler 1986; Lee 1999; Mitchell & Mitchell 1999) (Figs. 8.2 and 8.3). Both the reliability and validity of this assessment have been questioned (Dreyfuss et al 1994; Egan et al 1996; Sturesson et al 2000; van der Wurff et al 2000a,b).

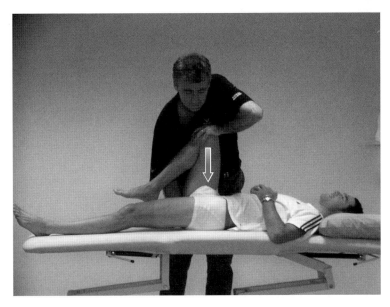

Figure 8.1 • Pain provocation test.

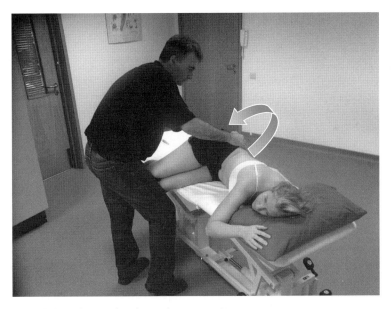

Figure 8.2 • Treatment technique for restricted sacral movement.

Several studies have shown that the individual tests have poor reliability, but perhaps there may be more promise in using a composite of tests in assessment, as happens clinically (Cibulka et al 1988; Cibulka & Koldehoff 1999; Fritz et al 1992; Tong et al 2006). The validity of these tests has been questioned on two fronts. Some investigators query the specificity of the tests because a high proportion of the pain-free population test positive, but this may simply be an indication that dysfunction can occur with or without pain. Others point to the fact that very little joint motion has been identified in movement studies of weight-bearing active movement, and suggest that the therapist's impression of joint movement is an illusion (Sturesson et al 2000). Unfortunately, the studies on motion have not

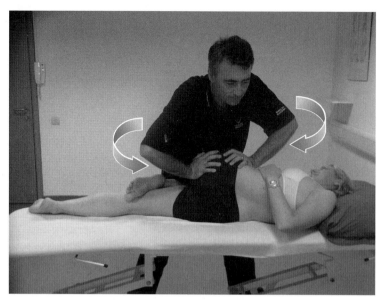

Figure 8.3 • Muscle energy technique for backward sacral torsion.

looked at the tests as they are performed clinically, and therefore, it is not clear that the results apply. Further work is warranted since these are commonly used clinical tools.

Recently, another test of SIJ dysfunction has evolved, the active straight leg raise test (ASLR). This test involves asking the patient to report on the effort involved in lifting each leg 5 to 20 cm off the bed from a relaxed supine position (Mens et al 1999). The ASLR is considered positive if the subject's perceived effort is altered when a compressive force is applied to the pelvis to stabilize the SIJ (Mens et al 1999; O'Sullivan & Beales 2007a). The test has been shown to be reliable and valid in discriminating between those with pregnancy-related pelvic pain and those without pain (Mens et al 2001). Moreover the perceived effort correlates well with the severity of symptoms and the degree of disability (Mens et al 2002), and it has been shown to correspond to hip flexion force output in that group of patients (de Groot et al 2006). It has been proposed that the ASLR identifies deficits in local muscle control, a proposition supported by the fact that aberrant muscle recruitment strategies have been identified in subjects with SIJ pain who test positive on these tests resolve on manual compression of the pelvis, and evidence that motor control rehabilitation strategies can resolve both the aberrant muscle activity and the effort of the ASLR manoeuvre (O'Sullivan et al 2002; O'Sullivan & Beales 2007a).

It has been suggested that the ASLR may be a valid tool with which to monitor the improvement of patients through treatment and rehabilitation (O'Sullivan & Beales 2007a; Stuge et al 2004a,b).

Manual therapy

Manual therapy may involve manipulation or mobilization techniques to resolve movement restrictions and soft tissue techniques to improve muscle function. Whilst widely accepted as being beneficial, at least in the short term (O'Sullivan & Beales 2007b; Stuge et al 2003; Tullberg et al 1998), the nature of the effect of manual therapy is the subject of some debate. Traditional descriptions suggest that mobilization can correct the alignment of the joint if it is applied in a direction to oppose asymmetries of position (Bourdillon et al 1992; DiGiovanna & Schiowitz 1997; Fowler 1986; Lee 1999; Mitchell & Mitchell 1999). This concept that the effect of treatment will be direction-specific, i.e. that it will vary depending on the direction of the applied manual force, is not without merit. For example, it is known that stability of the pelvis is direction-specific. The ligaments connecting the innominate to the sacrum are arranged in such a way that movement of the joint in one direction serves to compress and stabilize the pelvis, and the opposite movement disengages joint compression

(Snijders et al 1993a,b; Vleeming et al 1990a,b). Specifically, a relative posterior rotation of the innominate or nutation of the sacrum increases joint compression and posterior rotation decompresses the joint. Research on the ASLR has shown that joint compression can alter the recruitment of the lumbopelvic musculature (O'Sullivan et al 2002; O'Sullivan & Beales 2007a), and therefore it seems reasonable to propose that, if manual techniques can indeed alter the alignment and orientation of the joint, they may create changes in the activation of the surrounding musculature, to the potential benefit of the patient.

However, there is no evidence that manipulation and mobilization can change the position of the SIJ. In fact, X-ray imaging of implanted metalwork has demonstrated the opposite, i.e. no change in joint position after treatment, as measured in standing (Tullberg et al 1998). Interestingly, a palpation-detectable change in the position of the bony landmarks of the pelvis has been demonstrated when subjects have been reassessed in non-weight-bearing positions (Ellis et al 2003). One possible explanation for these apparently conflicting results is that, rather than altering the position of the joint per se, manual therapy may create a change in the directional strain upon the pelvis that is associated with changes in the activity of the surrounding trunk and pelvic musculature. The directional strain may be what is detected as asymmetries of pelvic position on clinical assessment (O'Sullivan & Beales 2007b).

Neuromuscular effects such as this have been demonstrated in recent research on manipulation. Manipulation of the SIJ has been shown to improve the feed-forward activation of the anterolateral abdominal muscles in an asymptomatic group (Marshall & Murphy 2006) and to improve the activation of the vastii and knee extensor torque in a group of patients with anterior knee (Suter et al 1999). These are intriguing results, but unfortunately both studies included only immediate post-intervention measures so there is no indication of the longevity of these effects.

The mechanism of these neuromuscular responses may be explained by a study on the porcine SIJ. Stimulation of the joint capsule and joint produced a response in the surrounding musculature and the muscles involved in the response varied, depending on the location of the stimulus (Indahl et al 1999). This suggests that the SIJ and its capsule play a role in the regulation of the activity of the surrounding musculature. Indahl et al (1999) suggested that abnormal loading on these structures in the dysfunctional pelvis may mediate the aberrant patterns of neuromuscular control seen in patients and that manual therapy may normalize the loads on the joint, capsule, and surrounding ligaments. The challenge to the therapist is to choose the treatment most likely to benefit the patient. Traditionally this has been done by a manual evaluation of the pelvis, an assessment that has, by and large, been shown to have poor inter-tester reliability (Potter & Rothstein 1985; van der Wurff et al 2000a). A recently suggested alternative is to perform techniques in a trial-and-error fashion, and to be guided by the patient's response (Horton & Franz 2007).

Rehabilitation

There is a growing body of literature to guide rehabilitation of the painful pelvis, although it focuses almost exclusively on pregnancy-related and postpartum pelvic pain. Various exercise protocols have been investigated. More general and strengthening exercise has not been shown to be of benefit. In pregnancy-related pain for example, exercise regimes incorporating strengthening exercises for the abdominals and gluteal muscles (Elden et al 2007), a home exercise regime of exercises performed with a ball between the knees in sitting, standing, and 4-point kneeling position with movements of the arms and legs (Nilsson-Wikmar et al 2005), and submaximal lateral pull-downs, standing leg-press, sit-down rowing, and curl-ups (Nilsson-Wikmar et al 2005), have been investigated with no measurable benefit. A general exercise class was also shown to provide no benefit with regard to function or pain (Dumas et al 1995). In postpartum pain, the efficacy of an exercise programme incorporating trunk-curl exercises and bridging, and one incorporating diagonal trunk-curls and diagonal extension (lifting one shoulder and the opposite leg off the supporting surface from a prone lying starting position), have been assessed with no measurable benefit compared to no exercise (Mens et al 2000). However, more specific exercise programmes that focus on the initiation of pelvic floor and anterolateral abdominal muscle activation do show promise. In a study of postpartum pelvic pain, Stuge et al (2004b) showed that a 20-week intervention that initially focused on specific activation of the transverse abdominal muscles produced significant benefits with respect to pain, functional status, and health-related quality of life compared to an intervention that did not include such specific stabilizing exercises. The group who performed the specific stabilizing exercises maintained their improvement, and were significantly better at both the 1- and 2-year follow-ups. An improvement in pain with a specific stabilizing exercise intervention has also been demonstrated in pelvic pain during pregnancy, but there is no indication of the longevity of that improvement (Elden et al 2005).

Conclusion

There is a growing understanding of the way in which disorders of the pelvis manifest and clinical tools for their assessment are developing. Disruptions to the neuromuscular control of the trunk and pelvis seem strongly related to the development of dysfunction in the area and rehabilitation principles for their management are being defined. It seems clear from the evidence to date that rehabilitation must specifically target the recruitment of the anterolateral abdominals and pelvic floor muscles.

Whilst there is a general acceptance that manual therapy to the pelvis can be of benefit, there is little consensus on the nature of its effect, and as yet, no evidence of long-term benefit. The improvements in neuromuscular function that have been noted with manual therapy interventions may indicate that it can provide a window of opportunity for the restoration of more normal neuromuscular function when combined with rehabilitation. The ASLR appears to be an appropriate test for these changes in neuromuscular function.

8.1   Acupuncture in pelvic dysfunction

Jennie Longbottom

Within the sporting world, a staggering 58% of UK professional soccer players have reported a history of sports-related groin injury (Karlssonn et al 1994). Much of the pain experienced in such cases is referred from adjacent or even remote myofascial and articular structures, and involves extensive release, muscle re-education, and functional restoration of the entire complex of shortened muscles. It must also be considered that myofascial trigger points (MTrPts) in the region of the abdominal muscles and pelvis can cause abnormal function in the visceral organs that has a somatovisceral effect, and that may mimic gynaecological conditions or symptoms presented to general surgeons, such as vomiting and diarrhoea. King et al (1991) found that 70% of subjects with pelvic pain reported complete or significant relief of their symptoms when the musculoskeletal dysfunction found during physiotherapy assessment was evaluated and treated. MTrPts may have a profound effect on urinary dysfunction, where those along the suprapubic rim involving the insertions of rectus abdominus, internal oblique, and transversus muscles can cause increased sensitivity, and spasms of the urinary bladder and sphincter, resulting in urgency, frequency, urinary retention, and pain. How many male patients are given the diagnosis of prostatitis without adequate attention to and assessment of the myofascial component before more invasive medical testing is offered? Both MTrPt needling and muscle energy techniques may be effective in relieving pain and discomfort, restoring normal muscle length, and facilitating rehabilitation. This comprehensive clinical reasoning approach to pain with myofascial origins may make it possible to provide relief and management of the pelvic region without surgical or diagnostic intervention.

Although athletic injuries around the hip and groin occur less commonly than injuries in the extremities, they can result in extensive rehabilitation time and considerable cost (Anderson et al 2001). Accurate diagnosis and treatment plans are essential, together with adequate management of pain-propagating structures in order to facilitate re-education and rehabilitation. Pelvic anatomical, biomechanical, and pain-propagating structures are amongst the most complex in the musculoskeletal system, offering many challenges to management protocols. A multidisciplinary approach is often necessary for optimal management of complex athletic injuries (Anderson et al 2001) (Table 8.1).

Table 8.1 Common disorders of hip and groin region

Acute injuries	Treatment priority
Muscle strain	Prevention
Trigger point dysfunction	Pain modification Muscle imbalance re-education
Contusions	Minimize bruising and muscle spasm Prevention of haematoma formation Rest and NWB Rehabilitation
Avulsions and apophyseal Injuries	More common in skeletal immaturity Reduce tenderness and swelling Rehabilitation
Hip dislocations and subluxations	Pain relief PWB 6–8 weeks Rehabilitation
Acetabular labral tears and loose bodies	Pain modification PWB 4 weeks Local anaesthetic injection Surgical option
Proximal femur fractures	Surgical management Rehabilitation
Insidious Onset	
Sports hernia and athletic pubalgia	Pain modification Address pelvic imbalance Rehabilitation
Osteitis Pubis/ Bursitis	Pain modification Address instability of Pubic Symphysis SIJs Rehabilitation
Snapping hip syndrome	Pain modification Rest Trigger point deactivation ITB, TFL
Osteoarthritis	Treatment involving pain propagating structures L1-L3
Lumbar and SI disorders	Address any nerve entrapment/ compression of nerves from trigger points
Entrapment of nerve structures	

Adapted from Anderson et al (2001).

Table 8.2 Pelvic Meridians and He Sea Points

Meridian	Anatomical supply	He Sea point
Spleen	Medial aspect leg, groin Anterior medial aspect abdominal wall	SP9
Stomach	Anterior aspect of Groin Anterior abdominal Wall Chest Face	ST36
Liver	Medial aspect of leg and Groin Anterior lateral aspect abdominal wall and Chest	LIV8
Kidney	Posterior medial aspect of foot and leg groin Anterolateral aspect Stomach and Chest	KID10
Conception Vessel (Ren)	Pubic Symphysis Anterior abdominal and Chest	CV6
Bladder	Posterior aspect of Cervical, Thoracic, and Sacrum Posterior lateral aspect of lower limb	BL40
Gall Bladder	Lateral aspect of lower limb, hip trunk Shoulder, neck, and head	GB34

The scope for acupuncture intervention in cases of acute and chronic pain management is extensive and will facilitate enhanced speed of rehabilitation. The pelvis has extensive meridian involvement, and a number of significant acupuncture points are available to improve blood flow, facilitate phagocytic activity, and restore muscle length (Lundeberg 1998) (Table 8.2). The complete pattern of muscle and joint dysfunction should be addressed to successfully treat subjects with hip and groin pain. Rehabilitation should generally be complete within 10 weeks if patients adhere to stretching and muscle imbalance regimes. Reoccurrence is not common and usually involves further injury, especially if abnormal foot mechanics are contributing to the problem and have not been addressed.

The presentation of pelvic and low back pain (LBP) is even more common in pregnancy (Kvoring et al 2004). Traditionally, needling has been contraindicated during the first trimester of pregnancy in acupuncture and physiotherapy (AACP 2004). However, within the past few years, there has been a growing demand from patients seeking acupuncture to address musculoskeletal pain management during pregnancy (Boylan 2006; Lee 2005; Manheimer et al 2008; Rouse 2008), and as a means of offering safe alternatives to medicinal management (Betts 2006;

Laing 2006; Roemer 2000). As yet, there is no evidence that acupuncture can harm a healthy pregnancy (Roemer 2000). Therefore, physiotherapists who have been trained in the management of acupuncture within pregnancy should consider this modality as a safe and effective management of pain for the pregnant patient.

The incidence of women who experience pelvic pain and LBP in pregnancy ranges from 24 to 90% for different population samples in both retrospective and prospective studies (Endersen 1955; Ostgaard & Andersson 1991). It was commonly regarded that since pregnancy has a limited time span, it was better to leave the condition to resolve or to treat it postpartum because overzealous intervention may constitute a danger to the foetus (Heckman & Sassard 1994). In fact, the evidence now suggests that management of musculoskeletal dysfunction, pain, and joint limitations is essential during pregnancy in order to facilitate an easier birth and prevent the development of chronic postpartum conditions (Ostgaard & Andersson 1992), a position supported by a growing number of studies indicating that acupuncture is safe and effective technique for the management of pelvic pain (da Silva et al 2004; Elden et al 2005) (Table 8.3).

Table 8.3 Acupuncture and pain in pregnancy

Date	Study	RCT	Outcome
2008	Elden et al	Standard care + acupuncture (n = 125), Standard care + stabilizing exercises (n = 131) Standard care (n = 130).	No difference in Rx groups Irrespective of modality, regression of pelvic girdle pain occurs in the great majority of women within 12 weeks after delivery.
2008	Manheimer et al Systematic Review	8 trials (1305 participants)	Acupuncture superior to standard care
2007	Pennick et al Systematic Review	8 trials (1305 participants)	Acupuncture 60% improvement Standard care 14%
2006	Lund et al	Needling techniques Superficial (n = 22) Deep (n = 25)	No differences between superficial and deep acupuncture stimulation modes were observed.
2005	Kim et al	n = 386 Standard care (n = 130) Standard care + acupuncture (n = 125)	Acupuncture + stabilizing exercises superior to standard care
2004	da Sailva et al	Acupuncture group (n = 61) Standard care (n = 27) Control (n = 34)	Acupuncture 78% pain decrease Standard care = 15% pain decrease ($p < 0.0001$)

Case Study 1

Cathie Morrow

Introduction

A 62-year-old female presented to the clinic with acute on chronic SIJ dysfunction caused by a hypomobile L5–S1 facet joint. The subject's X-ray findings highlighted lower lumbar osteoarthritis. The present case report concentrates on the use of acupuncture to aid pain relief when used in addition to manual therapy since there is evidence that acupuncture, in combination with other conventional therapies, relieves pain and improves function better than the conventional therapies alone (Furlan 2005; Thomas et al 2005). Treatment included manual therapy and a home exercise regime, but the most dramatic reduction in pain occurred when

acupuncture was introduced. Both local and distal points were used for the best effect (Bowsher 1998).

Subjective assessment

A 62-year-old female yoga instructor presented for physiotherapy with left-sided SIJ pain of 3-year duration and reported worsening symptoms over the past 2 months (Table 8.4). On examination, her pain was located over the SIJ. She described it as an intense ache with occasional sharp pain on movement and rated as 70/100 on the Visual Analogue Scale (VAS) (White 1998). She rated the severity as moderate and she was not taking any analgesics; irritability was reported as

(Continued)

Case Study 1 (Continued)

Table 8.4 Presenting Problems

Problem	Aim of treatment
Sacroiliac pain	Reduce pain
Sleep disturbance	Improve sleep pattern
Leg cramps	Reduce cramps
Reduced function	Improve function

moderate. The subject described cramping sensations down the posterior aspect of her left leg and mentioned that her feet always felt cold. Her symptoms were aggravated when she moved from sitting to standing, and were particularly severe first thing in the morning, lasting for a maximum of 2 hours. The symptoms were eased after 30 minutes of heat packs and hot baths. She experienced sleep disturbance, only managing a maximum of 5 hours sleep a night, which indicated an inflammatory element to her pain.

The subject's past medical history included a fall 15 years previously that had resulted in a fractured coccyx, followed by a further fall onto a hard stone floor 3 years before. She had received osteopathic treatment and acupuncture in the past, but had gained little benefit from the treatment. There were no other medical problems, no signs of cauda equina syndrome or cord compression and all red-flag questioning was negative. X-rays highlighted reduced disc space at L5–S1 with some osteophytic lipping.

Objective assessment

The objective assessment identified the following:
- The subject's lumbar range of movement (ROM) was limited in flexion; her fingertips could only reach to the upper third of her thigh.
- Extension was limited; her fingertips could only reach her gluteal crease.
- SIJ tests revealed a hypomobile left sacrum on her ilium.
- Her ASLR test was to 80° on the left and 90° on the right.
- Neurological testing was unremarkable.
- Peripheral pulses were present.
- Palpation revealed a deeper right sacral sulcus that increased on extension.
- A stiff left L5–S1 facet joint at early ROM.
- There was pain on palpation locally over the left SIJ, at early ROM.

Clinical impression

A diagnosis of left backward sacral torsion was made, the left sacrum being held back by a stiff left L5–S1 facet joint (Figs. 8.4 and 8.5).

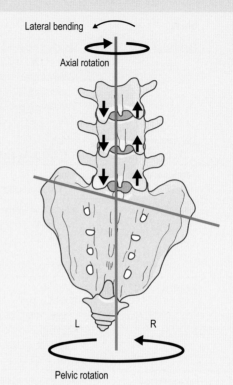

Figure 8.4 • Sacral torsion.

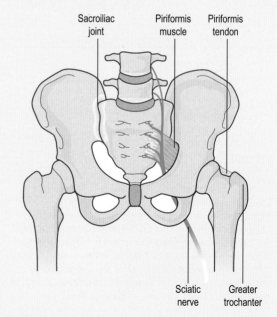

Figure 8.5 • L5–S1 impact on pelvis.

(Continued)

Case Study 1 (Continued)

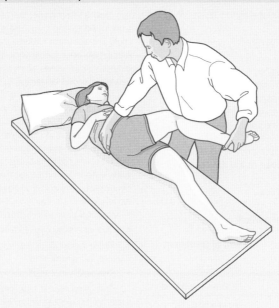

Figure 8.6 • Mobilizing treatment technique for the ilium.

Although the subject had suffered from long-standing symptoms of SIJ, this episode was classed as an acute flare-up. She had an inflammatory component to her symptoms highlighted by sleep disturbance, and pain and stiffness first thing in the morning. The condition was classed as nociceptive pain (Baldry 1993).

Manual therapy

The first four treatment sessions took place at weekly intervals and consisted of:

- Rotation mobilizations to the left L5–S1 facet in order to reduce joint hypomobility;
- Muscle energy techniques employed to improve the backward sacral torsion (Fig. 8.6); and
- A home exercise programme including core stability work and mobilizing exercises.

Subjective outcome

The subject reported the following outcomes. Her pain reduced to 600/100 (VAS), but remained variable. She still experienced difficulty teaching yoga. Her sleep pattern improved, but she complained of feeling lethargic during the day, indicating that she probably was not experiencing true rapid eye movement during the night. The amount of pain was still an issue first thing in the morning, but lasted only for 30 minutes.

Objective outcome

The subject's lumbar flexion had increased enough to allow her to touch the lower third of her thigh. Palpation revealed stiffness at half-range over the L5–S1 facet,

and pain was still reproducible on palpation of the left SIJ at half range.

Although her symptoms had improved, it was felt that acupuncture should be used as an adjunct to manual therapy to aid pain relief (Watkin 2004) (Table 8.5). This option was discussed in detail with the subject. She was very sceptical, having undergone acupuncture in the past with little relief. Both segmental and extrasegmental acupuncture points were chosen for the most effective pain relief (Bowsher 1998) (Table 8.6). Points to aid relaxation and improve sleep were also used following the manual therapy intervention, and she was advised to complete her home exercises as normal.

Post acupuncture subjective outcome

Following acupuncture intervention, the following subjective markers were reported:

- Her pain had reduced from 60/100 to 30/100 (VAS);
- She reported deep sleep for 15 hours;
- She had doubled the number of yoga classes taught every week;
- She was now able to sit cross-legged on the floor for the first time in 18 months;
- She was still complaining of occasional cramps; and
- She remained sore first thing in the morning.

Post acupuncture objective outcome

The following objective markers were observed:

- Lumbar ROM of flexion allowed her to reach her upper third of tibia;

(Continued)

Case Study 1 (Continued)

- Palpation of L5–S1 facet joint was tender at 3/4 of range; and
- There was increased sacral mobility on kinetic testing.

Further points were added once it was known that the subject was a good responder. These were indicated to reduce leg cramps and inflammation. The same manual treatment as previously was carried out along with the acupuncture points listed in Table 8.7.

The following subjective outcomes were reported by the patient: pain had reduced to 20/100 (VAS),

leg cramps had gone, the feet felt warmer, function continued to improve. The subject reported taking two high-impact yoga classes with no side effects, and that sleep had been undisturbed for a week. The following objective outcomes were observed: the subject's lumbar flexion allowed fingertips to reach the ankle, full vertebral ROM, and palpation at the L5–S1 facet provoked no pain. The SIJ kinetic tests joint movement was normal, and an ASLR of 90° was achieved.

Subjective and objective signs continued to improve; therefore, manual treatment and acupuncture points were kept the same, as was treatment time. Following four combined manual and acupuncture treatments, the subject's overall improvements were as follows:

- Reduction in pain from 70/100 to 10/100 (VAS);
- She was sleeping up to 7 hours a night;
- There were no further incidents of leg cramps and her feet felt warm; and
- She was teaching four yoga classes a week.

This case report highlights the value of combined treatments and the value of acupuncture as a pain-modulating intervention when used within manual therapy management.

Table 8.5 Acupuncture Intervention

Problem	Aim of treatment
Deficient Qi	Increase Qi
Reduced blood flow	Increase blood flow
Excessive heat (inflammatory)	Reduce heat
Excessive cold (OA and Osteopenia)	Reduce cold

Table 8.6 Acupuncture Point Rationale

Segmental points	Outcome	Clinical reasoning
HJJ L5–S1 (bilateral) BL25 (bilateral) BL28 (left)	De Qi achieved. Better quality movement lumbar flexion. Easier putting socks on.	Used to influence pain-gate mechanism. Improve local blood supply. Reduces inflammation (Hecker et al 2001).
Extrasegmental points SP6 (left) LIV3 (bilateral)		Regulates Qi and blood flow through pelvis. Calms mind and assists sleep. Reduces inflammation (Hecker et al 2001).

Table 8.7 Subsequent acupuncture rationale

Points used	Outcome	Clinical reasoning
HJJ L5–S1 (bilateral)		
BL25 (bilateral) BL28 (left) BL40 (left) BL62 (left) SP6 (left) LIV3 (bilateral)	De Qi achieved. Improved flexibility with SIJ kinetic tests. Felt more comfortable getting dressed.	Segmental pain gate inhibition. He Sea point improves circulation to lower leg, reduces cramp. Descending inhibition. Calms the mind (Hecker et al 2001).

Case Study 2

Daniel Christopher Martin

Introduction

The following case study describes the treatment of a 24-year-old rugby player with chronic groin pain. The symptoms resulted in severe pain and movement restriction, and interfered with everyday functional activities. A treatment regime incorporating acupuncture as an adjunct to other physiotherapy modalities was utilized. The regime brought positive results and allowed the player to return to competitive rugby.

Subjective assessment

The subject presented with an 18-month history of groin pain. He had already undergone an inguinal release in an attempt to resolve the condition, and when he was reviewed 4 months later, he was given some postoperative physiotherapy. He continued to experience pain and had difficulty with activities of daily living (ADL), especially turning in bed and sitting up without pain. His pain was constant through the day. The subject had no significant past medical history. He described the pain as moderate to severe, (VAS) 50/100, depending on the type of activity. Driving for longer than 20 minutes resulted in a VAS of 80/100. The main aggravating factor was twisting and turning activities.

Objective assessment

The objective assessment of the subject revealed the following:
- Pelvic asymmetry with anterior tilt on the left ilium and sacrum;
- A reduced range of movement of the lumbar spine;
- Tight muscle groups especially hip flexors, abductors, and rotators in left and right limbs;
- Marked muscular bulk asymmetry with the left side dominant over right;
- A positive resisted adduction squeeze test (Fig. 8.7);
- A positive hip impingement greater on the left than on the right;
- Active MTrPts in the adductors, as well as the rectus abdominus and iliopsoas muscles;
- A negative cough impulse;
- The Flexion, Abduction and External Rotation (FABER) (Fig. 8.8) test positive on bilateral testing (left greater than right); and
- A bilateral positive result on the Trendelenberg sign (Fig. 8.9).

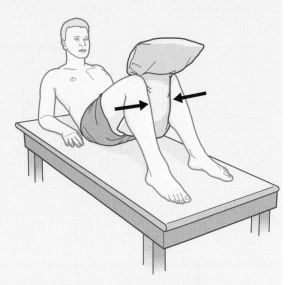

Figure 8.7 • Squeeze test.

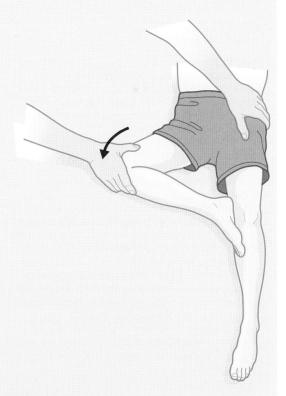

Figure 8.8 • Faber test.

(*Continued*)

Case Study 2 (Continued)

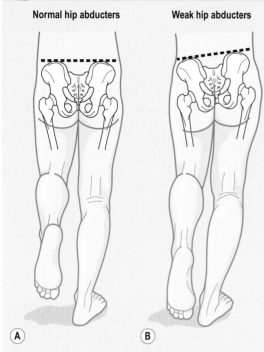

Normal hip abducters | Weak hip abducters

(A) (B)

Figure 8.9 • Trendelenberg test.

Diagnosis

From the subjective and objective assessments, a diagnosis of chronic osteitis pubis was reached. The most probable causes were gluteal muscle weakness and core deficit leading to excessive adductor spasm and shear on the pubic symphysis.

Osteitis pubis is a condition that has been poorly understood until recently, and as a result, poorly treated. Once the condition has been labelled, the prescribed treatment invariably involves prolonged rest. Unfortunately, this treatment is frequently met with a recurrence of pain once the offending activity has been recommended. Osteitis pubis is defined as a pathological process involving the pubic bone and pubic symphysis (Brukner & Khan 2002). The inflammation of the symphysis can lead to sclerosis and bony changes within the region. The factors thought to contribute to the condition include muscle spasm in the adductor and abdominal muscle groups, and shearing forces across the pubic symphysis (Rodriguez et al 2001).

The clinical signs of osteitis pubis are as follows:
- Pain on passive hip abduction;
- Pain and weakness with resisted adductor contraction;
- A positive squeeze test;
- Pain on resisted hip flexion;

- Adductor muscle guarding on passive combined hip external rotation and abduction; and
- Pain on resisted hip flexion adduction in the Thomas test position.

A progressive return to activity is supported by manual therapy, including spinal mobilization; massage therapy to the psoas, adductor, and abdominal muscle groups; and neural stretches. This needs to be accompanied by an aggressive and progressive abdominal strengthening program. The first six sessions focused on stretching and soft tissue mobilization of hip flexors, adductors, gluteal and oblique abdominal muscles. The subject was given a stretching programme. Over the 6 weeks he showed a marked improvement in symptoms, scoring 30/100 on the VAS, reporting no pain during ADL. He also demonstrated improved muscle ROM. At this stage, the subject was still having problems with attempting any gluteal muscle strengthening work, and was unable to perform a side-lying gluteal exercise because of pain inhibition from his perineum. Pelvic floor and core strengthening was introduced alongside the ongoing flexibility program. A return to function was also advocated and a walk-jog programme was implemented. The subject was given instructions about ensuring that he did not aggravate pubic pain during the programme.

The patient had improved over the preceding 3 weeks and was able to jog for 15 minutes without significant post-running effects. The squeeze test was positive, and he reported ongoing tightness and soreness through the adductor muscles. Acupuncture was not considered as the first line of treatment because of the significant biomechanical and structural problems that the subject was experiencing; however, acupuncture is extremely effective for the treatment of MTrPts and alleviating muscle spasm. This would prove to be particularly useful for relieving the adductor issues around the subject's pelvis.

The subject presented with a chronic condition that may well have led to changes in bony and muscle tissue over the 18 months of its course. Over a period of time, a patient's pain mechanisms change, and therefore, it is important to adapt the focus of acupuncture intervention to reflect the changing physiology of pain presentation. The aim of acupuncture was to balance the dysfunctional physiological mechanisms within the relevant tissues and central nervous system. The overriding pain mechanism was nociceptive pain, which has been demonstrated to respond positively to acupuncture treatment (Lundeberg et al 1988). The other possible contributor to the pain mechanism may have been centrally evoked pain. The chronicity of the problem could have led to sensitization of the spinal cord and areas of the sensory cortex in the brain; however, should the appropriate biomechanical issues resolve

(Continued)

Case Study 2 (Continued)

Table 8.8 Trigger point rationale

Muscles needled treatments	Outcome
Adductor longus & pectineus MTrPts	Improved AST
Adductor longus proximally (2 points) & pectineus muscles MTrPts	Improved power on gluteal muscle testing in side lying
Adductor longus proximally (3 points) & pectineus muscles MTrPts	Improved power on gluteal muscle testing in side lying

Notes: AST, adductor squeeze test.

themselves then this pain mechanism will become less of an issue. There has been research to suggest that slow-healing musculoskeletal conditions might be related to inhibition of the sympathetic nervous system (SNS), leading to trophic changes in target tissues (Bekkering & van Bussel 1998). Again, the subject displayed few SNS symptoms, but this would be something to be mindful of should his condition begin to plateau. Ceccherelli et al (2002) has suggested that deep acupuncture was more effective than more superficial techniques in the more chronic conditions, and thus deep MTrPt needling was again applied to maximize local effects.

The subject was given a positive diagnosis of myofascial pain syndrome (MFPS) as a part of his osteitis pubis and it was decided that acupuncture would be the most appropriate way of deactivation of the positive MTrPt (Table 8.8), and restoration of muscle length for full rehabilitation to be achieved. Diagnosis of the MTrPt was made through the production of the following signs on palpation: sensitivity to touch; the presence of a taut band in the muscle; palpation of an active trigger point; reproduction of pain on palpation of MTrPt; and propagation of the pain pattern on active needling.

Physiological research suggests that damaged fibril structures at the site of active MTrPt and degenerative changes in I bands in addition to capillary damage and disintegration of the myofibrillar network (Travell & Simons 1983) may contribute to the pain. In this present case the subject's taut bands and local tenderness are thought to be caused by decreased circulation and resulting ischaemia via sustained sarcomere shortening. Other mechanisms that shorten the actin and myosin complex include the traumatic release of calcium either from the sarcoplasmic reticulum or from a failure to restore adenosine triphosphate. Without the calcium release, the actin and myosin complex becomes

shortened and muscle dysfunction results (Travell & Simons 1983).

In trigger point needling, one of the main keys to treatment is deactivating the dysfunctional end-plate. It has been hypothesized that an accurately placed needle provides a localized stretch to the contracted microscopic structures, which disentangle the myosin filaments. Manipulation of the needle is theorized to assist in the effect of straightening the collagen fibres (Langevin 2001). Group II fibres will register a change in total fibre length, which will activate the gate-control system by blocking nociceptive input from the MTrPt and alleviate pain (Baldry 2001). In the presence of chronic pain, local needling is very much a priority. Acupuncture is a form of sensory stimulation that causes a barrage of A-delta (Aδ) afferent nerve activity at the segmental level, causing excitation of inhibitory interneurones in the dorsal horn, ultimately reducing the transmission of painful signals at the spinal segment.

The gluteus medius muscle power and adductor squeeze tests in side lying were used as the two main outcome measures, because they have good intrarater reliability (Lee 2004). These two markers were also useful ways for the subject to assess how his functional improvement was progressing.

Osteitis pubis is a common disorder for many in the sporting fraternity, and the condition involves myofascial dysfunction and inflammation. It can be difficult to treat and requires a holistic approach, incorporating pain relief and rehabilitation. Acupuncture is an extremely effective modality for the treatment of chronic musculoskeletal conditions. Acupuncture has been demonstrated to be a useful adjunct to traditional physiotherapy treatments for osteitis pubis. The present subject had eight sessions of MTrPt needling and his pain, function, and running time were greatly improved (Table 8.9). He has since played two full competitive games of rugby without return of symptoms.

(Continued)

Case Study 2 (Continued)

Table 8.9 Acupuncture Treatment Progression

Trigger point treatment	Outcome
Treatments 1–3 (weeks 1–2) Adductor longus Pectineus	Increased function Negligible soreness
Treatments 4–6 (weeks 3–4) Adductor longus ×2 Points Pectineus	Side-lying gluteus medius muscle test pain free Increased running Increased core stability Light functional weight regime started
Treatments 7–8 (weeks 5–6) Adductor longus ×3 points Pectineus	Negative gluteal muscle test Negative AST Running 30 mins Agility work ×10 mins

References

Acupuncture Association of Chartered Physiotherapists Safety Guidelines (AACP), 2004.

Adams, M.A., Bogduk, N., Burton, K., et al., 2002. The Biomechanics of Back Pain. Churchill Livingstone, Edinburgh.

Anderson, K., Strickland, S., Warren, R., 2001. Hip and Groin Injuries in Athletes. Am. J. Sports Med. 29 (4), 521–533.

Baldry, P.E., 1993. Acupuncture, Trigger Points and Musculoskeletal Pain, 2nd edn. Churchill Livingstone, London.

Baldry, P.E., 2001. Myofascial Pain and Fibromyalgia Syndromes. Churchill Livingstone, Edinburgh.

Bekkering, R., van Bussel, R., 1998. Segmental acupuncture. In: Filshie, J., White, A.R. (Eds.), Acupuncture in Medicine: A Western Scientific Approach. Churchill Livingstone, Edinburgh.

Betts, D., 2006. A review of research into the application of acupuncture in pregnancy. J. Chin. Med. 80, 50–55.

Bjorklund, K., Bergström, S., 2000. Is pelvic pain in pregnancy a welfare complaint? Acta Obstet. Gynecol. Scand. 79, 24–30.

Bourdillon, J.F., Day, E.A., Brookhout, M.R., 1992. Spinal Manipulation, 5th edn. Butterworth-Heinemann, Oxford.

Bowsher, D., 1998. Mechanisms of acupuncture. In: Filshie, J., White, A. (Eds.), Medical Acupuncture: A Western Scientific Approach. Churchill Livingstone, Edinburgh, pp. 69–82.

Boylan, M., 2006. Acupuncture and stabilising exercises important adjuncts in relieving pelvic girdle pain. Journal of the Australian Traditional-Medicine Society 2 (4), 207.

Brukner, P., Khan, K., 2002. Clinical Sports Medicine, 2nd edn. McGraw-Hill, New York.

Buyruk, H.M., Stam, H.J., Snijders, C.J., et al., 1999. Measurement of sacroiliac joint stiffness in peripartum pelvic pain patients with Doppler imaging of vibrations (DIV). Eur. J. Obstet. Gynecol. Reprod. Biol. 83 (2), 159–163.

Ceccherelli, F., Rigoni, M.T., Gagliardi, G., et al., 2002. Comparison of superficial and deep acupuncture in the treatment of lumbar myofascial pain: A double blind randomised controlled stud. Clin. J. Pain. 18 (3), 149–153.

Cibulka, M.T., Koldehoff, R., 1999. Clinical usefulness of a cluster of sacroiliac joint tests in patients with and without low back pain. J. Orthop. Sports Phys. Ther. 29 (2), 83–89.

Cibulka, M.T., Delitto, A., Koldehoff, R.M., 1988. Changes in innominate tilt after manipulation of the sacroiliac joint in patients with low back pain. An experimental study. Phys. Ther. 68 (9), 1359–1363.

Damen, L., Buyruk, H.M., Guler-Uysal, F., et al., 2001. Pelvic pain during pregnancy is associated with asymmetric laxity of the sacroiliac joints. Acta Obstet. Gynecol. Scand. 80 (11), 1019–1024.

Damen, L., Buyruk, H.M., Guler-Uysal, F., et al., 2002. The prognostic value of asymmetric laxity of the sacroiliac joints in pregnancy-related pelvic pain. Spine 27 (24), 2820–2824.

da Silva, J., Nakamura, M., Cordeiro, J., et al., 2004. Acupuncture for low back pain in pregnancy—a prospective, quasi-randomised, controlled study. Acupunct. Med. 22 (2), 60–67.

de Groot, M., Pool-Goudzwaard, A.L., Spoor, C.W., et al., 2006. The active straight leg raising test (ASLR) in pregnant women: Differences in muscle activity and force between patients and healthy subjects. Man. Ther. 13 (1), 68–74.

DiGiovanna, E.L., Schiowitz, S., 1997. An Osteopathic Approach to Diagnosis and Treatment, 2nd edn. Lippincott-Raven, Philadelphia.

Dreyfuss, P., Dreyer, S., Griffin, J., et al., 1994. Positive sacroiliac screening tests in asymptomatic adults. Spine 19 (10), 1138–1143.

Dreyfuss, P., Michaelsen, M., Pauza, K., et al., 1996. The value of medical history and physical examination in diagnosing sacroiliac joint pain. Spine 21 (22), 2594–2602.

Dumas, G.A., Reid, J.G., Wolfe, L. A., 1995. Exercise, posture, and back pain during pregnancy. Clin. Biomech. 10 (2), 104–109.

Egan, D., Cole, J., Twomey, L., 1996. The standing forward flexion test: an inaccurate determinant of sacroiliac joint dysfunction. Physiotherapy 82 (4), 236–242.

Elden, H., Ladfors, L., Olsen, M., et al., 2005. Effects of acupuncture and stabilizing exercises as adjuncts to standard treatment in pregnant women with pelvic girdle pain: randomized single blind controlled trial. Br. Med. J. 330 (7494), 761.

Elden, H., Ostgaard, H.C., Fagevik-Olsen, M., et al., 2007. Treatments of pelvic girdle pain in pregnant women: adverse effects of standard treatment, acupuncture and stabilising exercises on the pregnancy, mother, delivery and the fetus/neonate. Complement. Altern. Med. 8, 1–13.

Ellis T, Beck M Gautier E et al,. 2003 In Title, M., Helfet, D., Kellam, J. (Eds.), Fractures of the pelvis and acetabulum, 3rd edn. Lippincott, Williams and Wilkinson, Philadelphia.

Endersen, E., 1955. Pelvic pain and Low Back Pain in pregnant women: an epidemiological study. Scand. J. Rheumatol. 24, 135–141.

Fortin, J.D., Dwyer, A.P., West, S., et al., 1994a. The Sacroiliac joint: pain referral maps upon applying a new injection/arthrography technique. Part I: asymptomatic volunteers. Spine 19 (13), 1475–1482.

Fortin, J.D., April, C.N., Ponthieux, B., et al., 1994b. The Sacroiliac joint: pain referral maps upon applying a new injection/arthrography technique. Part II: clinical evaluation. Spine 19 (11), 1483–1489.

Fowler, C., 1986. Muscle energy techniques for pelvic dysfunction. In: Grieve, G.P. (Ed.), Modern manual therapy of the vertebral column. Churchill Livingstone, Edinburgh.

Fritz, J., Delitto, A., Vignovic., et al., 1992. Centralization phenomenon and status change during movement testing in patients with low back pain. Arch. Phys. Med. Rehabil. 81 (1), 57–61.

Furlan, A.D., Van Tulder, M.W., Cherkin, D.C., et al., 2005. Acupuncture and dry needling for low back pain: an updated systematic review with the framework of the Cochrane collaboration. Spine 30 (8), 944–963.

Gifford, L.S., Butler, D.S., 1997. The integration of pain sciences into clinical practice. J. Hand. Ther. 10 (2), 87–95.

Hecker, H.U., Steveling, A., Peuker, E., et al., 2001. Color atlas of acupuncture. Thieme, New York.

Heckman, J., Sassard, R., 1994. Musculo-skeletal considerations in pregnancy. J. Bone. Joint Surg. 76, 1720–1730.

Horton, S.J., Franz, A., 2007. Mechanical diagnosis and therapy approach to assessment and treatment of derangement of the sacroiliac joint. Man. Ther. 12 (2), 126–132.

Hungerford, B., Gilleard, W., Hodges, P., 2003. Evidence of altered lumbopelvic muscle recruitment in the presence of sacroiliac joint pain. Spine 8 (14), 1593–1600.

Indahl, A., Kaigle, A., Reikeras, O., et al., 1999. Sacroiliac joint involvement in activation of the porcine spinal and Gluteal musculature. J. Spinal. Disord. 12 (4), 325–330.

Jacob, H.A.C., Kissling, R.O., 1995. The mobility of the sacroiliac joint in healthy volunteers between 20 and 50 years of age. Clin. Biomech. 10 (7), 352–361.

Karlssonn, J., Sward, L., Kalebo, P., et al., 1994. Chronic groin pain in athletes. Sports Med. 17, 141–148.

King, P.M., Myers, C.A., Ling, F.W., et al., 1991. Musculoskeletal factors in chronic pelvic pain. J. Psychosom. Obstet. Gynaecol. 12, 87–98.

Kristiansson, P., Svardsudd, K., von Schoultz, B., 1996. Back pain during pregnancy. A prospective study. Spine 21, 702–709.

Kvoring, N., Holmberg, C., Grennert, L., et al., 2004. Acupuncture relieves pelvic and low back pain in late pregnancy. Acta Obstet. Gynecol. Scand. 83 (3), 246–250.

Laing, L., 2006. Acupuncture and IVF. Blue Poppy Press, Boulder, CO.

Langevin, H.M., Churchill, D.L., Cipolla, M.J., 2001. Relationship of acupuncture points and meridians to connective tissue planes. Anatomical Record Part B. New Anat. 268 (6), 265.

Laslett, M., Young, S.B., April, C. N., et al., 2003. Diagnosing painful sacroiliac joints: a validity study of a McKenzie evaluation and sacroiliac provocation tests. Aust. J. Physiother. 49 (9–11), 89–97.

Laslett, M., McDonald, B., Tropp, H., et al., 2005a. Agreement between diagnoses reached by clinical examination and available reference standards: a prospective study of 216 patients with lumbopelvic pain. British Medical Council Musculoskeletal Disorders 9, 6–28.

Laslett, M., Aprill, C.N., McDonald, B., et al., 2005b. Diagnosis of sacroiliac joint pain: validity of individual provocation tests and composites of tests. Man. Ther. 10 (3), 207–218.

Lee, D., 1999. The pelvic girdle: an approach to the examination and treatment of the lumbopelvic hip region, 2nd edn. Churchill Livingstone, Edinburgh.

Lee, D., 2004. The Pelvic Girdle: An Approach to the Examination and Treatment of the Lumbopelvic-Hip Region, 3rd edn. Churchill Livingstone, Edinburgh.

Lee, H., 2005. Promising results for acupuncture in pelvic girdle pain during pregnancy. Focus on Alternative and Complementary Therapies 10 (3), 208–209.

Lundeberg, T., 1998. The physiological basis of acupuncture. MANZ/PANZ Annual Conference Christchurch, New Zealand.

Lundeberg, T., Hurtig, T., Lundeberg, S., et al., 1988. Long term results of acupuncture in chronic head and neck pain. Pain Clin. 2, 15–31.

Maigne, J.-Y., Aivaliklis, A., Pfefer, F., 1996. Results of sacroiliac double block and the value of sacroiliac pain provocation tests in 54 patients with low back pain. Spine 21 (16), 1889–1892.

Manheimer, E., Pirotta, M.V., White, A.R., 2008. Acupuncture for pelvic and back pain in pregnancy: a systematic review. Am. J. Obstet. Gynecol. 193 (3), 254–259.

Marshall, P., Murphy, B., 2006. The effect of sacroiliac joint manipulation on feed-forward activation times of the deep abdominal musculature. J. Manipulative. Physiol. Ther. 29 (3), 196–202.

Mens, J.M., Vleeming, A., Snijders, C.J., et al., 1999. The active straight leg-raising test and mobility of the pelvic joints. Eur. Spine J. 8 (6), 468–473.

Mens, J.M., Snijders, C.J., Stam, H.J., 2000. Diagonal trunk muscle exercises in peripartum pelvic pain:

a randomised clinical trial. Phys. Ther. 80 (12), 1164–1173.

Mens, J.M., Vleeming, A., Snijders, C.J., et al., 2001. Reliability and validity of the active straight leg raise test in posterior pelvic pain since pregnancy. Spine 26 (10), 1167–1171.

Mens, J.M., Vleeming, A., Snijders, C.J., et al., 2002. Validity of the active straight leg raise test for measuring disease severity in patients with posterior pelvic pain after pregnancy. Spine 27 (2), 196–200.

Mens, J., Inklaar, H., Koes, B.W., et al., 2006. A new view on adduction-related groin pain. Clin. J. Sport Med. 16 (1), 15–19.

Mitchell, Fr., Mitchell, P.K.G., 1999. The muscle energy manual, vol. iii: Evaluation and treatment of the pelvis and sacrum. MET Press, East Lansing, MI.

Nilsson-Wikmar, L., Holm, K., Oijerstedt, R., et al., 2005. Effect of three different physical therapy treatments on pain and activity in pregnant women with pelvic girdle pain: a randomized clinical trial with 3, 6, and 12 months follow-up postpartum. Spine 30 (8), 850–856.

Ostgaard, H., Andersson, G., 1991. Prevalence of low back pain in pregnancy. Spine 16, 549–552.

Ostgaard, H., Andersson, G., 1992. Post partum low back pain. Spine 17, 53–55.

Ostgaard, H.C., Andersson, G.B., Karlsson, K., 1991. Prevalence of back pain in pregnancy. Spine 16, 549–552.

O'Sullivan, P.B., Beales, D.J., 2007a. Changes in pelvic floor and diaphragm kinematics and respiratory patterns in subjects with sacroiliac joint pain following a motor learning intervention: A case series. Man. Ther. 12 (3), 209–218.

O'Sullivan, P.B., Beales, D.J., 2007b. Diagnosis and classification of pelvic girdle pain disorders—Part 1: A mechanism based approach within a biopsychosocial framework. Man. Ther. 12 (2), 86–97.

O'Sullivan, P.B., Beales, D.J., Beetham, J.A., et al., 2002. Altered motor control strategies in subjects with sacroiliac joint pain during the active straight-leg-raise test. Spine 27 (1), E1–E8.

Petersen, T., Olsen, S., Laslett, M., et al., 2004. Intertester reliability of a new classification system of patients for patients with

non-specific low back pain. Aust. J. Physiother. 50, 85–94.

Pool-Goudzwaard, A., van Dijke, G.H., van Gurp, M., et al., 2004. Contribution of pelvic floor muscles to stiffness of the pelvic ring. Clin. Biomechics. 19 (6), 564–571.

Potter, N.A., Rothstein, J.M., 1985. Intertester reliability for selected clinical tests of the sacroiliac joint. Phys. Ther. 65 (11), 1671–1675.

Richardson, C.A., Snijders, C.J., Hides, J.A., et al., 2002. The relation between the Transversus abdominals muscles, sacroiliac joint mechanics, and low back pain. Spine 27 (4), 399–405.

Rodriguez, C., Miguel, A., Lima, H., et al., 2001. Osteitis Pubis Syndrome in the professional soccer athlete: A case report. J. Athl. Train 36 (4), 437–440.

Roemer, T., 2000. Medical Acupuncture in Pregnancy, 2nd edn. Thieme, Stuttgart.

Rouse, S., 2008. The use of acupuncture in the physiotherapy treatment of pelvic pain in pregnancy. J. Acupunct. Assoc. Chart. Physiotherapists 1, 67–72.

Schwarzer, M.D., Aprill, C.N., Bogduk, N., 1995. The sacroiliac joint in chronic low back pain. Spine 20 (1), 31–37.

Slipman, C.W., Jackson, H.B., Lipetz, J. S., et al., 2000. Sacroiliac joint pain referral zones. Arch. Phys. Med. Rehabil. 81 (3), 334–338.

Smidt, G.L., Wei, S.H., McQuade, K., et al., 1997. Sacroiliac motion for extreme hip positions. A fresh cadaver study. Spine 22 (18), 2073–2082.

Snijders, C.J., Vleeming, A., Stoeckart, R., 1993a. Transfer of lumbosacral load to iliac bones and legs. Part 1: Biomechanics of self-bracing of the sacroiliac joints and its significance for treatment and exercise. Clin. Biomech. 8 (6), 285–294.

Snijders, C.J., Vleeming, A., Stoeckart, R., 1993b. Transfer of lumbosacral load to iliac bones and legs. Part 2: Loading of the sacroiliac joints when lifting in a stooped posture. Clin. Biomech. 8 (6), 295–301.

Snijders, C.J., Ribberts, M.T., de Bakker, H.V., 1998. EMG recordings of abdominal and back muscles in various standing postures: validation of a biomechanical model on sacroiliac joint stability. J. Electromyogr. Kinesiol. 8 (4), 205–214.

Snijders, C.J., Hermans, P.F., Kleinrensink, G.J., 2006. Functional

aspects of cross-legged sitting with special attention to piriformis muscles and sacroiliac joints. Clin. Biomech. 21 (2), 116–121.

Stuge, B., Hilde, G., Vollestad, N., 2003. Physical therapy for pregnancy-related low back and pelvic pain: a systematic review. Acta Obstet. Gynecol. Scand. 82 (11), 983–990.

Stuge, B., Laerum, E., Kirkesola, G., et al., 2004a. The efficacy of a treatment program focusing on specific stabilising exercises for pelvic girdle pain after pregnancy: A randomised controlled trial. Spine 29 (4), 351–359.

Stuge, B., Veierod, M.B., Laerum, E., et al., 2004b. The efficacy of a treatment program focusing on specific stabilising exercises for pelvic girdle pain after pregnancy: a two-year follow-up of a randomised clinical trial. Spine 29 (10), E197–E203.

Sturesson, B., Selvik, G., Uden, A., 1989. Movements of the sacroiliac joints a roentgen stereophotogrammetric analysis. Spine 14 (2), 11162–11165.

Sturesson, B., Uden, A., Vleeming, A., 2000. A radiostereometric analysis of movements of the sacroiliac joints during the standing hip flexion test. Spine 25 (3), 364–368.

Suter, E., McMorland, G., Herzog, W., et al., 1999. Decrease in quadriceps inhibition after sacroiliac joint manipulation in patients with anterior knee pain. J. Manipulative. Physiol. Ther. 22 (3), 149–153.

Thomas, K.J., MacPherson, H., Ratcliffe, J., et al., 2005. Longer term clinical and economic benefits of offering acupuncture care to patients with chronic low back pain. Health Technol. Assess. 9 (332), iii–iv, ix–x, 1–109.

Tong, H., Oscar, G., Heyman, G., 2006. Interexaminer reliability of three methods of combining test results to determine side of sacral restriction, sacral base position, and innominate bone position. J. Am. Osteop. Soc. 106 (8), 464–468.

Travell, J.G., Simons, D.G., 1983. Myofascial Pain and Dysfunction: The Trigger Point Manual, Vol. i: Upper Limb. Williams and Wilkins, Baltimore.

Tullberg, T., Blomberg, S., Branth, B., et al., 1998. Manipulation does not alter the position of the sacroiliac joint. A roentgen stereophotogrammetric analysis. Spine 23 (10), 1124–1128.

van der Wurff, P., Hammier, R., Mines, W., 2000a. Clinical tests of the sacroiliac joint. A systematic methodological review. Part I: reliability. Man. Ther. 5 (2), 30–36.

van der Wurff, P., Meynes, W., Hagmeijer, R., 2000b. Clinical tests of the sacroiliac joint. A systematic methodological review. Part 2: Validity. Man. Ther. 5 (2), 89–96.

van der Wurff, P., Buijs, E.J., Groen, G. J., 2006. Intensity mapping of pain referral areas in sacroiliac joint pain patients. J. Manipulative. Physiol. Ther. 29 (3), 190–195.

van Wingerden, J.P., Vleeming, A., Buyruk, H.M., et al., 2004. Stabilisation of the sacroiliac joint in vivo: verification of muscular

contribution to force closure of the pelvis. Eur. Spine J. 13 (3), 199–205.

Vleeming, A., Stoeckart, R., Volkers, A.C.W., et al., 1990a. Relation between form and function in the sacroiliac joint. Part 1: Clinical anatomical aspects. Spine 15 (2), 130–132.

Vleeming, A., Stoeckart, R., Volkers, A.C.W., et al., 1990b. Relation between form and function in the sacroiliac joint. Part 2: Biomechanical aspects. Spine 15 (20), 133–136.

Vleeming, A., Wingerden, J.P., van Dijkstra, P.F., et al., 1992a. Mobility in the SI joints in old people: A kinematic and radiologic study. Clin. Biomech. 7, 170–176.

Vleeming, A., Buyruk, J.M., Stoeckart, R., et al., 1992b. Towards an integrated therapy for peripartum pelvic instability: A study of the biomechanical effects of pelvic belts. Am. J. Obstet. Gynecol. 166 (4), 1243–1247.

Watkin, H., 2004. Back pain: an integrated approach in primary care. Acupunct. Med. 22 (4), 203–206.

White, A., 1998. Measuring pain. Acupunct. Med. 16 (2), 83–87.

Young, S., Aprill, C.N., Laslett, M., 2003. Correlation of clinical examination characteristics with three sources of chronic low back pain. Spine 3 (6), 460–465.

The hip

9

Jennie Longbottom

CHAPTER CONTENTS

Introduction

The hip joint is a multiaxial ball-and-socket, synovial joint that connects the head of the femur and the pelvic acetabulum. The head of the femur forms approximately two-thirds of a sphere and is covered with hyaline cartilage (Nicholls 2004). Twenty-two muscles cross the hip in order to stabilize the joint and move the femur during locomotion. It is has evolved to operate under loads exceeding three times the weight of the body, and is controlled by muscles of enormous power and extraordinary accurate coordination (Strange 1965). Any excess or unstable load may damage both soft tissue and joint structures, depending on the position of the joint at the time (Sims 1999). Many problems of the hip complex show movement dysfunctions of the joint, in combination with the lumbar spine, sacroiliac joint, neurodynamic structures, and muscular systems (Hengeveld & Banks 2005), all of which need accurate assessment before appropriate and effective interventions are chosen.

Soft tissue injuries

The hip is an integral component in load transference during upper and lower limb performance, with approximately 30% of hip pain in young adults remaining without clear diagnosis. Controversial diagnoses such as acetabular tear, femoro-acetabular impingement syndrome, instability, and osteoarthrosis (OA) are referred to (Nicholls 2004). In sport, the hip joint has been attributed to contributing between 0.5 and 14% of athletic injuries (Reid 1988; van Mechelen et al 1992) and adductor muscle-related groin pain is a common presentation in the athlete. Hölmich (2007) reviewed 207 cases of groin pain in the sporting population; 18% of all cases occurred in runners. From a clinical standpoint, sports-related groin pain can be classified into four clinical subgroups (Hölmich 2007):

- Adductor-related groin pain;
- Abdominal-related groin pain;
- Pubic symphysis stress reaction; and
- Hip-related groin pain.

High-velocity eccentric muscle contractions may injure muscles and tendons, or damage may be done by oblique, explosive forces with sudden movement bursts (Sharma & Maffulli 2005). The potential for certain muscles to be injured is greater for some

© 2010 Elsevier Ltd.
DOI: 10.1016/B978-0-443-06782-2.00009-8

Table 9.1 Muscle activity in running phases

Phase of running	Muscle activity	Plane of activity % muscle activity	Motion required
Swing	Iliopsoas	Saggital plane quadriceps iliopsoas hamstrings 84% concentric and eccentric muscle activity.	Hip flexion increases with speed
End of swing	Gluteus maximus	Transverse plane external hip rotators 6.4% of concentric and eccentric muscle activity.	Decelerates hip flexion and internal rotation; increases with speed.
Start of stance	Gluteus maximus	Transverse plane external hip rotators 6.4% of concentric and eccentric muscle activity.	Extension of hip
Late swing to early middle stance	Gluteus medius	Frontal Plane	Provides adductor stability; prevents adduction of hip prior to and after foot contact.
	Tensor fascia lata	Gluteus medius tibialis anterior 18.9% of concentric and eccentric muscle activity.	More active with sprinting.

Adapted from Sahramann (2001).

than others, multijoint muscles being at greater risk because of their potential stretch over two joints. An accurate diagnosis and an assessment of the presenting muscle strain will rely on:

- The nature of the presenting injury;
- Gait analysis;
- Palpation;
- Muscle stretching; and
- The elimination of differential pathologies or the inclusion of current pathologies.

The goals of therapeutic intervention are to assist new muscle fibre growth and muscle fibre alignment, and reduce adhesion formation (Niemuth 2007). Numerous studies have documented the role of the hip muscles during running using electromyography (EMG) analysis to describe muscle activity in the swing and stance phases of running (Knuesel et al 2005; Sahraman 2001) (Table 9.1).

A common source of pain in runners is iliotibial band syndrome (ITBS), which is caused by repetitive friction of the iliotibial band sliding across the lateral femoral condyle. Fredericson et al (2000) hypothesized that weakness of the gluteus medius muscle causes overfiring and tightness of the tensor fascia lata (TFL) and ITBS, resulting in significant weakness of the hip abductors of the injured leg in injured runners.

In the acute stages of injury, gentle concentric strengthening activity is preferred, and as recovery is achieved, eccentric strengthening is particularly effective in promoting new collagen, reversing chronic degenerative tendon changes (LaStayo et al 2003), and promoting increased circulation for enhanced tenocyte and myocyte activity (Khan 1999).

Rehabilitation of proprioception is essential to avoid re-injury and return the patient to full function, especially the athlete. Repeated movements and sustained postures alter tissues that control the characteristics of movement, causing movement impairment (Sahramann 2001). Two main categories of movement impairment syndromes have been described: femoral and hip syndromes.

Femoral syndromes

These are believed to be impairments of accessory motions, which cause irritation of tissues. Femoral syndromes occur because of either excessive accessory motion or when accessory motion is occurring when it should not.

Hip syndromes

These are impairments of physiological motions that produce pain in muscles associated with the movement.

Detailed examination in order to identify and rectify movement impairment syndromes reveals a number of positive findings necessary for accurate confirmation of the diagnosis. A diagnosis of movement impairment using a variety of tests will identify the movement direction that must be corrected; these include:

- Hip alignment;
- Movement patterns;
- Muscle length;
- Muscle strength;
- Muscle stiffness;
- Pattern of muscle recruitment; and
- Presence of joint susceptibility to movement in a specific direction (Sahramann 2001).

The growth in the number of individuals participating in organized sport has contributed to an increase in the prevalence of hip-related injuries. Rehabilitation of the injured athlete requires knowledge of the physical and psychological demands on the patient, made by the sport and his or her expectation (Konin & Nofsinger 2007). Capsular and ligamentous injuries are not as commonly seen as musculotendinous injuries, but may arise from trauma and overuse, requiring arthroscopic diagnosis (Baber et al 1999). Amongst the acute problems encountered are:

- Acetabular labrum tears (Fitzgerald 1995; Ikeda et al 1988; McCarthy et al 2003);
- Acetabular rim syndrome (Ito et al 2001; Klaue et al 1991; Reynolds et al 2007);
- Instability and sprained ligamentum teres (Bellabarba et al 2007); and
- Loose bodies (Villar 1992).

Stress fractures develop as a result of the weakening and subsequent failure of the bone. With regard to the hip, individuals who progressively increase the duration of repetitive impact loading to the lower limb are most at risk to injury (Kahan et al 1994). Korpelainen et al (2001) found that those who were at highest risk were individuals with high longitudinal arches; leg length inequalities; excessive forefoot varus; and menstrual irregularities.

Diagnosis involves careful examination of all capsular movement patterns. Currently trial periods of non-weight-bearing for up to 3 months are advocated for patients with acute intra-articular dysfunction (Fitzgerald 1995; Ikeda et al 1988). In the acute stage the aim is to reduce weight bearing, relieve pain and inflammation, maintain range of movement, and maintain aerobic fitness. Overactivity in any of the hip muscles would increase compression forces on the joint. Both TFL and ITB overactivity demonstrate increased stress distributions in the cartilage of the superior part of the joint, which may lead to degeneration (Kummer 1993). The piriformis and obturator externus muscles may provide forces capable of producing posterior joint wear, whilst iliopsoas and rectus femoris muscles which have direct connections with the anterior capsule of the hip may demonstrate anterior joint wear (Sims 1999).

Muscle weakness or shortening as a result of an active trigger point (TrPt) in the gluteus medius may affect the hip abductor vector, causing a Trendelenberg gait, whilst fatigue may bring about a change in the muscular synergies, leading to adverse handling of repetitive impact loads (Mizrahi et al 1997). Therefore it is important to identify any musculoskeletal dysfunction and modulate pain in order to facilitate rehabilitation, and prevent further abnormal forces contributing to the more extensive pain of OA or joint changes later in life.

Osteoarthrosis

Osteoarthrosis is the most common reason for total hip and total knee replacement among adults aged over 30 years, and symptomatic hip OA occurs in approximately 3% of the UK population (Felson & Zhang 1998). Mechanical factors are of importance in the aetiology of OA; there is increasing evidence that an abnormal labrum is implicated in the early onset of OA (Ferguson et al 2003). In a normal hip, the capsule has no limiting effect other than at the end range positions; however, it has been argued that a person with capsular restriction, in attempting to walk normally, increases hip joint loads by stretching the tight capsule (Crowninshield et al 1978). Therefore, the hip is subjected to dynamic loads on impact as well as dynamic forces of equilibrium in single-leg stance; alterations in one component may affect another.

There has been limited research into the effectiveness of physiotherapy for OA hip, but in recent years, there have been an increasing number of randomized controlled trials (RCTs) evaluating the effect of exercise therapy (Hoeksma et al 2004; Tak et al 2005; van Baar et al 1998), manual therapy (Hoeksma et al 2004), acupuncture (Stener-Victorin et al 2004), and self-management (Heuts et al 2005). The effects of long-term exercise have yet to be demonstrated (Tak et al 2005; van Baar et al 1998).

Hoeksma et al (2004) focused on specific manipulations and mobilization of the joint, as well as exercise therapy involving active exercises to improve muscle function and joint motion. The treatment period was 5 weeks (nine sessions). The primary outcome was general perceived improvement (GPI) after treatment; secondary outcomes included reduced pain, and increased hip function, walking speed, range of movement (ROM), and quality of life. No major differences were found in baseline characteristics between the study groups, with 81% improvement in the manual therapy group and 50% in the exercise group. Patients in the manual therapy group had significantly better outcomes on pain, stiffness, hip function, and ROM, indicating that the effects of manual therapy, endured after 29 weeks, and that it was superior to the exercise therapy programme in patients with OA of the hip. Manual therapy techniques such as joint mobilizations, stretching, and joint traction/distraction appear to offer improvements in quality of life, function, and walking tolerance.

The European League against Rheumatism (EULAR) and the UK-based, multidisciplinary MOVE consensus group have developed recommendations for the management of OA hip based on the best available scientific evidence (Roddy et al 2004; Zhang et al 2005). The consensus is that strengthening, aerobic, and proprioceptive exercises are recommended, but the recommendations identify the need to increase research into the most effective exercise programme for OA hip with reference to compliance, effectiveness on land versus water, and individual versus group exercise (Roddy et al 2004; Zhang et al 2005).

In a survey of current practice for the management of OA hip in Republic of Ireland, French (2007) found limited evidence for a number of physiotherapy interventions, recommending that the role of education and self-management should be investigated further. Despite manual therapy being virtually unresearched, it was used by 96% of respondents in this survey.

Puett and Griffin (1994) reviewed 15 controlled trials on non-medicinal and non-invasive therapies for hip and knee OA, and concluded that exercises reduced pain and improved function, but the optimal exercise regime has not been determined.

Active and passive ROM has been considered an important part of rehabilitation for patients with OA as a means of regaining joint mobility and function (Biloxi 1998; Prentice 1992). Deyle et al (2000) evaluated the effectiveness of manual therapy and exercise therapy in OA knee. The treatment involved eight clinical visits, which produced a 52% improvement in function, stiffness, and pain, as measured by the Western Ontario and McMaster Universities Osteoarthritis Index (WOMAC), and a 12% improvement in walk test scores. Falconer et al (1992) found improvements in motion (11%), pain (33%), and gait speed (11%) over 4–6 weeks after 12 sessions of exercise combined with manual therapy for patients with clinically diagnosed OA knee.

A combination of manual therapy and supervised exercise appears to be more effective than no formal intervention on improving walking distance, and alleviating pain, dysfunction, and stiffness in patients with OA, helping to defer or decrease the need for surgical intervention.

Proprioceptive deficits contribute to functional instability, which could ultimately lead to further microtrauma and re-injury (Lephart et al 1997). Thus, incorporating a proprioceptive element into a physical therapy programme is suggested for joint disorders. Sensorimotor training to promote proprioceptive acuity and muscle contraction for patients with lower limb OA has been advocated since 1990 particularly for the re-education of the proprioceptors (Sharma et al 1997; Vad et al 2002). A therapeutic exercise programme incorporating sensory input to facilitate dynamic joint stabilization may retrain altered afferent pathways to enhance the proprioception of joint movement and improve a patient's function. However, until now, there has been no standard training protocol available. Closed-chain exercise has been shown to give a better result with respect to facilitating proprioceptors than open-chain exercise (Beard et al 1994; Fitzgerald 1997). The exercises should be performed in various positions throughout the full ROM since the different afferent responses have been observed in different joint positions (Lephart et al 1997).

Acupuncture intervention

Treatment for OA is largely symptomatic, including analgesics, non- steroidal anti-inflammatory drugs (NSAIDs), glucosamine, topical analgesics such as capsaicin cream, and exercise, behavioural interventions, and surgical treatment (Felson et al 2000). No drug treatment is without risks and adverse effects; thus, non-pharmacological interventions are attractive.

Kwon et al (2006) conducted a systematic review and meta-analysis of acupuncture for peripheral joint

OA, suggesting on the basis of best-evidence synthesis that the data evidence for manual acupuncture could be classified as fairly strong. Manual acupuncture appeared to reduce pain compared to waiting list controls and sham acupuncture, thus suggesting analgesic effects beyond a placebo response. Electroacupuncture (EA) was found to be superior to NSAID on the visual analogue scale (VAS) and WOMAC outcomes.

Stener-Victorin et al (2004) evaluated 45 patients, aged between 42 and 86 years who had radiographic changes consistent with OA of the hip. Those with pain related to motion load and ache were selected. The subjects were randomly allocated to EA, hydrotherapy, both in combination with patient education, or patient education alone. The outcome measures were the Disability Rating Index, the Global Self Rating, and the VAS. Assessments were taken before the intervention and immediately after the last treatment, and later, at 1, 3, and 6 months. Electroacupuncture and hydrotherapy, both in combination with patient education, induce long-lasting effects, as shown by reduced pain and ache, and by increased functional activity and quality of life, as demonstrated by differences in pre- and post-treatment assessments. Pain related to motion and pain on load was reduced up to 3 months after the last treatment in the hydrotherapy group and up to 6 months in the EA group. Ache during the day was significantly improved in both the EA and hydrotherapy groups up to 3 months after the last treatment. Ache during the night was reduced in the hydrotherapy and EA groups up to 3 and 6 months after the last treatment, respectively. Disability in functional activities was improved in the EA and hydrotherapy groups up to 6 months after the last treatment. Quality of life was also improved in EA and hydrotherapy groups up to 3 months after the last treatment. There were no changes in the education group alone. In conclusion, EA and hydrotherapy, both in combination with patient education, induce long-lasting effects, reduced pain and increased functional activity and quality of life, as demonstrated by differences in the pre- and post-treatment assessments.

The principle aims of acupuncture are to modulate pain and inflammation; improve circulation to the hip joint; and maintain muscle length and strength. Initially treatment should be aimed at segmental (Table 9.2) inhibition and pain-gate mechanisms whilst aiding blood flow and stimulating an anti-inflammatory response. Local segmental points on the Bladder channel will facilitate segmental dorsal horn inhibition, whilst distal points corresponding to the dermatome involvement (Fig. 9.1) will encourage a descending inhibitory response. Here a choice of points may be available, depending on the pain pattern.

With the enormous muscle bulk running over the hip joint, the myofascial element should not be ignored. Resolution of associated trigger points will often reduce pain and facilitate muscle imbalance re-education; pain and abnormal function may often be attributed to myofascial trigger points (MTrPts). If the patient presents with both myofascial and articular dysfunction rehabilitation is generally steady and progressive (Whyte-Ferguson & Gerwin 2005). Myofascial involvement commonly involves the following muscles:

- Quadratus lumborum;
- Gluteus minimus;
- Tensor fascia lata;
- Piriformis;
- Abdominal oblique;
- Iliopsoas;
- Pectineus; and
- Semimembrinosis.

The exact aetiology and pathophysiology of MTrPts remain unknown. The MTrPts have been described as having a characteristic EMG pattern termed spontaneous electrical activity (SEA) (Chen et al 2001). This SEA is characterized by continuous low-level EMG activity with superimposed large-amplitude spikes (Simmons et al 1995). Some EMG studies have recorded SEA active MTrPts in both humans (Hubbard & Berkoff 1993) and rabbits (Chen et al 2001). Contemporary opinion is that SEA is the result of acetylcholine leakage from the motor end-plate. The magnitude of this leakage is at a sufficient level to create a mini depolarization of the postsynaptic junction and result in the contraction of a small number of muscle fibres rather that the whole muscle (Huguenin et al 2005). Continued acetylcholine release and subsequent muscle contraction are thought to reduce the oxygen supply to the muscle, and consequently, an ischaemic environment ensues in which there is insufficient adenosine triphosphate (ATP) available to initiate release of the actin-myosin complex.

Chen et al (2001) found that the SEA in rabbit MTrPts could be reduced with needling. In comparison to controlled needling, needling of the active

Table 9.2 Segmental innervation and acupuncture points

Segmental innervation	Segmental acupuncture points	Dermatome points
Anterior hip joint capsule is innervated by sensory articular branches from the femoral nerve L2 L3	BL23 BL24 HJJ @ L2/L3 GV4 @ L2 ST30 + ST31	GB31 ST34 SP12 LIV11
Anteromedial innervation is determined by the articular branches of the obturator nerve	LIV11 LIV10 SP11 SP10	SP11 SP10
Posterior hip joint and capsule. The sciatic nerve	BL25 BL26	GB30 GV3 HJJ@ L5/S1
Posteromedial section of the hip joint capsule is innervated by articular branches of the anterior rectus femoral nerve	BL25 BL26	BL53 BL54
Posterolateral section of the hip joint capsule innervated by superior gluteal nerve	BL26 BL27	KID10 BL36 BL37
S1-S3 sciatic nerve	BL27 BL28 BL29	BL36 BL37 BL40 BL60 BL62

Notes: BL, Bladder; HJJ, Huatuojiaji; GV, Governor Vessel; ST, Stomach; LIV, Liver; SP, Spleen; KID, Kidney.

TrPt in the rabbit resulted in significantly lower normalized SEA in 7 out of 9 rabbits. Although this study primarily provides evidence for the efficacy of MTrPt needling in reducing SEA, it remains unknown whether reducing SEA is required to achieve pain relief. The study by Chen et al (2001) did not measure pressure-pain threshold pre- or post-treatment. To date, there is insufficient evidence to support or refute a reduction in SEA in MTrPt acupuncture.

In addition to a peripheral effect on the motor end-plate, MTrPt injection has been shown to activate diffuse noxious inhibitory control (DNIC). Fine et al (1988) investigated the effects of administering the opioid antagonist naloxone in MTrPt injections. The study found that MTrPt injections were effective in improving ROM and pressure-pain scores. The administration of 10 mg naloxone

significantly reversed the effects of the MTrPt injections. The findings of this study would suggest that central opioid activation is an underlying mechanism in the pain relief obtained from MTrPt injections.

Activation of DNIC and the subsequent release of opioids has been shown to reduce nociceptive transmission to higher centres at the spinal cord level (Fine et al 1988). It is possible that the reason why some studies fail to demonstrate a difference between placebo and MTrPt is that the placebo needling is of sufficient level of stimulus to activate DNIC. Furthermore, the clinical improvement from manual, soft tissue MTrPt therapy may also share the same pathway for its analgesic effects with acupuncture. Clinically, it is relevant to consider what level of stimulus is effective in activating DNIC and achieving pain relief in subjects with MTrPt, rather

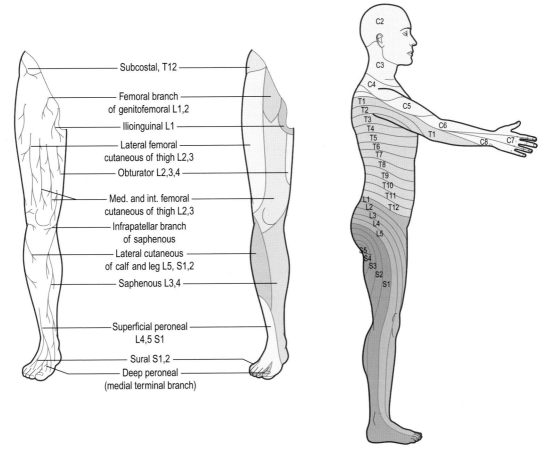

Figure 9.1 • Segmental and dermatome innervation.

than debating whether the stimulus is a placebo or a real treatment (Smith & Crowther 2002).

The sympathetic nervous system (SNS) has also been implicated in MTrPts. In an animal model Chen et al (1998) demonstrated that phentolomine reduced the SEA in rabbit MTrPts when compared with a control injection of saline. Although direct extrapolation of this finding to human subjects is limited, the study provides some preliminary data that suggest that sympathetic activity may contribute to myofascial MTrPt pain.

Clinically, it was hypothesized that the increased physiological demand on the muscle created an energy crisis where insufficient ATP was present to initiate skeletal muscle relaxation.

ATP is required for two processes of skeletal muscle relaxation. The first requirement for ATP is to decouple the myosin head from the actin molecule. Secondly, ATP is required to actively pump Ca^{2+} from the cytoplasm into the sarcoplasmic retinaculum. A reduction in active transport of Ca^{2+} by the calcium pump results in reduced Ca^{2+} concentrations in the sarcoplasmic reticulum. Reduced levels of sarcoplasmic Ca^{2+} have been suggested to prevent the actin and myosin attachment (Schwellnus et al 1997).

Bengtsson et al (1986) found reduced levels of high-energy phosphate bonds and increased levels of low-energy phosphate bonds in the MTrPt sites compared to non-tender muscle locations. Although these findings go some way to supporting the energy crisis theory, the above authors failed to show that any differences were demonstrated by product levels of anaerobic metabolism.

As an alternative to the energy crisis hypothesis, changes in spinal reflex and supraspinal control of the alpha motor nerve may be responsible for the development of the adductor muscle hypertonicity observed in athletes. Spinal control of the alpha motor nerve is essential for muscle relaxation (Schwellnus 1997). Under normal physiological conditions, excitatory input from the motor cortex, extrapyramidal, and muscle spindles must be decreased before muscle relaxation can occur (Gong 1993). Experimental evidence from animal studies show that, under fatigued conditions, type 1a muscle spindle afferent firing increases and type 1b Golgi tendon afferent firing decreases (Nelson & Hutton 1985). It would appear that muscle fatigue at the spinal level increases alpha motor activity as a result of the combination of increased type 1a and reduced type 1b afferent activity.

The evidence is inconclusive as to whether MTrPt needling is effective. In a systematic review and meta-analysis of RCTs, Tough et al (2009) found limited evidence that deep needling directly into MTrPts has an overall treatment effect when compared with standardized care. Whilst the result of the meta-analysis of TrPt needling, when compared with placebo controls, does not attain statistical significance, the overall direction could be compatible with a treatment effect of dry needling on MTrPt pain. However, the limited sample size and poor quality of the seven studies included highlights and supports the need for larger scale, good quality, and placebo-controlled RCTs in this field.

The use of acupuncture, whether using MTrPt or traditional Chinese acupuncture points, as means of reducing pain, and as precursors to manual and exercise therapy, appears to offer some enhancement of successful rehabilitation programmes for the management of pain in OA, although the research evidence is sparse and larger, placebo-controlled, pragmatic RCTs are required.

Case Study 1

Anonymous

Introduction

A 20-year-old male decathlete presented to a sports medicine department complaining of a 3-week history of left-sided adductor groin pain. The subject recalled that while attending a training camp, he had developed pain in his left groin following javelin practice. During this training session, the athlete was instructed by his coach to increase his approach speed and increase the height of his leg crossover. The subject could not recall any acute injury during the training session; however, approximately 30 minutes after the session he developed mild pain and tightness in the left groin. The athlete had competed the previous weekend in the 400-m, pole vault and discus without any impact on his performance; however, he felt decidedly apprehensive about competing in further hurdles and high jump training because of the risk of re-injury.

The main symptom that the subject reported was intermittent sharp left groin pain, rated as 60/100 on the VAS, when he was turning over in bed, coughing, or attempting to jump (see Fig. 9.2). His functional limitations were an inability to undertake high jump, javelin, and hurdle training at a level of less than 65% of the required intensity level. His goals were to resume full training; and compete in the national under-23 decathlon championships in 6 weeks. The following investigations involving an ultrasound scan were performed; no muscle injury was detected, with no evidence of posterior abdominal wall disruption or positive cough impulse.

The clinical presentation suggested that the athlete had presented with myofascial adductor-compartment-related groin pain. Although this implied an adductor muscle injury, the lack of a clear mechanism of injury during the training session and the negative ultrasound scan findings negated this hypothesis.

The following treatment plan was discussed:
• Deactivate active MTrPts;
• Strengthen the adductor muscle;
• Improve hip mechanics in both the passive and active ranges; and
• Manage training intensity to minimize continued adductor hypertonicity.

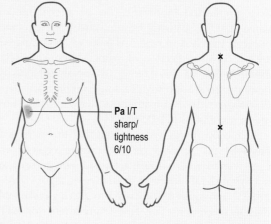

Pa l/T sharp/ tightness 6/10

Figure 9.2 • Body chart showing location of symptoms.

(Continued)

Case Study 1 (Continued)

The clinical presentation of the subject backed the diagnosis of adductor-related groin pain. The main clinical findings supporting the hypothesis of adductor compartment pain were discomfort on resisted contraction and palpation of the adductor compartment. The main negative clinical test that would further support the diagnosis of adductor-related groin pain were the negative Pubic Symphysis Stress Test; normal hip examination; symmetry; non-provocative neurodynamic tests; and the negative lumbar spine and sacroiliac joint pain provocation tests (Table 9.3).

The clinical history and ultrasound scan results did not support the clinical findings of an adductor muscle injury. The majority of these injuries occur with an eccentric hip abduction combined with hip external rotation, and most athletes are able to recall the exact moment of injury (Brukner & Khan 2007).

Considering the aforementioned factors, an alternate explanation for the subject's symptoms had to be considered. The clinical presentation was more in keeping with active MTrPts in adductor longus and magnus muscles. The requirement of the athlete to increase the speed of his approach run in the coronal plane, coupled with a loss of hip extension, would necessitate an increase in adductor muscle recruitment to achieve the desired movement pattern.

MTrPt needling was not used during the first three treatment sessions. Initially, post isometric inhibitory soft tissue techniques with digital ischaemic pressure were used to treat the adductor muscle MTrPt. Although these techniques resulted in an immediate reduction in pain during the adductor squeeze test, there was no carryover into the next treatment session, with the subject reporting only a short-term improvement following therapy. Based on the clinical presentation, it was decided to include MTrPt needling into the management of this adductor-related groin pain. Needling was selected to deactivate the active MTrPt in the adductor muscles, which reproduced the subject's symptoms.

This athlete was seen on six occasions. The first three treatment sessions comprised local soft-tissue techniques to the adductor muscles and implementation of a rehabilitation programme. Although the subject demonstrated an immediate improvement in isometric hip adduction strength, as measured by the pressure

Table 9.3 Assessment

Observation	Lordotic posture Increased tone lumbar erector spinae Reduced gluteal bulk and tone
Functional assessment	Overhead squat reduced hip flexion range Lateral lunge left reproduced pain Single leg squat left increased knee adduction
Neural provocation testing	Femoral and obturator nerve tests L = R No abnormal mechanosensitivity detected
Active range of motion	Reduced lumbar extension 80%R2 No pain reproduction Reduced hip extension on left in comparison to right
Muscle length tests	Rectus femoris, iliotibial band restricted on right Adductor longus limited on left because of muscle guarding
Palpation	Hypertonicity of adductor compartment with active trigger points reproducing pain adductor longus and adductor magnus. No abdominal wall or pubic symphysis tenderness
Special tests	−ve Pubic Symphysis Stress test −ve SIJ pain provocation and active SLR −ve hip impingement and acetabular labrum testing +ve adductor squeeze test 60° = P1 180 mmHg +ve adductor squeeze at 0° P1 = 40 mmHg −ve eccentric sit-up with rotational variations

(Continued)

Case Study 1 (Continued)

Table 9.4 Acupuncture Selection

Treatment	Location	Outcome
1	Adductor magnus Adductor longus	Reduced pain on groin pressure cuff testing 220 mmHg
2	Adductor longus Adductor magnus	Pressure cuff score 280 mmHg before pain onset
3	Adductor magnus, two locations Adductor longus Bicep femoris	Groin pressure cuff scores = 300 mmHg

cuff, this progress was not carried over into subsequent treatment sessions. Moreover, adductor muscle hypertonicity was still evident in comparison to the subject's other side and he still reported a restricted ability to undertake his hurdle and jumping sessions. Following the first session of acupuncture, his pain-free adduction power improved to 220 mmHg. More importantly, this progress was carried over into following treatments (Table 9.4). Following two further sessions the subject was pain-free on muscle testing and his strength had returned to the level measured on pre-season

testing. He reported that he was in full training at 100% intensity. Clinical examination revealed that there was no adductor muscle hypertonicity in comparison to the contralateral muscle group.

Discussion

To date, only one study has investigated the use of MTrPt needling in the elite sports population (Huguenin et al 2005). This report investigated placebo and needling of gluteal MTrPt in athletes with posterior thigh pain. Both needling techniques resulted in subjective improvements in the levels of gluteal and hamstring tightness during running. Objectively, the straight leg raise test and internal hip rotation range remained unchanged. The findings of the above study would suggest that both active and placebo needling techniques might have a central neural mechanism underpinning their effect. Huguenin et al suggested that this might be as a result of activation of descending noxious inhibitory control.

Delta fibre stimulation could explain why the MTrPt needling was more effective than soft-tissue techniques in reducing the present subject's groin pain. Delta fibre stimulation has been shown to produce the most effective stimulus for segmental inhibition of pain (Bars & Willer 2002). Potentially, MTrPt needling could have resulted in a larger number of A-delta (Aδ) fibres being stimulated than those in soft-tissue techniques; this would result in a more intense noxious stimulus to the central nervous system. Bars and Willer found that the intensity of the peripheral stimulus would appear to be more important than the mode of stimulus delivery in the activation of DNIC mechanisms.

 ## Case Study 2

Sharon Helsby

Introduction

A 55-year-old woman presented with an 8-week history of right lateral hip pain. The subject could not recall any trauma associated with the onset of her symptoms, but reported that the pain had gradually been getting worse. After 5 weeks of having symptoms, which showed no signs of resolving, she saw her general practitioner who prescribed NSAIDs, which helped to settle the pain slightly, and sent the subject for a hip X-ray. The X-ray confirmed a diagnosis of right hip moderate OA and she was referred to an orthopaedic consultant.

The diagnosis was confirmed and the subject was given the option of a hydrocortisone injection for temporary relief, a Birmingham hip resurfacing operation, or conservative treatment, which comprised of NSAIDs

and physiotherapy. She was not keen on having surgery and opted for the conservative approach, so she was referred to physiotherapy.

Subjective assessment

On initial presentation the subject reported an intermittent deep ache in the lateral aspect of her right hip; she described the ache as 60/100 on VAS. The symptoms were at their worst first thing in the morning, on rising, at which time she also felt stiffness. The pain and stiffness settled as she started walking and were completely gone following her morning shower. The subject's symptoms were aggravated throughout the day by activities such as getting into and out of a car and walking for periods more than 15 minutes.

(Continued)

Case Study 2 (Continued)

Table 9.5 Acupuncture treatment protocol

Treatment	Local points	Distal points	Outcome measures
1	piriformis MTrPt[R]	LI4[B]	Decreased tenderness on palpation of piriformis VAS 50/100 Right internal rotation 15° Right abduction ISQ
2	GB29[R] GB30[R] GB43[R]	LI4[B]	VAS 40/100 Right internal rotation 15° Right abduction 35°
3	GB29[R] GB30[R] GB43[R]	LI4 [B]	VAS 30/100 Right internal rotation 15° Right abduction 35°
4	GB29[R] GB30[R] GB43[R]	LI4[B] GB34[B]	VAS 30/100 Right internal rotation 20° Right abduction 40°
5	GB29[R] GB30[R] GB43[R]	LI4[B] GB34[B]	VAS 20/100 Right internal rotation 20° Right abduction 40°

Notes: B, bilateral; R, right.

She was currently able to continue her job as a secretary since this did not aggravate her symptoms. However, the subject had stopped going to the gym, which she usually attended twice a week, because she found that the symptoms were increased immediately following the session, especially when she used the treadmill.

Objective assessment

On observation, the subject had a normal gait pattern with some mild gluteus maximus wasting on the right. Hip active range of movement on the right was limited by pain and stiffness into internal rotation (5°) and abduction. (30°); all other hip movements were full and pain free. Passive ROM equalled that of the active limitation, with a bony end-feel on abduction and a springy end-feel on internal rotation. Both abduction and internal rotation reproduced the subject's symptoms.

Muscle power was reduced to 4/5 on the Oxford Scale on abduction, and internal rotation and extension. Specifically, the right gluteus maximus and medius muscles were weak on muscle testing to 4/5. Furthermore, palpation revealed local tenderness and muscle spasm provocation over the piriformis muscle on the right side.

Treatment regime

Physiotherapy treatment began with advice and education about the subject's condition, including self-help strategies

and adaptions to lifestyle. The subject was also given a home exercise programme of stretching and strengthening exercises in order to help stabilize the hip joint.

There had been no change in VAS or ROM at this point and therefore, the first acupuncture session concentrated upon deactivation of active MTrPt in piriformis muscle (Table 9.5), which was restricting internal rotation and produced a positive pain referral pattern on palpation.

Clinical reasoning

Acupuncture was chosen as the treatment modality primarily for its analgesic properties in the treatment of pain (Tiquia 1996). During acupuncture, peripheral terminals of nociceptors in the skin are stimulated, which in turn release vasodilative substances such as calcitonin gene-related neuropeptide and histamine, leading to vasodilation and increased blood flow to the local area (Sato et al 2000). A further reason for choosing acupuncture, as a treatment modality is that there are many available research studies that form a reliable evidence base supporting its use as a pain-relieving modality for a variety of musculoskeletal disorders. Furthermore, a few studies specifically support the effectiveness of acupuncture for OA of the hip (Haslam 2001); many more support its effectiveness on OA of the knee (Barlas 2005; Berman et al 2004; Linde et al 2005; Sherman & Cherkin 2005; Tillu et al 2001).

(Continued)

Case Study 2 (Continued)

Initially, MTrPt acupuncture into the piriformis muscle bulk was performed at the location of the MTrPt, as described by Cummings (2000). Meridian acupuncture along the Gall Bladder channel was chosen for local use, with variable distal points. The Gall Bladder meridian is said to have an influence on muscles and tendons, the courses of which pass over the lateral and posterior aspects of the hip (Haslam 2001). Large Intestine 4 (LI4) was chosen as a distal point because of its general pain-relieving influence (Ellis 1994). Bilateral needling was carried out for the distal points since this method has been shown to be more effective than a unilateral approach because of the resulting bilateral stimulation of the ascending and descending spinal pathways involved in pain modulation (Tillu et al 2001). Manual stimulation was carried out twice throughout each session to maintain de Qi.

Outcome

Following the first session, the subject responded with a decrease in local tenderness in the right piriformis muscle, a 10/100 (VAS) reduction in local pain on the VAS and a 10° improvement in internal rotation with no change to her abduction.

Following the next five sessions, all outcome measures improved. By the sixth session her VAS score had improved from her original rating of 60/100 to 20/100. The subject's active ROM had also improved significantly on internal rotation, which was originally 5°, but improved to 20° by the sixth session. Her range of abduction had also improved from 30° to 40°.

By the last session the subject had also reported improvements to her functional ability and reported less intense stiffness in the mornings, which also resolved more quickly than before treatment. She also reported to be able to walk for periods longer than 30 minutes before pain came on, instead of the original 15 minutes. Other symptoms, such as getting into and out of her car, had also settled post-treatment. Furthermore, the subject had returned to the gym on a twice-weekly basis, but concentrated on non-weight-bearing activities with no problems.

Discussion

Positive results were gained from the acupuncture protocol employed, in terms of both the subject's VAS scale and her active ROM. However, only a total of six sessions were carried out. Meng et al (2003) highlighted 10 sessions of acupuncture as being effective as a standard frequency of treatments, although this study was carried out on chronic low back pain patients. Therefore, further improvements to VAS and active ROM may have continued had more sessions been employed.

The chosen acupuncture protocol used points on the gall bladder meridian for local application. Although this brought about benefits to the VAS and active ROM, other meridians or local points could have been considered. Haslam (2001) used Ah Shi points around the greater trochanter in a north, south, east, and west formation and produced good results. Haslam (2001) also used Stomach 44, which is not only a distal point, but also one that Ellis (1994) reported as having a strong pain-relieving influence. Another point that could have been considered was Bladder 23 because this offers a segmental approach to anterior hip pain.

The positive outcome from combining acupuncture and manual therapy in the present case study not only aided in pain modulation, but also facilitated further rehabilitation and a consequent return to function and exercise.

Case study 3

James Thomson

Introduction

This presentation seeks to develop a rationale for the use of acupuncture in a case study involving the treatment of a runner presenting with symptoms consistent with piriformis origin. The physiology and reasoning behind the use of acupuncture is explored, along with a record of the progress of treatment, discussion of the different means by which acupuncture facilitated the development of diagnosis and broadened the outlook of the physiotherapist with regards to both the uses of acupuncture and the importance of treatment which is not necessarily confined to a medical mode of thinking.

Acupuncture has evolved in Western medical practice from its original roots in traditional Chinese medicine (TCM) to become one of the most pervasive elements of the management of neuromusculoskeletal pain in the primary healthcare setting (Kam et al 2002). Whilst it may remain the subject of some controversy, the clinical benefits have been studied across a variety of contexts, including shoulder pain (Gunn & Milbrandt 1977; Tukmachi 1999); back pain (Ernst & White 1998); temporomandibular joint dysfunction (Aung 1996); and osteoarthritis of the knee (Berman et al 2004). Acupuncture has not been without its critics and unfortunately research has predominantly examined acupuncture in patient groups assumed to be homogenous, despite the fact that patients presenting to physiotherapy departments are far removed from this

(Continued)

Case Study 3 (Continued)

factor. The use of clinical reasoning models and more appropriate treatment rationales may ensure that an evidence base develops, which is not only specific to the postulated effects of acupuncture, but which has direct influences on our reasoning (Bradnam 2002, 2003).

The present case study discusses the rationale for the use of acupuncture in the management and diagnosis of a combination of piriformis TrPt combined with mechanical lumbar and pelvic pain in a runner. The treatment performed could not be considered consistent with a strictly scientific rationale, but was successful partly because the training of the therapist had included the implicit guidance that a key part of the use of acupuncture included following clinical hypotheses and pursuing possible sources of TrPt dysfunction in the area. As such, acupuncture proved a key method in confirming these hypotheses.

Subjective assessment

The subject was a 40-year-old female working as a secretary in local government; a sedentary occupation. She had been a successful club athlete, retiring at the time of the birth of her first child, but had since taken up running again and had completed a number of fun runs over the past few years, together with running most evenings. Whilst running one month before her appointment, she experienced a sharp stabbing pain down the back of her right thigh, followed by pins and needles, which settled within 5 minutes. She continued with her running schedule, occasionally experiencing the same symptoms, for 2 weeks. At this time she began to feel a constant 'niggly' ache in her right buttock, after a few hours of sitting at work. This ache became worse and at the time of presentation (one month on) was a 60/100 on the VAS. The pain was centred in her buttock, radiating to her posterior thigh and was aggravated by sitting and running. Her general practitioner had diagnosed a lumbar facet joint irritation and administered 'keep moving' advice and a course of NSAIDs with little effect.

Objective assessment

The key objective markers are demonstrated in Table 9.6. The presentation was confusing as to whether presenting pain was emanating from a muscular origin with postural dysfunction in the lumbar spine, or a piriformis referral, approximating both an L5 and S1 facet joint irritation with a corresponding referral pattern. The distal symptoms experienced whilst running could have been more consistent with either piriformis syndrome or a nerve root involvement. The initial treatment plan was to initiate abdominal contractions through exercise, utilizing the core stability model involving the recruitment of transversus and multifidus. A temporary abdominal brace was used until such time as the subject's own core

Table 9.6 Main objective markers

Marker	Interpretation
20° anterior pelvic tilt ASIS and PSIS angle	Muscular dysfunction, issues with lumbar biomechanics
Poor abdominal muscle tone	As above
Bilateral pronating forefoot position	Increased work of hip lateral rotators in running
SLR (L) clear SLR (R) slight radiation in right posterior thigh	Indicative of either nerve root tension or piriformis trigger points.
Lumbar ROM pain free	No real help to diagnosis
Hip ROM full Combined hip flexion and adduction reproduced pain pattern	Activation of trigger points?
Palpation of taut band of piriformis muscle	Muscle twitch
Reproduction of pain pattern	Needle grasp
	Pain propagation

stability was sufficiently strong enough and the spine had achieved a good neutral position, to resume running (Tsao & Hodges 2002).

Clinical reasoning for acupuncture

Treatment was compounded with some clinical doubt as to whether the subject's symptoms were lumbar, pelvic, ergonomic, biomechanical, or related to TrPts. Using Bradnam's (2003) clinical reasoning model, acupuncture was used to aid diagnosis, relieve pain, and serve as a potential precursor to muscle imbalance exercises. An increasing understanding of the pathophysiology of pain, particularly with regards to how it is initiated and why it persists, is now leading to more selective use of acupuncture in its treatment (Bradnam 2003) and to address the following pain mechanisms:

- Stimulation of nociceptive pathways, release of histamines, and stimulation of nerve endings (Wu et al 1999);
- Activation of anti-nociceptive pathways in the hypothalamus (Sato et al 1986); and
- Pre- and post-synaptic inhibition through production of endogenous opioids, histamines, endorphins, serotonin and dopamine, beta-endorphins, and cortisol (Longbottom 2008).

More specific to the present case study is the use of acupuncture in pain relief through the stimulation of TrPts.

(Continued)

Case Study 3 (Continued)

It is interesting to note that a close correlation has been explored between TrPts points and acupuncture points, despite their derivation in such different philosophies (Melzack et al 1977). The deeper pistoning method used within TrPt needling has been postulated as resultant from stimulation of underlying pathological processes, linked by Melzack (1977) to nodules of fibrous tissue. With the presentation of biomechanical abnormalities, e.g. bilateral pronating foot position and anteriorly tilted pelvis, combined with the repetitive running, had possibly caused either an acute strain or more likely a repetitive strain insult to the piriformis muscle, consistent with the findings of Andersen et al (1995), that repetitive movements in a fixed, or slightly awkward posture were often sufficient to initiate myofascial pain.

Within the pathophysiological approach, the formation of TrPts is thought to be a result of one of two initial processes.

- Overuse or disuse injury results in dysfunction in the motor endplate, leading to continuous release of small amounts of acetylcholine into the synaptic cleft and permanent depolarisation of the muscle (Hubbard & Berkoff 1993).
- It has also been suggested that damage to the sarcoplasmic reticulum causes the same continuous muscle contraction through increased calcium deposition (from Hecker et al 2008).

The result of both these processes is the continuous contraction of actin and myosin filaments, the production of contractile, painful knots in the muscle, and compression of the blood supply, leading to the classic 'energy crisis' as described by Travell and Simons (1992). This repeating process leads to nociceptive pain and increased sympathetic activity. TrPt needling is thought to alter significantly the motor end-plate, resulting in a stretch in the dysfunctional muscle fibres that will ultimately lead to realignment of muscle fibres (Langevin 2001). In terms of specific research, there appears to be a lack of well-controlled randomized controlled trials to advocate use (Cummings & White 2001). However, this review did advocate the use of dry needling as an adjunct to treatment, although no significant benefit over placebo was demonstrated.

Acupuncture point rationale and use

Thomas (1997) considers several parameters important in initiating a positive clinical response to acupuncture intervention, these include:

- Site of needle insertion;
- Intensity of stimulation;
- Duration of treatment;
- Timing of intervention relative to tissue healing; and
- Mode of stimulation.

Two TrPts were selected within the piriformis muscle after manual palpation revealed a contractile knot,

Table 9.7 Rationale for use of acupuncture points

Point	Location	Rationale
TrPt 1	Along the line of piriformis, close to insertion	Needle grasp Referral of patient pain pattern.
TrPt 2	Close to the muscle origin	Needle grasp Referral of patient pain pattern
BL54	3 Cun lateral to sacral hiatus	Local acupuncture point
GB30	Lateral side of hip, on line connecting the greater trochanter and sacral hiatus	Local point for posterior hip pain

taut band, and patient pain propagation (Hecker et al 2008) (Table 9.7). On needling in the first session, twitch response was not elicited (Hong 1994), but during sessions 2 and 3 a localized twitch was evident. This is considered by Hong (1994) and in Travell and Simons (1992) as important both to confirm needle placement and as it appears to improve treatment outcome.

Also considered were acupuncture points Gall Bladder 34 (GB34) and GB39, which may have been used as a segmental approach to the lumbar pain presented by the subject; using a clinical reasoning model, with focus on the myofascial pain presentation, allowed the clinician to reassess to determine whether more extensive global pain relief was indeed necessary following this initial intervention. In terms of intensity and duration, caution was used in the initial session, but once patient compliance was achieved, treatments were more robust in subsequent sessions, with improved outcomes.

The subject demonstrated improvement in the frequency and intensity of symptoms, although manual and exercise intervention, incorporating a phased running regime and ergonomic and muscle imbalance interventions to further assist in return to full function, is ongoing.

Outcomes

Acupuncture and TrPt intervention was commenced at treatment 2, following the establishment of an advice and exercise regime (Table 9.8). Two TrPts were deactivated within piriformis, whilst GB30 was added in order to enhance the spinal, segmental inhibition of pain and possibly reduced treatment soreness. The reported, subjective pain at this treatment was 60/100 VAS. At treatments 1 and 2, the same procedure was repeated. As palpable tender knots and taut bands remained, deep

(Continued)

Case Study 3 (Continued)

Table 9.8 Outcome measurements and results

Session	Points used	Outcome (initial)	Outcome (7 days)
1	Nil-established exercise regime		
2	GB30 TrPts 1 and 2	Some pain exhibited during treatment. Piriformis stretching exercise given	VAS 60/100
3	GB30 TrPts 1 and 2	Deep, bruising sensation. Lasted 3 days piriformis stretches	VAS 30/100 painful when running
4	GB30 TrPts 1 and 2	Treatment soreness for one day	VAS 0/100 at rest 30/100 on stretching piriformis

piriformis muscle stretching exercises were added at this stage and VAS reduced to 30/100. At the final treatment 4, the TrPts were treated, the patient reported a VAS of 0/100 at rest, 30/100 when stretching.

At time of writing, the treatment was ongoing, with increased hip stretching and lower quadrant muscle imbalance work. One of the key areas of improvement has been the ability of the subject to adhere to a good, effective stretching regime. Her VAS improved significantly with three sessions, whilst further interventions, addressing the biomechanics and ergonomics will hopefully restore muscle imbalance and facilitate her return to normal function whilst minimizing the incidence of repeated trauma.

References

Andersen, J.H., Kaergaard, A., Rasmussen, K., 1995. Myofascial Pain in different occupational groups with monotonous repetitive work. Pain 3, 57.

Aung, S.K., 1996. The treatment of temporomandibular joint dysfunction and distress: a Chinese traditional medical approach. Am. J. Acupunct. 24 (4), 255–267.

Baber, Y., Robinson, A., Villar, R., 1999. Is diagnostic arthroscopy worthwhile? J. Bone Joint Surg. 81B, 600–603.

Barlas, P., 2005. Encouraging results for the efficiency of acupuncture on Osteoarthritic knee pain. Focus on Altern. Complemen. Ther. 10 (2), 123–124.

Bars, D., Willer, J., 2002. Pain modulation triggered by high-intensity stimulation: implication for acupuncture analgesia? Int. Congr. Ser. 1238, 11–29.

Beard, D., Dodd, C., Trundle, H., et al., 1994. Proprioception enhancement for anterior cruciate ligament deficiency. J. Bone Joint Surg. 76B, 654–659.

Bellabarba, C., Sheinkop, M., Kua, K., 2007. Idiopathic hip instability: an unrecognised cause of coxa saltans in the adult. Clin. Orthop. Relat. Res. 355, 261–271.

Bengtsson, A., Henriksson, K.G., Larsson, J., 1986. Reduced high-energy phosphate levels in the painful muscles of patients with primary fibromyalgia. Arthritis Rheum. 29 (7), 817–821.

Bensoussan, A., 1990. The vital meridian. Churchill Livingstone, Edinburgh.

Berman, B.M., Lao, L., Langenberg, P., et al., 2004. Effectiveness of acupuncture as adjunctive therapy In Osteoarthritis of the knee: A randomised controlled trial. Ann. Intern. Med. 21, 141.

Biloxi, M., 1998. Orthopaedic manual physical therapy document describing advanced clinical practice. Am. Academy of Orthopaedic Manual Physical Therapists.

Bradnam, L., 2002. Western acupuncture point selection: A scientific clinical reasoning model. J. Acupunct. Assoc. Chartered Physiotherapists March, 21–28.

Bradnam, L., 2003. A proposed clinical reasoning model for Western acupuncture. New Zealand J. Physiother 31, 40–45.

Brukner, P., Khan, K., 2007. Clinical sports medicine, 3rd edn. McGraw Hill, Sydney.

Chen, J.T., Chen, S.M., Kuan, T.S., et al., 1998. Phentolamine effect on the spontaneous electrical activity of active loci in a myofascial trigger spot of rabbit skeletal muscle. Arch. Phys. Med. Rehabil. 79 (7), 790–794.

Chen, J.T., Chung, K.C., Hou, C.R., et al., 2001. Inhibitory effect of dry needling on the spontaneous electrical activity recorded from myofascial trigger spots of rabbit skeletal muscle. Am. J. Phys. Med. Rehabil. 80 (10), 729–735.

Crowninshield, R., Johnston, R., Andrews, J., et al., 1978. A biomechanical investigation of the human hip. J. Bone Joint Surg 69A, 1021–1031.

Cummings, M., 2000. Piriformis syndrome. Acupunct. Med. 18 (2), 108–121.

Cummings, M., White, A., 2001. Needling therapies in the management of myofascial trigger point pain: a systematic review. Arch. Phys. Med. Rehabil. 82 (7), 986–992.

Deyle, G.D., Henderson, N.E., Matekel, R.L., et al., 2000. Effectiveness of manual physical therapy and exercise in osteoarthritis of the knee. A randomized, controlled trial. Ann. Intern. Med. 132 (3), 173–181.

Ellis, N., 1994. Acupuncture in clinical practice, 1st edn. Chapman and Hall, London.

Ernst, E., White, A., 1998. Acupuncture for back pain; a meta-analysis of randomised control trials. Int Arch Med 158, 2235–2241.

Falconer, J., Hayes, K.W., Chang, R.W., 1992. Effect of ultrasound on mobility in osteoarthritis of the knee: a randomized clinical trial. Arthritis Care Res. 5, 29–35.

Felson, D., Zhang, Y., 1998. An update on the epidemiology of knee and hip osteoarthritis with a view to prevention. Arthritis Rheum. 41, 1343–1355.

Felson, D., Lawrence, R., Hochberg, M., et al., 2000. Osteoarthritis: new insights: Part 2 treatment approaches. Ann. Intern. Med. 33, 726–737.

Ferguson, S., Bryant, J., Ganz, R., et al., 2003. An in vitro investigation of the acetabular labral seals in hip joint mechanics. J. Biomech. 36 (2), 171–178.

Fine, P.G., Milano, R., Hare, B.D., 1988. The effects of myofascial trigger point injections are naloxone reversible. Pain 32 (1), 15–20.

Fink, M.G., Wipperman, B., Gehrke, A., 2001. Non-specific effects of traditional Chinese acupuncture In Osteoarthritis of the hip. Complemen. Ther. Med. 9 (2), 82–89.

Fitzgerald, G., 1997. Open versus closed kinetic chain exercise: issues in rehabilitation after anterior cruciate ligament reconstructive surgery. Phys Ther 77, 1747–1754.

Fitzgerald, R., 1995. Acetabular labrum tears. Clin. Orthop. Relat. Res. 311, 60–68.

Fredericson, M., Cookingham, C.L., Chaudhari, A.M., et al., 2000. Hip abductor weakness in distance runners with iliotibial band syndrome. Clin. J. Sport Med. 10 (3), 169–175.

French, H., 2007. Physiotherapy management of osteoarthritis of the hip: a survey of current practice in acute hospitals and private practice in the Republic of Ireland. Physiotherapy 93, 253–260.

Gong, D., Liang, C., Lai, X., et al., 1993. Effects of different acupuncture manipulation on plasma estradiol, testosterone and cortisol in patients with kidney deficiency. Zhen Ci Yan Jui 18 (4), 253–256.

Gunn, C.C., Milbrandt, W.E., 1977. Tenderness at motor points: an aid in the diagnosis of pain in the shoulder referred from the cervical spine. J. Am. Osteopath. Assoc. 77 (3), 196–212.

Haslam, R., 2001. A comparison of acupuncture with advice in Osteoarthritis of the hip: a randomised controlled trial. Acupunct. Med. 19 (1), 19–26.

Hecker, H.U., Steveling, A., Peuker, E., et al., 2008. Trigger and acupuncture points of the piriformis muscle. In: *Color atlas of acupuncture*. Stuttgart: Thieme.

Hengeveld, E., Banks, K., 2005. Maitland peripheral manipulation, 4th edn. Elsevier, Butterworth Heinemann, Tortonto.

Heuts, P., de Bie, R., Drietelaar, M., et al., 2005. Self-management in osteoarthritis of the hip or knee: a randomised clinical trial in a primary healthcare setting. Health Technicians Assessment 9, 1–114.

Hoeksma, H., Dekker, H., Ronday, A., et al., 2004. Comparison of manual therapy and exercise therapy in osteoarthritis of the hip: a randomised clinical trial. Arthritis Rheum. 51, 722–729.

Hölmich, P., 2007. Long-standing groin pain in sportspeople falls into three primary patterns, a 'clinical entity' approach: a prospective study of 207 patients. Br. J. Sports Med. 41, 247–252.

Hong, C., 1994. Lincoaine injection versus dry needling to myofascial trigger point: the importance of the twitch response. Am. J. Phys. Med. Rehabil. 73, 256–263.

Hubbard, D., Berkoff, G., 1993. Myofascial trigger points show spontaneous needle EMG. Spine 18, 1803–1807.

Huguenin, L., Brukner, P.D., McCrory, P., et al., 2005. Effect of dry needling of gluteal muscles on straight leg raise: A randomized, placebo controlled, double blind trial. Br. Med. J. 39, 84–90.

Ikeda, T., Suzuki, S., Okada, Y., et al., 1988. Torn acetabular labrum in young patients. J. Bone Joint Surg. 70B, 13–16.

Ito, K., Minka-II, M., Leunig, M., et al., 2001. Acetabular impingement and the cam effect. J. Bone Joint Surg. 83B, 171–176.

Kahan, J., McClennan, R., Burton, D., 1994. Acute bilateral compartment syndrome of the thigh induced by exercise: A case report. J. Bone Joint Surg. 76A, 1068–1071.

Kam, E., Eslick, G., Campbell, A., 2002. An audit of the effectiveness of acupuncture on musculoskeletal pain in primary health care. Acupunct. Med. 20 (1), 35–38.

Khan, K., 1999. Histopathy of common tendinopathies. Sports Med. 27 (6), 393–408.

Klaue, K., Durnin, C., Ganz, R., 1991. The acetabular rim syndrome: a clinical presentation of dysplasia of the hip. J. Bone Joint Surg. 73B, 423–429.

Knuesel, H., Geyer, H., Seyfarth, A., 2005. Influence of swing leg movements on running stability. Hum. Mov. Sci. 24 (4), 532–543.

Konin, J., Nofsinger, C., 2007. Physical therapy management of athletic Injuries of the hip. Oper. Tech. Sports Med. 15 (4), 204–216.

Korpelainen, R., Orava, S., Karpakka, J., et al., 2001. Risk factors for recurrent stress fractures in athletes. Am. J. Sports Med. 29 (3), 304–310.

Kummer, B., 1993. Is the Pauwels theory of hip biomechanics still valid? A critical analysis based on modern methods. Ann. Anat. 175, 203–210.

Kwon, Y.D., Pittler, M.H., Ernst, E., 2006. Acupuncture for peripheral joint osteoarthritis: a systematic review and meta-analysis. Rheumatology 45 (11), 1331–1337.

Langevin, H.M., Vaillancourt, P., 1999. Acupuncture: does it work and, if so, how? Seminal Clin. Neuropsychiatry. 4, 167–175.

LaStayo, P., Woolf, J., Woolf, M., 2003. Eccentric muscle contractions: their contribution to injury prevention, rehabilitation and sport. J. Orthop. Sports Phys. Ther. 33, 557–571.

Lephart, S., Incivero, D., Giraldo, J., et al., 1997. The role of proprioception in the management and rehabilitation of athletic injuries. Am. J. Sports Med. 25 (130), 137.

Linde, K., Weidenhammer, W., Streng, A., et al., 2005. Acupuncture for osteoarthritic pain: an observational study in routine care. Rheumatology 45 (2), 22–27.

Longbottom, J., 2008. The mechanisms of acupuncture analgesia in acupuncture for pain relief. Acupunct. Assoc. Chart. Physiotherapists course notes 2 (2.1), 16.

McCarthy, J., Barsoum, W., Puri, L., et al., 2003. The role of hip arthroscopy in the diagnosis and treatment of hip disease. Clin. Orthop. Relat. Res. 406, 38–47.

Melzack, R., Stillwell, D.M., Fox, E.J., 1977. Trigger points and acupuncture points for pain: correlations and implications. Pain 3, 3–23.

Meng, C.F., Wang, D., Ngeow, J., et al., 2003. Acupuncture for chronic low back pain in older patients: a randomized, controlled trial. Rheumatology 42 (12), 1508–1517.

Mizrahi, J., Voloshin, A., Russek, D., et al., 1997. The influence of fatigue on EMG and impact acceleration in running. Basic Appl. Myol. 7, 111–118.

Nelson, D., Hutton, R., 1985. Dynamic and static stretch responses in muscle spindle receptors in fatigued muscle. Med. Sci. Sports Exerc. 17 (4), 445–450.

Nicholls, R., 2004. Intra-articular disorders of the hip in athletes. Phys. Ther. in Sport. 5 (1), 17–25.

Niemuth, P., 2007. The role of hip muscle weakness in lower extremity athletic Osteoarthritis. Arthritis Rheum. 40, 1518–1525.

Prentice, W., 1992. Techniques of manual therapy for the knee. J. Sports Rehabil. 8, 161–189.

Puett, D.W., Griffin, M.R., 1994. Published trials of nonmedicinal and noninvasive therapies for hip and knee osteoarthritis. Ann. Intern. Med. 121 (2), 133–140.

Reid, D., 1988. Prevention of hip and knee injuries in ballet dancers. Sports Med. 6, 295–307.

Reynolds, D., Lucas, J., Klaue, K., 2007. Retroversion of the acetabulum: a cause of hip pain. J Bone Joint Surg. 81B, 281–288.

Roddy, E., Zhang, W., Doherty, N., et al., 2004. Evidence based recommendations for the role of exercise in the management of osteoarthritis of the hip or knee: the MOVE consensus. Rheumatology 44, 67–73.

Sahramann, S., 2001. Diagnosis and treatment of movement impairment syndromes. Mosby, London.

Sato, T., Usami, S., Takeshige, C., 1986. Role of the arcuate nucleus of the hypothalamus as the descending pain inhibitory system in acupuncture point and non-point produced analgesia. In: Studies on the mechanism of acupuncture analgesia based on animal experiments. Showa University Press, Tokyo.

Sato, A., Sato, Y., Shimura, M., et al., 2000. Calcitonin gene-related peptide produces skeletal muscle vasodilation following antidromic stimulation of unmyelinated afferents in the dorsal roots in rats. Neuroscience 283, 137–140.

Schwellnus, M.P., Derman, E.W., Noakes, T.D., 1997. Aetiology of skeletal muscle 'cramps' during exercise: A novel hypothesis. J. Sports Sci. 15 (3), 277–285.

Sharma, P., Maffulli, N., 2005. Tendon injury and tendinopathy. J. Bone Joint Surg. 87 (1), 187–202.

Sharma, L., Pai, Y., Holtkamp, K., et al., 1997. Is knee joint proprioception worse in the arthritic knee versus the unaffected knee in unilateral knee osteoarthritis? Arthritis Rheum. 40 (8), 1518–1525.

Sherman, K.J., Cherkin, D.C., 2005. Acupuncture modestly beneficial treatment for osteoarthritis of the knee. Focus on Altern. Complemen. Ther. 10 (2), 121–122.

Sims, K., 1999. Assessment and treatment of osteoarthritis of the hip. Man. Ther. 4, 139–144.

Smith, C., Crowther, C., 2002. The placebo response and effect of time in a trial of acupuncture to treat nausea and vomiting in early pregnancy. Complemen. Ther. Med. 10 (4), 210–216.

Stener-Victorin, E., Kruse-Smidje, C., Jung, K., 2004. Comparison between electro-acupuncture and hydrotherapy, both in combination with patient education and patient education alone, on the symptomatic treatment of osteoarthritis of the hip. Clin. J. Pain 20, 179–185.

Strange, F., 1965. The hip. Heinemann Medical Books, London.

Tak, E., Staats, P., van Hepsen, A., et al., 2005. The effects of an exercise programme for older adults with osteoarthritis of the hip. J. Rheumatol. 3, 1106–1113.

Thomas, M., 1997. Acupuncture studies on pain. Acupunct. Med. 15 (1), 23.

Tillu, A., Roberts, C., Tillu, S., 2001. Unilateral versus bilateral acupuncture on knee in advanced osteoarthritis of the knee: a prospective randomised trial. Acupunct. Med. 19 (1), 15–18.

Tiquia, R., 1996. Traditional Chinese medicine: a guide to its practice. Choice Books (Australian Consumers Association), Marriokville, Australia.

Tough, E.A., White, A.R., Cummings, T.M., et al., 2009. Acupuncture and dry needling in the management of myofascial trigger point pain: a systematic review and meta-analysis of randomised controlled trials. Eur. J. Pain 13 (1), 3–10.

Travell, J.G., Simons, D.G., 1992. Myofascial pain and dysfunction: the trigger point manual, vol. ii: the lower extremities. Williams and Wilkins, Baltimore.

Tsao, H., Hodges, P., 2002. Persistence of improvements in postural strategies following motor control training in people with recurrent low back pain. J. Electromyogr. Kinesiol. 18 (4), 559–567.

Tukmachi, E., 1999. Frozen shoulder: a comparison of western and traditional Chinese approaches and a clinical study of its acupuncture treatment. Acupunct. Med. 17, 9–21.

Vad, V., Hong, H., Zazzali, M., et al., 2002. Exercise recommendations in athletes with early osteoarthritis of the knee. Sports Med. 32, 729–739.

van Baar, M., Dekker, J., Oostendorp, R., et al., 1998. The effectiveness of exercise therapy in patients with osteoarthritis of the hip or knee; a randomised controlled trial. J. Rheumatol. 25, 2432–2439.

van Mechelen, W., Hlobil, H., Zijilstra, W., et al., 1992. Is range of motion of the hip and ankle joint related to running injuries? Int. J. Sports Med. 13, 605–610.

Villar, R., 1992. Hip arthroscopy. Butterworth Heinemann, Oxford.

Whyte-Ferguson, L., Gerwin, R., 2005. Hip and groin pain: the disordered hip complex in: clinical mastery of myofascial pain. Lippincott Williams and Wilkins, Philadelphia 271–301.

Wu, H.G., Zhou, L.B., Pan, Y.Y., et al., 1999. Study of the mechanisms of acupuncture and moxibustion treatment for ulcerative colitis rats in view of the gene expression of cytokines. World J. Gastroenterol. 5 (6), 515–517.

Zhang, W., Doherty, M., Arden, N., et al., 2005. EULAR evidence based recommendations for the management of hip osteoarthritis: report of a task force of the EULAR standing committee for international clinical studies including therapeutics. Ann. Rheum. 64, 669–681.

Anterior knee pain

10

Lee Herrington

Introduction

Anterior knee pain (AKP) is a common clinical presentation in musculoskeletal management in patients of all ages and activity levels. The categories of conditions that can be placed within the diverse grouping of AKP can be defined as involving pain; inflammation; and muscle imbalance and/or instability of any component of the extensor mechanism of the knee. This disturbance of the extensor mechanism of the knee is regarded as one of the commonest disorders of the knee, affecting between 5 and 15% of all patients reporting for treatment (Devereaux & Lachmann 1984; Kannus et al 1987; Milgrom et al 1991). Once present, it frequently becomes a chronic problem, forcing the patient to stop sport and other activities; the condition has long been regarded as the black hole of orthopaedics (Dye & Vaupel 1994). The classification of symptoms is confusing, with AKP being present in many clinical conditions. The commonest clinical conditions displaying symptoms of AKP are:

- Patellofemoral pain syndrome (PFPS);
- Patellar tendinopathy;
- Fat pad syndrome;
- Traction apophysitis (Osgood-Schlatters disease/ Sinding-Larsen-Johansson disease);
- Plica syndrome;
- Iliotibial band syndrome (ITBS); and
- Nerve entrapment.

In a retrospective review of patients attending a sports medicine clinic, AKP was found to be the primary presenting complaint in 29.2% of all running injuries (Taunton et al 2002), a figure very similar to the 28% found two decades earlier (Clement et al 1981). Of the patients found with AKP, in the Taunton et al (2002) study, 56.5% had PFPS, 28.8% had ITBS, and 16.4% had patella tendinopathy.

Even when a diagnostic label can be found for the condition, dealing with why a particular structure has become injured is the key to the successful

DOI: 10.1016/B978-0-443-06782-2.00010-4

treatment of this group of conditions. Furthermore, the varieties of pathologies that present under the umbrella of AKP often have similar signs and symptoms, which is a significant limiting factor when it comes to determining the exact underlying structural pathology. What may be more appropriate is to look at the potential causes of the AKP itself.

Tissue homeostasis, overload, and the presence of pathology

The presence of tissue homeostasis is a concept familiar to physiologists, but less so to musculoskeletal medicine clinicians. It could be defined as the process of actively maintaining a constant condition or balance within an internal (cellular) environment (Cannon 1929).

All musculoskeletal tissues are, to a greater or lesser extent, metabolically active. The purpose of this metabolic activity is to maintain a constant environment within the cellular structure of the tissues. When these cells are stressed (e.g. with exercise), a cascade of reparative physiological processes take place within the cell, in response to the damage that has occurred, in order to bring the cells back into a homeostatic state.

The tissue homeostasis model is as follows:

- If the stress is of an appropriate level, the cells will adapt to the repeated exposure of this stress and become stronger and more tolerant of the load placed upon them.
- If a single load of sufficient magnitude is applied to the tissue, or multiple repetitive loads, it is possible that, at least in the short term, the trauma caused to the tissue (disturbance of homeostasis) is beyond the ability of the tissue to cope with and therefore tissue damage (disturbance of homeostasis) will occur (Dye & Vaupel 1994; Dye 2005.

This model shows four distinct zones:

- The zone of subphysiological under-load;
- Homeostasis;
- Supraphysiological overload (Fig. 10.1); and
- Tissue failure.

By varying either the level of load or the frequency with which it is applied, the load placed on the tissues can move between these zones. Loading within the zone of homeostasis allows for tissue balance. Loading in the subphysiological underload

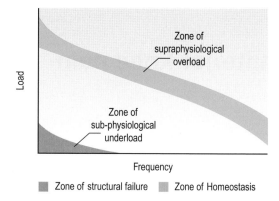

Figure 10.1 ● A schematic representation of the tissue homeostasis model. (adapted from Dye & Vaupel 1994; Dye, 2005.)

zone causes the tissues to atrophy and become less tolerant to load, since the tissues are understressed. Loading in the zone of supraphysiological overload is the most biologically significant. If loading is applied, but the tissue is given sufficient time to recover, the tissue will adapt to this new level of loading, i.e. it will get stronger. This will cause the barrier of the zone of homeostasis to move to the right; the tissues can now tolerate greater loads without becoming overly stressed. If sufficient time is not given for tissue recovery, tissue breakdown will occur, eventually leading to failure recognizable as injury.

The tissue homeostasis model can be used to describe why an injury has occurred; for instance, a single blow to the patella might generate sufficient force to be in the zone of tissue failure. Patients increasing their running distance may apply a low load with sufficient frequency to supraphysiologically overload the tissues, and if they run these distances frequently, not giving the tissues sufficient time to recover, this can lead to injury. Moviegoers knee is a common complaint of patients with AKP and can easily be explained by the tissue homeostasis model. Sitting for a prolonged period applies a sustained low load on the patella; this could be beyond the tissues' ability to cope with, hence provoking symptoms and pain.

Injuries caused by overloading of the tissue concerned are either acute and usually traumatic or chronic and long term, involving low loads that eventually cause the tissue to break down because of the dripping tap effect, of an overuse or, more correctly, an overload injury (Fig. 10.2).

The common feature of all of these factors is that they change the loading of the patellofemoral

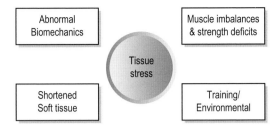

Figure 10.2 • Causes of altered loading.

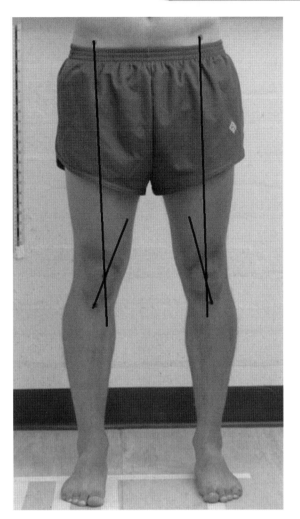

Figure 10.3 • Q angle.

joint (PFJ) and the surrounding structures. This can occur as a result of change in the magnitude of the load, which is influenced in turn by the degree of knee flexion and the amount of quadriceps force, relating directly to the PFJ, whereas distribution of the loading is related to patellar tracking, i.e. structural alignment and soft-tissue balance.

Abnormal biomechanics

A number of biomechanical factors can have a significant influence on the loading of the PFJ and other associated structures, the most significant of these being the quadriceps angle (Q-angle) and its relationship to asymmetrical loading of the patella and the surrounding supporting structures. Knowledge of the Q-angle (Fig. 10.3) and its effect on PFJ loading is important to understanding how abnormal biomechanics can affect the joint. The Q-angle represents the force vector (direction of pull) of the quadriceps during their contraction (Fig. 10.3). With optimal alignment of the tibia relative to the femur, the patella is drawn through the trochlear of the femur and the load is equally distributed across the articular surfaces of the patella. With altered suboptimal alignment of the tibia relative to the femur (or vice versa), contraction of the quadriceps can cause the patella to be drawn medially or laterally from its normal course; this will have the potential effect of increasing the stress and loading of the PFJ, and the structures associated with it. By increasing the Q-angle by 10°, significant load is increased on the lateral structures of the PFJ (Elias et al 2006). The Q-angle can be affected by the following mechanisms:

- Malalignment within the lower limb, such as anteriorly rotated pelvis;
- Femoral ante or retroversion;
- Tibial torsion; and
- Pronation of the foot.

Soft-tissue tightness and muscle weakness

A variety of soft tissues can influence the Q-angle by changing the relative position of the femur to the tibia. At the hip, shortened hip flexors, principally the rectus femoris, iliopsoas, and iliotibial band (ITB), can cause the pelvis to be held in an anteriorly rotated position and change the Q-angle. If the adductor muscles, principally the adductor longus, are short (or overactive), this will cause the femur to be held in an internally rotated and adducted position, increasing the Q-angle.

Through its attachment onto Gerdy's tubercle of the tibia, a short ITB can cause the tibia to be held in an externally rotated position, thereby moving the tibial tubercle laterally and so changing the Q-angle. If either the gastrocnemius or soleus muscles (the triceps surae complex) are short, this limits the ability of dorsiflexion at the ankle. In order to continue to allow full movement during gait, the foot will compensate for this lack of movement by pronating excessively, using dorsiflexion that occurs with mid-foot pronation, to compensate for the lack of movement at the ankle.

Pronation of the foot

If the foot overly pronates (i.e. the longitudinal arch becomes flattened), the leg will internally rotate excessively, causing the knee to point inwards, thus changing the Q-angle. Anterior pelvic rotation causes one leg to appear longer and the body must compensate for this. One way it typically compensates is to overly flatten (pronation) the foot. The foot of the longer leg, in an attempt to shorten it, thus changes the Q-angle, as the tibia is drawn into a more medially rotated position.

Muscle imbalances and strength deficits

Research into AKP has paid considerable attention to achieving increased activity and strength in the vastus medialis oblique muscle (VMO) with the aim of drawing the patella medially, and thus centralizing it against the pull of the laterally attached vastus lateralis muscle. The problem is that the majority of the literature has failed to report findings of either problems with the VMO in patients with AKP (Powers 1998) or a means of specifically training this muscle in isolation without simultaneously facilitating contraction in the rest of the quadriceps muscles (Herrington et al 2006).

A consistent feature of the research literature on the causes of AKP is that patients with AKP have been reported to have weak quadriceps on the whole (Mohr et al 2003), and a number of studies have demonstrated successful resolution of symptoms upon strengthening of the quadriceps muscles (Herrington & Al-Shehri 2007). Regardless of the position of the patella relative to the femur in the frontal plane, if the quadriceps does not contract appropriately, there will be a reduced area of contact between the articulating surfaces of the patella and the trochlear. Contraction of the quadriceps causes the patella to be seated deeper within the trochlear notch, maximizing the contact of the articular surfaces; any reduction serves to increase the stress per unit area of the PFJ, and subsequently increases loading.

A further group of muscles, whose weaknesses have been consistently reported within the literature to be associated with AKP, are the gluteal muscles (gluteus maximus, medius, and minimus) (Tyler et al 2006). Weakness of these muscles causes the thigh to drop into a more adducted and internally rotated position during weight-bearing, increasing the Q-angle and causing asymmetrical loading on the PFJ.

Training or environmental triggers

All of the above problems can be found in many members of the public who do not have AKP, suggesting that these predisposing factors require a trigger, which will affect the tissue in a negative way, reducing tolerance to loading. There are many potential triggers leading to change in tissue-load tolerance; for example:

- Direct contact trauma;
- Surgery;
- A change in loading brought about by new training shoes or boots;
- A change of training surface; and
- A rapid increase in loading following a period of de-training (decreased loading of the tissues, with loss of tolerance) caused by illness or holiday.

All of these above have the potential to shift the border of the zone of supraphysiological loading to the left (Fig. 10.2). The patient experiences loads that were previously tolerable, but now cause stress and the potential for injury (Dye 2005).

Sources of pain in and around the patellofemoral joint

There are a number of structures in and around the PFJ which, when subjected to load, could be the source of patellofemoral pain syndrome (PFPS). Dye et al (1998) found that palpation of the anterior synovium and fat pad elicited the strongest sensation of pain, followed by both the medial and lateral retinaculum, with the articular surface of the joint exhibiting least pain on probing. Biedert et al (2000) supported these findings, reporting the highest number of afferent nerve fibres to be in the medial and lateral retinaculum. Witonski and Wagrowska-Danielewicz (1999) found nerve fibres that were immunoreactive for substance P in the fat pad, retinacula, and synovium, but not in the articular cartilage of patients with PFP. The levels of these substance-P-positive nerve fibres in the retinaculum were significantly higher than those found in patients undergoing anterior cruciate ligament reconstruction or total knee replacement for osteoarthritis (OA).

The lateral retinaculum has been shown to have many histological features associated with PFPS, including:

- Nerve fibrosis and neuroma formation (Sanchi-Alfonso et al 1998);
- Increased numbers of unmyelinated nociceptive nerve fibres (Witonski & Wagrowska-Danielewicz 1999);
- Increased vascularity (Sanchi-Alfonso et al 1998);
- Peripatellar synovitis, which is considered to be one of the main sources of PFJ pain, with its high sensitivity to compression and probing (Dye et al 1998); and
- Histological changes found in symptomatic individuals (Arnoldi 1991).

Even though the articular cartilage does not appear to be the direct source of pain, it is potentially a major indirect source. Joenson et al (2001) demonstrated a significant positive association between the presence of articular cartilage lesions of the patella and PFPS (17 out of 24 patients assessed). Superficial cartilage lesions may lead to chemical or mechanical irritation of the synovium, or progress to subchondral bone erosion. Increases in intraosseous pressure of the PFJ subchondral bone could result in pain (Dye & Vaupel 1994), possibly secondary to transient venous outflow obstruction (Arnoldi 1991) that may be related to malalignment of the patella. Harilainen et al (2005) showed that specific malalignments (e.g. lateral tilt of the patella) predispose to patellofemoral cartilage lesion.

Intraosseous pressure can rise to 70 mmHg when the patella is compressed into the trochlear groove. Hejgaard & Arnoldi (1984) observed a significant relationship between increased PFJ intraosseous pressure and AKP in a study of 40 patients. Resting intraosseous pressure in painful patellae was 29 mmHg compared with 15 mmHg in pain-free subjects. Also, the painful knees showed a greater increase in pressure on maximum flexion (90 mmHg), compared with healthy knees (60 mmHg). In the PFJ, articular cartilage degeneration reported to be accompanied by venous engorgement within the patella and decreased venous outflow (Waisbrod & Treiman 1980).

Strategies for management

Pain relief

The most obvious way to relieve pain is to take away the stress causing the tissue to be overloaded. This can be done using the following approaches.

Changing the magnitude or distribution of the load

One very successful treatment method, which has been used to change the distribution of tissue loading, is taping. Patella taping has been shown significantly to reduce pain on numerous occasions (Aminaka & Gribble 2005), although the mechanism involved remains unclear (Warden et al 2008). It has been hypothesized that subtle changes in loading, and therefore, tissue homeostasis are brought about by small, but biologically significant changes in the patella position (Herrington 2006). Similar effects have also been attributed to using braces (Warden et al 2008).

In-shoe orthosis

The aim of the in-shoe orthosis is to change the magnitude or timing of foot pronation (Vicenzino 2004), which will in turn affect the degree and rate of tibial rotation, and load distribution through changes in the Q-angle outlined above.

The use of taping, bracing, and foot orthosis are likely to have an immediate effect on the patient's symptoms because of these treatments' potential to directly effect load distribution through altering tibial alignment, however subtly. A number of other methods are available to the therapist to modify the load distribution on structures in and around the anterior knee. By addressing the shortened soft tissues, muscle imbalances, and strength deficits outlined above, the distribution of load on structures will be changed. This process will take longer as neuromuscular and histological changes need to occur in the tissues through consistent exercise loading. This element of treatment involves accurately assessing the causes of altered loading, and addressing them with appropriate rehabilitation.

The majority of patients with AKP, particularly those with PFPS and patella tendinopathy (PT), demonstrate higher peak forces through the structures of the knee than normal subjects on landing, stair descent and other functional activities (Herrington et al 2005). This may be related to their inability to generate sufficient (or appropriately timed) force eccentrically in their quadriceps (Andersen & Herrington 2003) in order to decelerate these loads. By improving quadriceps strength, particularly eccentric strength, the magnitude of the loads being imparted on the structures of the knee can be reduced, thus reducing stress and pain.

Improving tolerance to load

Biological tissues have the ability to adapt to the loads to which they are exposed. As described earlier in Fig. 10.2, the application of supraphysiological loads to tissues will cause the loaded tissue to break down; if sufficient time is allowed for recovery, the tissue adapts to these repeated loads and becomes stronger. This is the overload principle that forms the central tenet of strength training

(Magee et al 2007) and the development of load tolerance in biological tissues. A significant element in the rehabilitation of patients with AKP is progressively loading the tissues, in order to improve the tolerance to load of the tissues and, in so doing, move the zone of homeostasis of the tissues to the right (Fig. 10.2). This explains the success of the numerous studies that have been carried out with non-specific quadriceps muscle training in a progressive manner, bringing about significant improvements in the pain levels and function of patients with AKP (Herrington & Al-Shehri 2007; Witvrouw et al 2000).

Conclusion

The management of AKP has always been regarded as difficult because the problem takes a prolonged period to resolve, and often reoccurs. Successful management of this group of conditions involves clearly identifying what is causing the pain, not only in terms of which structure has been irritated, but also in terms of what has changed within the loading dynamic of that tissue. Therefore treatment is a logical progression of this assessment, with pain relief involving decreasing the loading and removing any predisposing factors to abnormal loading. The tissue is then progressively loaded until it can tolerate the demands placed upon it by the patient.

10.1 Acupuncture in the management of knee pain

Jennie Longbottom

Whether the presenting knee disorder is that of an acute sports injury or has the chronicity of OA, most knee dysfunction has a myofascial element accompanying other structural pain-provoking mechanisms. Patients who demonstrate persistent knee pain following rehabilitation and progressive strengthening regimes cannot achieve full function unless the relevant trigger points (TrPts) are deactivated (Whyte-Ferguson & Gerwin 2005). In a study of discharged patients suffering from persistent knee pain after total-knee arthroscopy, an estimated 87.5% reduction in pain was achieved after an average of 12 sessions of manual trigger point (MTrPt) therapy, combined with TrPt injections (Feinberg & Feinberg 1998). Näslund et al (2002) conducted a randomized controlled trial to evaluate the effect of acupuncture treatment on idiopathic anterior knee pain (IAKP). Fifty-eight patients were randomly assigned to either deep or superficial acupuncture. Pain measurements on a Visual Analogue Scale (VAS) decreased significantly within both groups from 25/100 to 10/100 in the deep needling, acupuncture group, and 30/100 to 10/100 in the superficial needling group. The VAS remained significant after 3 and 6 months. This study demonstrated that both groups experienced significant sustained pain relief as a result of afferent needle stimulation or non-specific (placebo) effects.

Many of the myofascial pain presentation may be attributed to the presence of active TrPts; if TrPts are not addressed, patients will demonstrate a failure to progress with strengthening exercises and rehabilitation regimes. The quadriceps femoris (QF) group is the most common muscle group involved, referring pain to the anterior, lateral, and medial aspects of the knee, and lower thigh. Tight hamstrings often perpetuate the QF TrPts, hindering full extension of the knee and placing excessive loads on the QF group (Simons et al 1999). The characteristic of the vastus medialis (VM) dysfunctional muscle is that pain may be somewhat overlooked since shortening is not immediately apparent. With the presence of prolonged TrPt dysfunction, the initial pain phase can be followed by an inhibitory phase involving unexpected weakness and letting down of the knee joint, especially on climbing and descending stairs, sitting to standing,

or any spontaneous activity, even in the absence of a traumatic event (Simons et al 1999). Myofascial pain from the QF muscles may be present at night, misleadingly making the practitioner suspect that there is an inflammatory component (Reynolds 1981). This is slightly out of keeping with pain patterns in most TrPts, which are relieved by rest and off-loading of the affected muscles.

Establishing an accurate baseline and measuring the patient's status before and after intervention is important. Myofascial dysfunction is one of the contributing factors to altered knee biomechanics and instability, in addition to dysfunction of the cruciate–meniscus complex and the PFJ (Whyte-Ferguson & Gerwin 2005). Pain localized around the anterior aspect of the knee can originate from problems with the quadriceps complex, the patellofemoral or tibiofemoral joints, or the infra- and suprapatellar tendons (Bizzini et al 2003; Cook & Khan 2001; Grays 1964; Khan et al 1999). It has been reported that 75% of all cases of AKP can be correctly diagnosed (Khan et al 1999), but both PFPS and tendinopathy can be difficult to distinguish or may coexist (Fig. 10.4).

The action of needling active TrPts to reduce myofascial pain and increase the length of a dysfunctional muscle has a biomechanical component perceived by the operator, i.e. the presence of

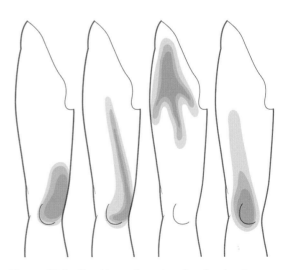

Figure 10.4 • Quadriceps femoris pain referral pattern.

needle grasp (Cheng 1987; Helms 1995), which is the contraction of skin and subcutaneous tissue achieved through the needle pulling on superficial collagen fibres. The mechanism of winding or pistoning the tissues (rapid in and out manipulation of the needle) may have the effect of gradually building up torque in the tissues, amplifying the friction force, and mechanical coupling between tissue and needle (Hibbler 1995). Once the needle has become coupled to the tissue, subsequent needle manipulation may pull on collagen fibres, resulting in deformation of the extracellular connective tissue matrix, which has the multifactorial effect of cell contraction, gene expression, secretion of paracrine or autocrine factors, and the subsequent neuromodulation of afferent sensory input (Langevin et al 2001). These are long-lasting effects, and may further explain why TrPt release may offer a permanent impact (Langevin 2007).

Itoh et al (2008) evaluated the effect of TrPt needling on pain and quality of life in OA knee patients as compared with acupuncture at standard points and sham acupuncture. A statistically significant difference was demonstrated between TrPt acupuncture, a standard acupuncture point protocol, using Stomach (ST) 34, ST35, Spleen (SP) 9, SP10, and Gall Bladder (GB) 34; and sham acupuncture, the results of which continued 5 weeks after treatment. The results suggest that TrPt needling may be more effective than standard point selection for OA of the knee. The patients in this study received five acupuncture treatment sessions, indicating that TrPt deactivation may produce greater activation of sensitized polymodal-type receptors, resulting in stronger pain relief than standard acupuncture alone (Kumazawa 1993).

Acupuncture excites receptors or nerve fibres in the stimulated tissue, which can also be physiologically activated by strong muscle contractions similar to the effect of protracted exercise (Andersson & Lundeberg 2002). Acupuncture and exercise produce rhythmic discharges in nerve fibres, causing the release of endogenous neurotransmitters, such as opioids, monoamines, and oxytocin, aiding regulation of the sympathetic nervous system (Andersson & Lundeberg 2002), and peripheral release of sensory neuropeptides, which may cause vasodilatory effects (Blom et al 1992). Näslund et al (2002) demonstrated pain-relieving benefits lasting over 6 months, from the use of electroacupuncture (EA) and superficial subcutaneous needling, on patients diagnosed with IAKP (Table 10.1).

Table 10.1 Acupuncture points and dermatomal innervation

Points	Segmental innervation
ST34	L2 to L4
ST36	L4 to L5
ST38	L4 to L5
SP9	S1 to S2
SP10	L2 to L3
GB34	L5 to S1

Notes: ST, Stomach; SP, Spleen; and GB, Gall Bladder.
Adapted from Näslund et al (2002)

The pain reduction was not significantly better for patients receiving deep acupuncture compared with the subcutaneous acupuncture, given twice-weekly over a total of 15 treatments.

Knee pain in the older population is a common disabling condition, with the most likely diagnosis being OA that has been shown by radiography to be present in 70% of community-dwelling adults with knee pain aged 50 years or more (Duncan et al 2006). A recent best-evidence summary of systemic reviews concluded that exercise therapy (i.e. strengthening, stretching, and functional exercises), compared with no treatment, is effective for patients with knee OA (Smidt et al 2005).

Foster et al (2007) found that true acupuncture, using local points SP9, SP10, ST34, ST35, ST36, Xiyan, and GB34 with deactivation of active TrPts, combined with distal points, Large Intestine (LI) 4, Triple Heater (TH) 5, SP6, Liver (LIV) 3, ST44, Kidney (KID) 3, Bladder (BL) 60, and GB41, did not show any greater therapeutic benefit than a credible control procedure (standard exercise advice) in patients with a clinical diagnosis of knee OA. Acupuncture provided no additional improvement in pain scores compared with a course of six sessions of physiotherapy-led advice and exercise. Again, patients received six acupuncture sessions over a period of 3 weeks.

The more significant effects of acupuncture pain relief in OA knee come from a variety of trials (Manheimer et al 2007; Streng 2007; Vas & White 2007) suggesting that between 10 and 12 treatments are required in order to achieve a significantly long-standing effect from acupuncture intervention with OA knee, something practitioners must take into account when offering this modality within the present primary and private healthcare setting. Every effort should be made to teach patients the use of transcutaneous electrical nerve stimulation (TENS) over significant acupuncture points according to the musculoskeletal pain presentation, in order to empower and self-manage this treatment whilst retaining the acupuncture model for pain management.

Case Study 1

Andy Reynolds

Introduction

Patellar tendinopathy causes substantial morbidity in professional athletes (Cook et al 2000), but continues to be a constant problem for therapists to combat (Cook & Khan 2001) since there is no defining evidence that supports one particular modality. Even the terminology has not been widely accepted because there are many different umbrella terms that incorporate AKP. As when treating any condition, diagnosis and pathology are paramount to success.

The term tendinopathy is defined as degeneration of the tendons, not inflammation; or tendinosis not tendinitis. Tendinosis is the disorientation of collagen, focal necrosis, and increased prominence of vascular spaces (Khan et al 1996, 1999). With this in mind, the traditional approach of wrongly treating tendon problems as inflammation and prescribing non-steroidal anti-inflammatory drugs (Dreiser et al 1991; Lecomte et al 1994), corticosteroids (Capasso et al 1997), cryotherapy (Molnar & Fox 1993), and rest (Ferretti et al 1985) have, unsurprisingly, been shown to be ineffective. In contrast, acupuncture (Crossley et al 2001; Jensen et al 1999), quadriceps strengthening (Werner 1995), and resistive brace/taping (Harrison et al 1999) have been shown effective.

Case Report

Subjective assessment

A 27-year-old semi-professional rugby player presented with an acute onset of left patellar pain. He recalled a feeling of discomfort during a game 2 weeks previously, and since this, he had experienced a rapid increase of symptoms. The subject had pain on walking and found it extremely uncomfortable to climb stairs, rating this activity 70/100 on the VAS. He had suffered no altered sensation; the site of the pain was localized to the patella. His discomfort was aggravated by any increase in activity but his sleep remained unaffected. He had been unable to train or play with the team during the previous week.

Objective assessment

On examination the left knee had full active range of movement, with pain starting at 90° of flexion remaining through end of range (EOR) at 115°. Range of passive flexion was slightly increased to 125°, but still painful from 90°. Extension was equal and pain-free when compared to the opposite side.

On testing maximum quadriceps power, pain over the tendon was constant throughout range, but no pain was elicited on maximum hamstring contraction. There was no obvious muscle atrophy in the QF or the hamstrings muscle groups. A complete physical assessment of the knee joint was carried out including all ligaments, the menisci, plica and fat pad, and neurology, which were all normal. On the opposite side, decreased QF length was noted on the left side; however, the Q-angles were equal. A double-legged wall squat aggravated pain from 20° of knee flexion, together with left foot forward lunge at 30°. The subject's gait and forefoot–hind foot biomechanics were within normal limits and required no further assessment.

Palpation of the apex of the left patella was exquisitely painful and the patient subject reported that this was the root of his pain. From both the subjective and objective history, the clinician's impression was that he had developed a patellar tendinopathy. The aims of the treatment were to:

- Reduce pain;
- Maintain the full length of knee extensor and hip flexion;
- Correct muscle imbalance and eccentric control/strengthening;
- Encourage patellar self-mobilizations; and
- Commence cryotherapy post-training.

Pain management

Pain management involved acupuncture and used traditional points for global pain modification combined with TrPt point deactivation of the adductor brevis, the vastus medialis, and the rectus femoris muscles (Table 10.2). A total of five acupuncture sessions were given involving a total treatment time of 30 minutes. For local pain deactivation, the focal TrPt was located and the needle inserted until muscle relaxation was achieved and pain propagation was eased (Fig. 10.5).

Clinical reasoning

Trigger point release used in the present case study adheres closely to the work of Simons et al (1999). Needling is thought to disrupt the abnormal motor end-plate where excess acetylcholine has built up, which is thought to be one of the causes of ischaemic referred pain. Needling will induce a localized stretch in the contracted actin and myosin filaments, disentangling the myosin from the Z-band and subsequent straightening of the collagen fibres (Langevin 2007). Insertion of a local needle into the skin, stimulation of A-beta (Aβ)

(Continued)

Case Study 1 (Continued)

Table 10.2 Treatment Protocol

Treatments	Points	Dermatome distribution	VAS score
1 & 2	ST35 Xiyan ST36 LIV3[B] Heding	L2–L4	70/100
3	BL23 BL24 BL40 ST35 Xiyan Heding	L2–L3 L2–L4	60/100
4	BL23 BL24 BL40 ST35 Xiyan Heding LI4, LIV3[B] TrPt to: VM RF AB	L2–L3 L2–L4	20/100
5	TrPt to: VM RF AB		0/100

Notes: VM, Vastus Medialis; RF, Rectus Femoris; AB, Adductor Brevis; B, bilateral.

afferent mechanoreceptors synapsing in laminae II of the dorsal horn (DH). Collateral branches from the DH then suppress the nociceptor cells of the A-delta (Aδ) and C pain fibres at the substantia gelatinosa (SG). This inhibits the normal transmission of information from this segmental level to the higher centres of the cortex. The stimulation of enkephalin is initiated at the SG, which also helps to suppress the C system cells at a local area via an enkephalinergic interneuron. It is also important to note that histamine and bradykinin are produced during this presynaptic phase. Impulses from the activation of the fast-twitch Aδ pain fibres travel up through the spinothalamic tract, which relays information to the periaqueductal grey matter, an area of the brain associated with pain modulation. Here the stimulation of serotonin (5HT) and noradrenalin causes the descending

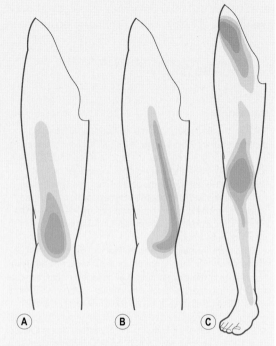

Figure 10.5 • Pain pattern of positive trigger points. (a) Rectus femoris. (b) Vastus medialis. (c) Adductor brevis.

neurons to pass through various subregions of the nucleus raphe and then into the DH, where enkephalin is generated. The action of inserting the needles also stimulates the body's pituitary and hypothalamus to secrete beta-endorphin.

Discussion

As a result of the use of acupuncture, an eccentric strengthening programme, patellar self-mobilizations, and lower limb stretches, within 2 weeks the subject's VAS had dropped from 70/100 to 0/100 at rest. This dramatic decrease in symptoms allowed him to resume rugby training within 3 weeks and take full part in a team match 4 weeks after commencing the treatment. Objectively, full range of movement with maximum strength and no discomfort was achieved. Both a full squat and lunge could be performed without pain, prior to commencing sport-specific training.

Throughout the present case study, a combination of clinical reasoning and evidence-based research using Western and traditional Chinese medical acupuncture in order to manage pain and subsequently enhance rehabilitation was employed whilst integrating manual, acupuncture, and exercise techniques in order to successfully manage the diagnosis of patellar tendinopathy.

(Continued)

Case Study 2

Melissa Johnson

Introduction

The following case study presents a 28-year-old female, 2 weeks after an anterior cruciate ligament (ACL) reconstruction. The subject presented with severe limitation of range of movement (ROM) throughout the knee joint and poor muscle activity as a result of prevailing fear and anxiety. Her fears and anxieties were restricting physiotherapy interventions, possible rehabilitation potential, and protocol management.

A treatment regime incorporating auricular seeds and acupuncture, as an adjunct to other physiotherapy modalities, was employed. Progress was assessed using the lower extremities function scale (LEFS) (Binkley et al 2001) and the pain catastrophization score (PCS) (Swinke-Meewise et al 2006) as a means of objective measurement of anxiety and fear following physiotherapy intervention. The subject responded well to both the auricular seeds and acupuncture as treatment moda-lities, facilitating the use of other physiotherapy treat-ment modalities previously not tolerated. Progress was made following a biweekly treatment programme using acupuncture, in combination with physiotherapy inclu-ding hydrotherapy, and manual and exercise therapy. For the purpose of the study the biweekly management occurred over an 8-week period, following which the subject joined an advanced lower limb class for ACL rehabilitation.

ACL reconstructions are a very common orthopaedic procedure, performed using part of the patella tendon or hamstring tendon to reconstruct the cruciate ligament. There is a great deal of research available into ACL reconstruction and the management of such, including physiotherapy intervention for all stages of rehabilitation (Beard & Dodd 1998). Experimental research has investigated the cruciate ligaments and the forces acting upon the reconstructed graft, through which initial closed-chain exercises and joint ROM guidelines were developed in order to protect the graft from damage or further injury incurred from functional or sporting use (Shelbourne & Nitz 1990). Subjects are encouraged to achieve full knee extension immediately postoperatively in order to prevent joint ROM complications and improve functional recovery (Bollen 2001). Postoperatively, it is common for protocol management to vary according to particular surgeon preference and experience, combined with the variations on chosen graft material and methods deployed. The protocol used included the following physiotherapy management:

0–2 weeks

- Restoration of full knee extension;
- Restoration of 90° of knee flexion;
- Restoration of normal gait pattern;
- Restoration of muscle imbalance; and
- Management of swelling and bruising.

The above can be achieved using therapy modalities such as hydrotherapy, manual mobilization techniques, and exercise therapy.

There is limited research on the use of acupuncture for ACL reconstruction. Most research articles have looked at the use of acupuncture in OA of the knee (Ezzo et al 2001). However, research is prevalent into the use of acupuncture for pain, mood, and relaxation that were deemed relevant to this case study. Through the use of magnetic resonance imaging (MRI), there is scientific evidence of brain activity gained from acupuncture needling (Kaptchuk 2002). Sensory stimulation in the periphery has shown to be effective in the treatment of pain and thus the use of acupuncture needling as a treatment modality targets peripheral sensory stimulation by influencing endogenous pain modulation (Lundeberg & Thomas 1996).

The use of auricular acupuncture using the Shenmen relaxation points has been shown to reduce significantly anxiety levels (Yang 2001). Much research has been undertaken into the use of auricular acupuncture for anxiety-related management in preoperative care, cessation of smoking, and other drug addictions and was cited in the Cochrane review (White et al 2006). Auricular seeds or needles can also be used as therapy in itself. Auricular seeds are used to reinforce acupuncture points located within the auricle and are stimulated by the patient, using mild acupressure at the chosen points. Their use can thus empower the patient whilst facilitating home management of pain, providing benefits when time constraints and appointment availability are a concern; there are also benefits for those persons intolerant of needles.

Subjective assessment

The subject was a 28-year old female who sustained a ruptured ACL in a fall when skiing 14 months previously; she was X-rayed, but no abnormalities were detected. The subject's knee was swollen, painful, and prevented full weight-bearing. On return to the UK she presented to her local hospital for further investigations. On physiotherapy assessment, she tested positive for ACL rupture that was later confirmed by MRI and surgery was planned. The subject underwent a preoperative rehabilitation programme to strengthen her musculature. The ACL repair was carried out using a patella tendon graft. She was discharged, fully weight-bearing as pain allowed, with crutches and placed in an extension splint for 2 weeks as part of the consultant protocol.

Objective assessment

Following removal of the extension splint physiotherapy was commenced and the objective assessment revealed:
- Active knee flexion 10°;
- Active knee extension minus 15°;

(Continued)

Case Study 2 (Continued)

- Compensating gait with hip movement and no knee extension which was limited by patient anxiety and fear of causing damage to the reconstructed ligament;
- Passive ROM impossible owing to fear and anxiety; and
- Fear of moving her knee, with resulting nausea.

Despite reassurance and empathy, the assessment was very limited; the patient was instructed on the current research and evidence for stability of the reconstruction, the successful protocol used, and the required movement allowed. The subject became very emotional about her anxieties and frustrations and thus rest, ice, compression, and elevation advice (RICE), plus the importance of isometric muscle exercises, were stressed and a further appointment was arranged for 3 days later.

Management plan

The following management plan was discussed and agreed with the subject:
- Address fear and anxiety using auricular seeds to stimulate relaxation and parasympathetic response of the central nervous system (CNS);
- Increase ROM within tolerance; and
- Engage and strengthen the muscle imbalance.

The validated outcome measurements, LEFS at initial assessment and PCS 27 at final assessment, were used in an attempt to demonstrate objectively the subject's response.

Treatment sessions

Education on the function and use of auricular therapy was given and auricular seeds applied to both ears. The subject was advised to acupressure the area for 2 minutes for approximately 5 times a day. On return, the patient reported a significant change in mood; she had been able firstly to get to sleep without worrying about further damage to the knee during the night. She reported sleeping throughout the night and she felt more relaxed and more positive about attending physiotherapy. Her mood was very different; she was very keen to have the knee assessed again and LEFS 20 and PCS 22 assessment revealed a drop in score (Table 10.3).

The patient commenced hydrotherapy after the first acupuncture treatment with home exercises of quadriceps and hamstring closed-chain muscle strengthening programme. Other treatment techniques used in the physiotherapy sessions included soft-tissue release work and manual mobilization techniques.

Outcomes

The subject reported the following outcomes:
- Improvement in mood and anxiety levels with full compliance to the rehabilitation programme;
- Full knee extension and 130° of knee flexion;

Table 10.3 Treatment plan and outcomes

Treatment	Points	Needle size	De Qi	Outcome
1	LI4, LIV3[B]	25 mm	Yes	LEFS: 14 PCS: 27
2	LI4, LIV3[B]	25 mm	Yes	LEFS: 20 PCS: 22
3	LI4, LIV3[B] GB34[B]	25 mm	Yes	LEFS: 27 PCS: 14
4	LI4, LIV3[B] SP9	25 mm	Yes	LEFS: 31 PCS: 11
5	LI4, L3[B]	25 mm	Yes	LEFS: 14 PCS: 27
6	LI4, LIV3, GB34[B] SP 9 SP10	25 mm	Yes	LEFS: 36 PCS: 8
7	LI4, LIV3[B] GB34[B] SP9, SP10	25 mm	Yes	LEFS: 41 PCS: 6
8	LI4, LIV3[B] GB34[B] ST34 ST44	25 mm	Yes	LEFS: 46 PCS: 4

Notes: B, bilateral; LEFS, lower extremities function scale; PCS, pain catastrophization score.

- Achieving 30 kg weight-resisted exercises for quadriceps;
- Ability to perform a single leg squat; and
- LEFS score was 46 (up from 14), PCS 4 (reduced from 27).

As of the final acupuncture treatment, she was entered into the advanced lower limb gym circuit class to continue her ACL rehabilitation. This class follows the subjects to final rehabilitation for a further 3 months, achieving full function, with a further 3 months rehabilitation to return to sport and former fitness levels.

Discussion

Acupuncture is becoming more widely used and accepted in Western medicine for the management of pain (Wu et al 1999). Through this research, a close relationship and link between anxiety and pain (Carr et al 2004) has been identified. This subject did not perceive pain to be the main limiting factor, but her anxiety and fears postoperatively were preventing rehabilitation

(Continued)

Case Study 2 (Continued)

and return to function. Research into the management of anxiety shows that by influencing the neurobiology and endogenous modulators, an opioid effect can be established, mirroring the acupuncture analgesic effect (Carr 2004).

Acupuncture has been shown to have central effect on the hypothalamus, stimulating an increase in levels of serotonin, oxytocin, and adrenocorticotropic hormone (ACTH) (Gollub et al 1999). The stimulation of the endocrine system and altered blood chemistry has a calming effect via stimulation of the parasympathetic nervous system, resulting in reduced blood pressure, stroke volume of the heart, and a general relaxation effect.

In traditional Chinese acupuncture (TCM), a sensation known as De Qi is produced when needling (Wang et al 1985), thought to be the resultant stimulation of Aβ, Aδ, and C fibres in the skin and muscle, ultimately leading to release of opioid peptides, causing an inhibition of nociceptive information transmitted from the dorsal horn in the spinal cord (Chan 1984; Wang et al 1985). The release of endorphins and leu-enkephalins produced by Aδ and Aβ fibre stimulation also acts to mediate nociceptive input of the C fibres (Melzack & Wall 1996). The gate theory proposed by Melzack and Wall (1996) is used commonly in Western acupuncture as it is recognized that the scientific physiological effects as described above occur when using distal points to utilize the most sensory aspects of the body, that is, the hands and the feet. Utilizing all four points, LI4 and LIV3 in both hands and feet, is referred to as the four-gate technique, used for pain modulation via the endogenous opiate system (Lundeberg 1995). This reinforces the hypothesis that acupuncture was used initially to allow the subject to become accustomed to the sensation of needling and De Qi, in an area outside of the affected hypersensitivity as a means of reducing anxiety concerning interactions around the knee.

Activation of ascending C fibre nociceptive input (from needling) not only stimulates the hypothalamus, but also the periaqueductal grey matter (PAG) and the pituitary; these, in turn and in collaboration, release serotonin, norepinephrine, histamine, bradykinin, endorphins, dopamine, and ACTH. Neurotransmitters such as the serotonin and endorphins result in a positive emotional response and are often used to lift mood, reflected in the subject's response and reduction in her PCS score.

It must also be noted that the use of acupuncture needling can also influence the limbic system via the effects on the endocrine and autonomic nervous system. The limbic system is involved in emotion, motivation, and emotional associated memory. Structures included in the limbic system (both cortical and subcortical) relevant to this case study include the amygdala involved in motivational stimuli to the cortex, such as those related to fear. It was this fear element that was most limiting to physiotherapy. Reassurance and education were insufficient in reducing anxiety and fear; it was not until acupuncture that a positive difference was reflected in the PCS.

Within TCM, acupuncture points are employed as a means of managing homeostatic balance, a balance between yin and yang, which may be paralleled in physiological explanation, as a balance between the sympathetic and parasympathetic nervous system.

This patient responded well to acupuncture and therefore, treatment was progressed by introducing more local points as her fear of injury subsided. Acupoint Spleen 9 (SP9), coupled with SP10 was used to reduce oedema and is referred to within TCM as cardinal local points for knee pain. Points used were to address the holistic requirements for this patient regarding her anxieties, mood, and physiological postoperative effects of pain and swelling, which were all contributing factors in inhibiting her rehabilitation.

Conclusion

This case study supports the use of acupuncture as an adjunct to other physiotherapy techniques in an attempt to treat the subject with a holistic approach, within an area that is not well researched. The limitations and efficacy of the results must therefore be taken into consideration within the context of a single case study. However, through utilizing the evidence in current research and the more quantitative data from MRI, in combination with clear clinical reasoning and understanding of the physiological effects of needling, one can cautiously credit the use of acupuncture and the auricular seeds in this case study, and further research must be encouraged as an integral part of unwrapping the effects of acupuncture beyond pain relief (Deadman 2003). A flexible working approach is encouraged within physiotherapy practice and therefore, integration of acupuncture within musculoskeletal management must be encouraged by offering treatment in the most effective way.

References

Aminaka, N., Gribble, P., 2005. A systematic review of the effects of therapeutic taping on patellofemoral pain syndrome. J. Athl. Train. 5 (40), 341–351.

Anderson, G., Herrington, L., 2003. A comparison of eccentric isokinetic torque production and velocity of knee flexion angle during step-down in patellofemoral pain syndrome patients and normal controls. Clin. Biomech. 18, 500–504.

Arnoldi, C., 1991. Patellar pain. Acta. Orthop. Scand. 62, 244.

Beard, D.J., Dodd, K.A., 1998. Rehabilitation following anterior cruciate ligament reconstruction: a randomized controlled trial. J. Orthop. Sport Phys. Ther. 27 (2), 134–143.

Biedert, R., Lobenhoffer, P., Lattermann, C., 2000. Free nerve endings in the medial and posteromedial capsuloligamentous complexes: occurrences and distribution. Knee Surgery, Sports Trauma and Arthroscopy 8, 68–72.

Binkley, J.M., Stratford, P.W., Lott, S.A., et al., 2001. The lower extremity functional scale (LEFS). J. Rheumatol. 28, 431–438.

Bizzini, M., Childs, J., Piva, S., et al., 2003. A systematic review of the quality of randomised controlled trials for patellofemoral syndrome. J. Ortho. Sports Phys. Ther. 33 (1), 4–20.

Blom, D., Davidson, I., Angmar-Mansson, B., 1992. The effect of acupuncture on salivary flow rates in patients with xerostomia. Oral Surg. Oral Pathol. 73, 298.

Bollen, S.R., 2001. Response of hepatic glucose out-put to electro-acupuncture stimulation in hind limb in anesthetized rats. Anatomic Neuroscience 115 (2), 7–14.

Cannon, W., 1929. Organization for physiological homeostasis. Physiol. Rev. 9 (3), 399–431.

Carr, E.C., Nicky Thomas, V., Wilson-Barnet, J., 2004. Patient experiences of anxiety, depression and acute pain after surgery: a longitudinal perspective. Int. J. Nurs. Stud. 42 (5), 521–530.

Chan, S.H., 1984. What is being stimulated in acupuncture? Evaluation of the existence of a specific substrate. Neurosci. Biobehav. Rev. 8 (1), 25–33.

Cheng, X., 1987. Chinese acupuncture and moxibustion. Foreign Language Press, Beijing.

Clement, D., Taunton, J., Smart, W., et al., 1981. A survey of overuse running injuries. Phys. Sports Med. 1 (9), 47–58.

Cook, J., Khan, K., 2001. What is the most appropriate treatment for patellar tendinopathy? Br. J. Sports Med. 35, 291–294.

Cook, J., Khan, K., Maffulli, N., et al., 2000. Overuse tendinosis, not tendinitis: part 2. Phys. Sportsmed. 6, 31–46.

Crossley, K., Bennell, K., Green, S., et al., 2001. A systematic review of physical interventions for patellofemoral pain syndrome. Clin. J. Sport Med. 1 (2), 103–110.

Deadman, P., 2003. Acupuncture in the West: keynote debate. Eur. J. Orient. Med. 4 (4), 6–10.

Devereaux, M., Lachmann, S., 1984. Patellofemoral arthralgia in athletes attending a sports injury clinic. Br. J. Sports Med. 18, 18–21.

Dreiser, R.L., Ditisheim, A., Sharlot, J., et al., 1991. A double blind, placebo controlled study of niflumic acid gel in the treatment of acute tendonitis. Eur. J. Rheumatol. Inflamm. 11, 38–45.

Duncan, R.C., Hay, E.M., Saklatvala, J., et al., 2006. Prevalence of radiographic osteoarthritis-it all depends on your point of view. Rheumatology 45, 757–760.

Dye, S., 2005. The pathophysiology of patellofemoral pain. Clin Orthod Res Revis 436, 100–110.

Dye, S., Vaupel, G., 1994. The pathophysiology of patellofemoral pain. Sports Med. Arthrosc. Revis. 2, 203–210.

Dye, S., Vaupel, G., Dye, C., 1998. Conscious neurosensory mapping of the internal structures of the human knee without intra-articular anaesthesia. Am. J. Sports Med. 26, 773–777.

Elias, J.J., Bratton, D.R., Weinstein, D.M., et al., 2006. Comparing two estimations of the quadriceps force distribution for use during patellofemoral simulation. J. Biomech. 39, 865–872.

Ezzo, J., Hadhazy, V., Birch, S., 2001. Acupuncture for osteoarthritis of the knee. Arthritis Rheum. 44 (4), 819–825.

Feinberg, B.I., Feinberg, R.A., 1998. Persistent pain after total knee arthroplasty: treatment with manual therapy and trigger point injections. J. Musculoskeletal Pain 6 (4), 85–95.

Ferretti, A., Puddu, G., Mariani, P., et al., 1985. The natural history of jumpers knee: patella or quadriceps tendonitis. Int. Orthop. 8, 239–242.

Foster, N.E., Thomas, E., Barlas, P., et al., 2007. Acupuncture as an adjunct to exercise based physiotherapy for osteoarthritis of the knee: randomised controlled trial. Br. Med. J. 335 (7617), 436.

Gollub, R.L., Hui, K.K., Stefano, G.B., 1999. Acupuncture: pain management coupled to immune stimulation. Acta Pharmacol. Sin. 20 (9), 769–777.

Gray, H., 1964. Grays' Anatomy—Descriptive and Applied, 34th edn. Longmans, Green and Co, London.

Harilainen, A., Lindroos, M., Sandelin, J., et al., 2005. Patellofemoral relationships and cartilage breakdown. Knee Surgery, Sports Traumatology and Arthroscopy 13, 142–144.

Harrison, E.L., Sheppard, M.S., McQuarrie, A.M., 1999. A randomized controlled trial of physical therapy treatment programs in patellofemoral pain syndrome. Physiother. Can. 51 (2), 93–100.

Hejgaard, N., Arnoldi, C., 1984. Osteotomy of the patella in patellofemoral pain syndrome. The significance of increased intraosseous pressure during sustained knee flexion. Int. Orthop. 8, 189–194.

Helms, J.M., 1995. Acupuncture Energetics—a Clinical Approach for Physicians. Medical Acupuncture Publishers, Berkeley.

Herrington, L., 2006. The effect of corrective taping of the patella on patella position as defined by MRI. Res. Sports Med. 14, 215–223.

Herrington, L., Al-Shehri, A., 2007. A controlled trial of open versus closed kinetic chain exercises for patellofemoral pain. J. Orthop. Sports Phys. Ther. 37, 155–160.

Herrington, L., Blacker, M., Enjuanes, N., et al., 2006. The effect of hip position, exercise mode and contraction type on overall activity of VMO and VL. Phys. Ther. Sport 7, 87–92.

Herrington, L., Malloy, S., Richards, J., 2005. The effect of patella taping on vastus medialis oblique & vastus lateralis: EMG activity and knee kinematic variables during stair descent. J. Electromyogr. Kinesiol. 15, 604–607.

Hibbler, J.M., 1995. Engineering mechanics, statistics and dynamics. Prentice-Hall, Englewood Cliffs, NJ.

Itoh, K., Hirota, S., Katsumi, Y., et al., 2008. Trigger point acupuncture for treatment of knee osteoarthritis—a preliminary RCT for a pragmatic trial. Acupunct. Med. 26 (1), 17–26.

Jensen, R., Gothesen, O., Liseth, K., et al., 1999. Acupuncture treatment of patellofemoral pain syndrome. J. Altern. Complement. Med. 5 (6), 521–527.

Jonsson, P., Alfredson, H., 2005. Superior results with eccentric compared to concentric quadriceps training in patients with jumper's knee: a prospective randomized study. Br. J. Sports Med. 39 (11), 847–850.

Kannus, P., Aho, H., Jarvinen, M., et al., 1987. Computerized recording of visits to an outpatient sports clinic. Am. J. Sports Med. 15, 79–85.

Kaptchuk, T.J., 2002. Acupuncture: theory, efficacy and practice. Am. Int. Med. 136 (5), 374–383.

Khan, K.M., Bonar, F., Desmond, T.M., et al., 1996. Patella tendinosis (jumpers knee): finding at histopathologic examination: UF & MR imaging. Victorian institute of sport tendon study group. Radiology 200 (3), 821–827.

Khan, K.M., Cook, J.L., Bonar, F., et al., 1999. Histopathology of common tendinopathy: update and implications for clinical management. Sport Med. 27 (6), 393–408.

Kumazawa, K., 1993. Polymodal receptor hypothesis on the peripheral mechanisms of acupuncture and moxibustion. Am. J. Acupunc. 21, 331–338.

Langevin, H.M., 2007. Connective tissue fibroblast response to acupuncture: dose-dependent effect of bidirectional needle rotation. J. Altern. Complement. Med. 13 (3), 355–360.

Langevin, H.M., Churchill, D.L., Cipolla, M.J., 2001. Mechanical signalling through connective tissue: a mechanism for the therapeutic effect of acupuncture. FASEB J. 15 (12), 2275–2282.

Lecomte, J., Buyse, H., Taymans, J., et al., 1994. The treatment of tendonitis and bursitis: comparison of Nimesulide and Naproxen sodium in a double blind parallel trial. European Journal of Rheumatology Information 14, 29–32.

Lundeberg, T., 1995. Pain Physiology and principles of treatment. Scand. J. Rehabil. Med. 32 (1), 13–42.

Magee, D., Zachazewski, J., Quillen, W., 2007. Scientific foundations and principles of practice in musculoskeletal rehabilitation. Saunders Elsevier, St Louis.

Manheimer, E., Linde, K., Lao, L., et al., 2007. Meta-analysis: acupuncture for osteoarthritis of the knee. Ann. Intern. Med. 146 (12), 868–877.

Melzack, R., Wall, P., 1996. Textbook of Pain. Penguin, London.

Milgrom, C., Finestone, A., Eldad, A., et al., 1991. Patellofemoral pain caused by overactivity. J. Bone Joint Surg. 73A, 1041–1043.

Mohr, K.J., Kvitne, R.S., Pink, M.M., et al., 2003. Electromyography of the quadriceps in patellofemoral pain with patellar subluxations. Clin. Orthop. Relat. Res. (415), 261–271.

Molnar, T., Fox, J., 1993. Overuse injuries of the knee in basketball. Clin. Sport Med. 12, 349–362.

Näslund, J., Näslund, U., Odenbring, S., et al., 2002. Sensory stimulation (acupuncture) for the treatment of idiopathic anterior knee pain. J. Rehabil. Med. 34 (5), 231–238.

Powers, C., 1998. Rehabilitation of patellofemoral joint disorders: a critical review. J. Orthop. Sports Phys. Ther. 28, 345–354.

Reynolds, M.D., 1981. Myofascial trigger point syndromes in the practice of rheumatology. Arch. Phys. Med. Rehabil. 62, 111–114.

Shelbourne, K.D., Nitz, P., 1990. Accelerated rehabilitation after anterior cruciate ligament reconstruction. Am. J. Sports Med. 18 (3), 528–534.

Simons, D.G., Travell, J.G., Simons, L.S., 1999. Myofascial pain and dysfunction: the trigger point manual, 2nd edn. Williams and Wilkinson, Baltimore.

Smidt, N., de Vet, H.C., Bouter, L.M., et al., 2005. Effectiveness of exercise therapy: a best-evidence summary of systematic reviews. Aust. Physiother. 51, 71–85.

Streng, A., 2007. Summary of the randomised controlled trials from the German model projects on acupuncture for chronic pain. J. Chin. Med. 83, 5–10.

Swinkels-Meewise, I.E., Roelofs, J., Oostendorp, R.A., et al., 2006. Acute low back pain: pain-related fear and pain catastrophysing influence on physical performance and perceived disability. Pain 120 (5), 36–43.

Taunton, J., Ryan, M., Clement, D., et al., 2002. Retrospective case-control analysis of 2002 running injuries. Br. J. Sports Med. 36, 95–101.

Thomas, M., Lundeberg, T., 1996. Does acupuncture work? Pain Clinic Updates 4, 1–4.

Tyler, T., Nicholas, S., Mullaney, M., et al., 2006. The Role of hip muscle function in the treatment of patellofemoral pain syndrome. Am. J. Sports Med. 34, 630–637.

Vas, J., White, A., 2007. Evidence from randomized controlled trials on optimal acupuncture treatment for knee osteoarthritis: an exploratory review. Acupunct. Med. 25 (1–2), 29–35.

Vicenzino, B., 2004. Foot orthotics in the treatment of lower limb conditions: a musculoskeletal physiotherapy perspective. Man. Ther. 9, 185–196.

Waisbrod, H., Treiman, N., 1980. Intra-osseous venography in patellofemoral disorders: a preliminary report. J. Bone Joint Surg. 62B, 454–456.

Wang, K., Yao, S., Xian, Y., et al., 1985. A study of the receptive field of acupoints and the relation between characteristics of needling sensory and group of afferent fibres. Sci. Sin. 28 (9), 963–971.

Warden, S., Hinman, R., Watson, M., et al., 2008. Patellar taping and bracing for the treatment of chronic knee pain: a systematic review and meta-analysis. Arthritis Rheum. 59, 73–83.

Werner, S., 1995. An evaluation of knee extensor and knee flexor torques and EMGs in patients with patellofemoral pain syndrome in comparisons with matched controls. Knee Surgery Sports Traumatic Arthroscopy 3 (2), 89–94.

White, A.R., Rampes, H., Campbell, J., 2006. Acupuncture and related interventions for smoking cessation. Cochrane Database Syst. Rev. 1, CD000009.

Whyte-Ferguson, L., Gerwin, R., 2005. Clinical Mastery in the Treatment of Myofascial Pain. Lippincott, Williams &Wilkins, Philadelphia.

Witonski, D., Wagrowska-Danielewicz, M., 1999. Distribution of substance P nerve fibres in the knee joint of patients with anterior knee pain: a preliminary report. Knee Surgery, Traumatology and Arthroscopy 7, 177–183.

Witvrouw, E., Lysens, R., Bellemans, J., et al., 2000. Intrinsic risk factors for the development of anterior knee pain in an athletic population. Am. J. Sports Med. 28, 480–489.

Wu, M.T., Hsieh, J.-C., Xiong, J., et al., 1999. Central nervous pathway for acupuncture stimulation: localization of processing with functional MRI imaging of the brain. Radiology 212 (1), 133–141.

Yang, S.M., 2001. Acupoint injections are as effective as droperidol in controlling early post-operative nausea and vomiting. Anaesthesiology 93 (3), 1178–1180.

Foot and ankle

Cherye Roche

Introduction

The foot and ankle must provide support and shock absorption whilst at the same time balancing the body. This requires both mobility to adapt to a varying terrain, stability to allow supported contact and push-off from the ground. Shock absorption occurs as a result of the dissipation of forces through complex movements at the foot, the ankle and imposed adaptation, mainly through rotation, in the lower extremity, namely at the knee, hip and pelvis. Dysfunction at the feet may thus have consequences throughout the entire body; the need for lower extremity compensation may result in more proximal pain, including low back pain.

(Souza 2001)

This chapter will focus on some of the most common conditions of the foot and ankle seen in physical medicine practice. However, there is also a brief discussion regarding the reasons biomechanical faults can be an underlying causes of chronic overuse syndromes in the local soft tissues, as well as how these contribute to chronic conditions further up the kinetic chain (Hertel 2000; Rose et al 2000; Ryan 1994).

The injuries and conditions of the foot and ankle commonly seen in a physical medicine practice can be categorized as both acute and traumatic, or chronic overuse problems; each is dependent on the mechanism of injury. Traumatic injuries involve a mechanism that is acute in nature and results in overloading of the bone or soft tissues, such that there is disruption of the area, resulting in erythema, oedema, pain, and immobility. This is referred to as macrotraumatic injury. Overuse injuries involve chronic and repetitive stress to the soft tissues supporting a joint. This stress to the muscles, tendons, and other connective structures results in minor disruption of the integrity of the tissues with resultant pain and swelling.

The initial plan of management for both categories of injury generally involves applying the PRICES protocol for the provision of the standard treatment regime. This acronym describes a treatment involving:

- Protecting the involved area from further injury;
- Rest of the part to allow healing and avoid further insult;
- Ice application to facilitate vasoconstriction and thereby decrease swelling;

© 2010 Elsevier Ltd.

DOI: 10.1016/B978-0-443-06782-2.00011-6

- Compression to further protect the area and keep swelling down;
- Elevating the part to facilitate lymphatic drainage to remove exudates and decrease swelling; and
- Support of the injured part with splints, wraps, and/or braces to facilitate immobility or partial mobility, and avoid further injury during the acute phase of healing (Souza 2001).

Additionally, patients are prescribed either prescription or over-the-counter anti-inflammatory medications to reduce further swelling and thereby relieve pain. Other sources of neutraceutical remedies are available, but are not discussed (Pizzorno et al 1997, 2005, Pizzorno & Murray 2007).

This chapter focuses on the complementary management of chronic overuse injuries, conditions, and syndromes of the foot and ankle commonly seen in physical medicine practices, including:

- Acute inversion sprains;
- Acute and chronic achilles tendinopathies;
- Plantar fasciitis;
- Metatarsalgia;
- Morton's neuroma; and
- Anterior and posterior tibial tendon disorders (shin splints).

Acute inversion sprain

The mechanism of injury for an acute ankle inversion sprain involves plantar flexion, inversion, and adduction of the foot relative to the ankle. When this motion occurs with excessive force, the anterior talofibular ligament is sprained. The sprain is graded as:

- Mild, first degree;
- Moderate, second degree; and
- Severe, third degree.

The most common mechanism of injury in ankle sprains is a combination of plantar flexion and inversion. The lateral stabilizing ligaments, which include the anterior talofibular, calcaneofibular, and posterior talofibular ligaments, are most often damaged, with sprains ranging in severity from grade I to grade III. The grade I sprain is characterized by stretching of the anterior talofibular and calcaneofibular ligaments. In the grade II sprain, the anterior talofibular ligament tears partially, and the calcaneofibular ligament stretches. The grade III

sprain is characterized by rupture of the anterior talofibular and calcaneofibular ligaments, with partial tearing of the posterior talofibular and tibiofibular ligaments.

The early management is pivotal to the effective rehabilitation of an ankle sprain. Early conservative treatment should consist of partial weight-bearing, cryotherapy, bandage compressions, and elevation above heart height with non-steroidal anti-inflammatory treatment and exercises to prevent loss of range of movement (ROM). Failing this, chronic pain, loss of ROM, and swelling can persist with potential joint instability. It is well established that effective ankle rehabilitation must involve four main components (Balduini et al 1987; Kerkhoffs et al 2002; Van der Wee et al 2006), ROM rehabilitation, progressive muscle-strengthening exercises, proprioceptive training, and activity-specific training, as functional stress stimulates the production and orientation of stronger replacement collagen with eccentric strengthening and conditioning of peroneal muscles providing additional support to the lateral ligaments (Glick et al 1976) and assisting in the prevention of reoccurrences.

The diagnosis will depend on the extent of the disruption of the ligament and the supportive lateral muscles and tendons, especially tibialis anterior and the peroneii. The problem often leads to chronic instability and recurrent minor sprains. In addition to the standard PRICES approach to the management of the resulting pain and swelling, there are also manipulative and mobilization techniques that have been shown (Peterson & Bergmann 2002; Whitman et al 2005) to restore normal intra-articular motion and enhance healing in both acute and chronic recurrent inversion ankle sprains (Gillman 2004).

Manipulation or mobilization is practised by manual therapists and has been shown to decrease joint pain and normalize function. The mechanisms of action are not well understood. Current theories propose that an imbalance of muscle activity is the source of pain. Manipulation can relieve this through reflexive actions and may be appropriate for early conservative care as part of a comprehensive treatment programme (Eisenhart et al 2007; Fryer et al 2002; Justus et al 2002). Eisenhart et al (2007) compared two groups of patients undergoing emergency ankle treatment in which one group was allocated to standard care and the other to standard care and osteopathic manipulation treatment (OMT). Both groups were found to have significant improvement, but the OMT group demonstrated significant ($f = 5.92$; $p = 0.2$) improvement in pain, oedema, and ROM.

An inversion sprain/strain injury can result in a talus that is mal-positioned and fixed in both anterior and lateral positions. Fig. 11.1 demonstrates one method for adjusting an anterolateral talus.

It has also been suggested that the incorporation of manipulation of the lumbar spine and pelvis, as well as the hip and knee, can help to ensure normal circulation and nerve integrity in order to optimize healing (Logan & Row 1995). It is important to note that extremity manipulation techniques require a great deal of skill and training in order to be applied safely in acute or chronic circumstances.

Achilles tendinopathies (acute and chronic)

The achilles tendon can sustain either acute traumatic or chronic overuse injuries depending on the mechanism of injury. An acute strain of the achilles tendon results from a rapid tensile stress placed on the tendon that causes tissue disruption (Fig. 11.2). Like the ankle sprain, this injury is graded as mild, moderate, or severe. Achilles tendinopathy is prevalent and potentially incapacitating in athletes involved in running sports. It is considered to be a degenerative, not an inflammatory condition (Kader et al 2002). Severe cases may respond to conservative care, but sometimes require surgical intervention. However, mild and moderate cases will respond to conservative care using the PRICES protocol. In addition, the use

of temporary heel lifts will relieve some of the tensile stress in the tendon during recovery. If a heel lift is to be used it is important to note that there should be a lift of equal size under both extremities to avoid an artificial leg length inequality and potential injury to the joints further up the kinetic chain.

The exact aetiology and pathogenesis of tendon pain is not fully understood (Alfredson 2005; Shalabi et al 2004) and is undergoing much research at present. Recent studies have shown that there may be a genetic predisposition to suffering from a tendinopathy (Harvie et al 2004; Kannus & Natri 1997). Multiple intrinsic and extrinsic risk factors have been associated with achilles tendon injuries; suggesting this condition is complex and interactions between gene–gene and gene–environment are probably involved in the aetiology of these conditions (September et al 2007).

In association with tendon degeneration, there appears to be signs of neural inflammatory markers

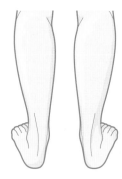

Figure. 11.2 • Medial Achilles tendon stress due to rearfoot valgus.

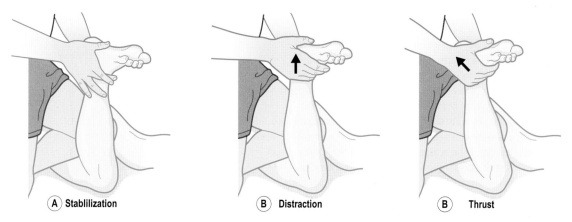

(A) Stablilization   (B) Distraction   (B) Thrust

Figure 11.1 • Sample extremity adjusting technique for an anterior and lateral talus (a) Stabilization; (b) distraction; (c) thrust.

in nerves in close proximity to affected tendons (Hart et al 1995). The well-known neurotransmitter and potent modulator of pain in the central nervous system, glutamate, is found in high levels in painful tendons, but not in normal tendons (Alfredson et al 2001). In conjunction with neurovascular ingrowths into painful tendons as demonstrated by Bjur et al (2005), there is now evidence that neural pathways and neovascularization are associated with the pain of tendinopathy rather than just a simple case of tissue degeneration.

There appears to be a lack of research consensus on the efficacy of management of this achilles tendinopathy, but the lack of suitable evidence in support of a given management method does not necessarily imply a lack of clinical effectiveness (Andres et al 2008).

The following interventions have been demonstrated as providing clinical effectiveness:

- *Mechanical conditioning*—Tendons respond to mechanical forces by adapting metabolism and structural reorganization (Hampson et al 2008). Tenocytes respond by altering gene expression patterns, protein synthesis, and cell phenotype to enhance healing (Wang 2006).
- *Eccentric loading*—The best evidence to date demonstrates that eccentric exercises are likely to be a useful management for achilles tendinopathy, but is insufficient to suggest it is superior or inferior to other forms of therapeutic exercise (Rompe et al 2007).

The initial occurrence of an achilles tendon strain can subsequently result in chronic strains and/or tenosynopathy. When this occurs, the practitioner must consider the possibility of an underlying biomechanical weakness contributing to the chronicity of recurrent achilles tendinopathies. Chronic achilles tendinopathy (CAT) may result from chronic overuse of the tendon as a result of an underlying biomechanical weakness in foot and ankle function. Excessive and prolonged pronation through the rear foot is an example of this type of underlying biomechanical foot fault. As a result, the calcaneous undergoes excessive eversion during the gait cycle, causing a valgus stress through the medial aspect of the calcaneus and the distal attachment of the achilles tendon. This ultimately results in pain, oedema, and sometimes crepitus from overuse of the tendon and yields a tendinopathy. This overuse injury may be resolved with the use of the PRICES protocol, but will be recurrent if there is an underlying biomechanical

weakness. The preferred option for the management of this condition is the addition of foot orthoses to the treatment plan (Alfredson & Lorentzon 2000). There is a further discussion of foot orthoses in the management of chronic overuse syndromes in the foot and ankle at the end of this chapter.

Plantar fasciitis

The plantar fascia is a connective tissue that is a cross between a tendon and a ligament. It attaches to the bottom of the heel and then spans the length of the foot, spreading out like a fan to connect with the distal metatarsals, as shown in Fig. 11.3. The function of the plantar fascia is to support the medial longitudinal arch (MLA) and control the pronation of that arch during normal gait.

When abnormal pronation occurs, the plantar fascia is repetitively and excessively stressed, causing a pain in the arch of the foot that is felt most keenly on the plantar and medial aspects of the calcaneus, at the calcaneal tubercle, although this pain can also extend along the full length of the foot. On histological examination, Lemont et al (2003) found increased fibroblasts, ground substance, and vascularity, but not significant inflammatory mediators.

In the light of any objective findings, including calf muscle length, talocrural hypomobility, forefoot

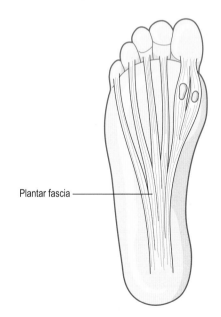

Plantar fascia

Figure 11.3 • Plantar fascia.

pronation, and heel pain, treatment is encouraged to include a multifaceted approach that addresses underlying anatomical and biomechanical conditions (Dyck & Boyajian-O'Neill 2004). This can be the case with either an overpronated or oversupinated foot (Souza 2001); a classic sign of this condition is severe pain on walking in the morning that dissipates once the patient is up and moving about.

Plantar fasciitis (PF) is very common among runners, walkers, aerobic dancers, and athletes involved in jumping sports. Its onset can be triggered by changes in the surface used for training or competition (e.g. from track to grass or vice versa), or a change in footwear. Another common trigger for PF is a change in training; the addition of hills, stairs, or sprints, for example, can cause overuse of the plantar fascia, leading to inflammation and injury. The patient will often report an increase or change in walking habit, over longer distances, wearing inappropriate footwear, or a change of walking surface (i.e. carpet to hardwood flooring).

If a patient develops PF for the very first time as a result of these changes in activity, the condition will usually respond readily to standard treatments. However, a recurrence of the condition despite treatment suggests that there is an underlying mechanical fault. The mechanism is similar to that discussed above and involves excessive or prolonged overpronation that causes stress to the plantar fascia at the calcaneal attachment.

In addition to the PRICES protocol for the relief of symptoms, spray and stretch techniques that block the reflex spasm and sensation of pain have also been shown to be effective in the conservative treatment of PF. Other techniques, such as cross-friction, ischaemic compression, heat, and manipulation, are effective on their own, or in combination with the spray and stretch technique. Considering the referral pattern of trigger points (TrPts) of the gastrocnemius/soleus to the foot, passive stretching of these muscles leads to a better prognosis and reduces the likelihood of recurrence. Acupuncture has also shown to be effective with treatment of TrPts associated with PF (Steinmetz 1999). Taping techniques have been shown to be one of the most reliable and effective short-term treatments if used correctly. These can also be used to predict the success of orthotics and are important indicator of the specific goals of orthotic therapy (Cornwall & McPoil 1999). The inclusion of functional orthotic therapy (FOT) has been demonstrated to be an effective addition to management plans for acute

and chronic PF (Bartold 2004; Dimou et al 2004; Martin et al 2001).

Metatarsalgia and Morton's neuroma

Pain in the forefoot is often associated with, and is a precursor to, Morton's neuroma. The patient will initially experience the insidious onset of forefoot pain that gets progressively worse if it goes untreated. If the condition is allowed to progress, this will eventually result in connective tissue formation (scarring) around the peripheral nerves of the foot, predominantly in the nerves between the second, third, and fourth digits of the foot. The patient may then experience paraesthesia in the toes along with secondary forefoot pain, referred to as entrapment neuralgia (Souza 2001).

The standard treatment involves the PRICES protocol with the addition of a metatarsal pad placed under the metatarsal arch to relieve pressure on the soft tissues between the distal metatarsals (Hassouna & Singh 2005; Nashi et al 1995). Footwear modifications may be required (e.g. a wider shoe) and wearing high-heeled shoes should be discouraged.

It is interesting to note that the underlying mechanism of this overuse injury is associated with overpronation through the rearfoot, midfoot, and forefoot changing the functional biomechanics of the metatarsal arch (Michaud 1997). Once again the incorporation of FOT along with pain management strategies can facilitate enhanced recovery.

Anterior and posterior tibial tendinopathy

Pain on the anterior or posterior aspect of the tibia is commonly referred to as 'shin splints'. The posterior tibial muscle and tendon are attached along the posterior and medial aspect of the tibia, passing posteriorly to the medial malleolus and underneath the MLA and attaching to the plantar aspect of the tarsal bones of the foot, allowing it to support the MLA like a stirrup. The anterior tibial muscle and tendon are attached along the anterolateral aspect of the tibia and insert into the superior aspect of the midtarsal bones. When the muscle and tendon contract, there is a lifting of the superior aspect of the tarsal bones that contributes to the support of the MLA.

When the MLA overpronates excessively, there is a consequent overstretching of the anterior and posterior tibialis muscles and tendons. The muscles and tendons exert tractional stress along the attachments to the tibia, causing disruption of the soft tissues of the tendon as well as the periosteum of the bone. Chronic irritation will eventually lead to a stress fracture of the tibia, secondary to the chronic stress on the periosteum. Clinically, this causes palpatory pain, particularly in the lower third of the tibia.

This type of injury is common in long-distance runners, but it is also frequently seen in other sports, especially those that involve jumping. As with PF, if an athlete develops this condition for the very first time following abrupt changes to training surfaces or methods, the problem will respond readily to standard treatment. However, if the condition is unresponsive to treatment, or recurs subsequently, then there may well be an underlying biomechanical weakness in the foot that will benefit from the inclusion of FOT in the treatment plan.

Bilateral asymmetrical pronation syndrome

The inquisitive practitioner will note that these overuse injuries are often unilateral, or at least worse on one side. Why then, when the patient presents with one of these overuse injuries, does this asymmetry occur? As they were walking or running with both feet, there must be an inherent asymmetry in the joint mechanics that predisposes one extremity to become symptomatic over the other.

As noted above, many of these conditions are secondary to overpronation of the rear foot, medial longitudinal arch, or forefoot, secondary to faulty foot mechanics. The diagram in Fig. 11.4 demonstrates how rear foot and forefoot varus deformity present in the non-weight-bearing phase of the gait cycle becomes a valgus stress as the foot and ankle go from an inverted to everted position with weight-bearing. When this occurs repetitively, excessively, or for a prolonged period during a single gait cycle, the result is overuse of the soft tissues.

This then is the underlying mechanism of the soft-tissue irritation in the plantar fascia that initially causes heel and arch pain; progressing to overstretching of the metatarsal arch and the development of metatarsalgia and eventually advances to Morton's neuroma. Overuse of the anterior and posterior tibial tendons causes shin splints; excessive stretch of the medial aspect of the achilles tendon results in tendinopathy; and ultimately, this varus (inversion) to valgus (eversion) motion also contributes to torsional forces up through the kinetic chain of the knee, hip, and pelvic and spinal joints to cause chronic soft-tissue injury and joint dysfunction in these more proximal regions. The diagram in Fig. 11.5 illustrates how the overpronation in the foot:

- Creates a torsion force in the femur;
- Drives the femur distally;
- Stretches the iliopsoas muscles;
- Tilts the pelvis down on the ipsilateral side; and
- Causes stress in the sacroiliac and lumbar facet joints.

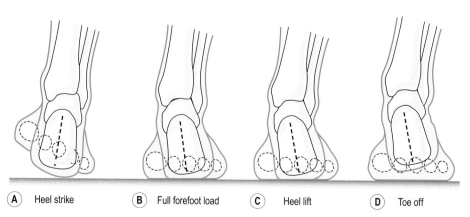

<table>
<tr><td>(A) Heel strike</td><td>(B) Full forefoot load</td><td>(C) Heel lift</td><td>(D) Toe off</td></tr>
</table>

Figure 11.4 • Stance phase motions. (a) Heel strike; (b) full forefoot load; (c) heel lift; (d) toe off.

Most patients will adapt throughout their lives to minor asymmetries, but if the asymmetry is more severe, or they engage in activities that cause repetitive strain to those structures, then the result is chronic tissue irritation, swelling, and pain.

Our first responsibility is to help patients with their discomfort using pain-reducing modalities as discussed as part of the PRICES protocol, together with other modalities such as electrotherapy, acupuncture, and taping. However, beyond this, we must consider whether there are underlying biomechanical faults in the feet that may inhibit healing or predispose the patient to recurrent symptoms; otherwise the patient becomes dependent on pain management care and has continual suffering because temporary relief has been offered without identifying the underlying cause of the chronicity and recurrence of the condition. As such, when

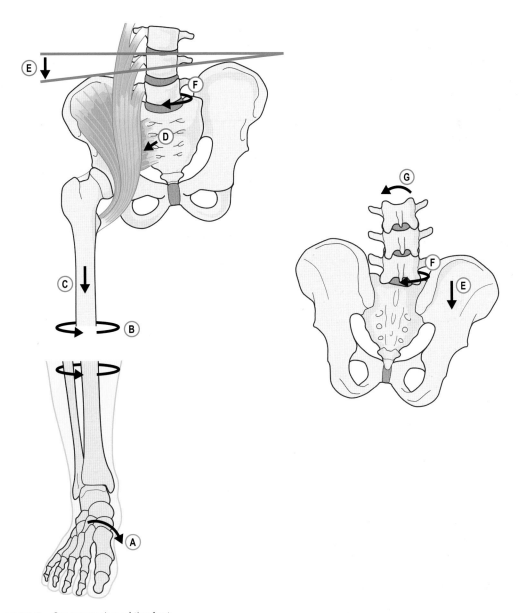

Figure 11.5 • Overpronation of the foot.

there is evidence of faulty foot mechanics, the practitioner may want to consider the inclusion of foot orthoses in the plan of management.

Foot orthoses

Foot orthoses, more commonly known as 'orthotics' (Fig. 11.6), are valuable tools for treating chronic overuse injuries in the weight-bearing joints of the body that result from faulty foot mechanics. In simple terms, orthotics are inserts placed in the shoe to support the joints and soft tissues of the foot. There are a wide variety of options, ranging from very simple foam arches, which are available over-the-counter, to highly sophisticated devices prescribed by musculoskeletal professionals who use such technological assessment tools as video gait and/or digital pressure plate analysis. Data such as this can quantify the nature and extent of the abnormal stress in the soft tissues of the feet. Fig. 11.7 illustrates a comparison of a normal pressure plate scan with that of an overpronating foot. The pressure sensors indicate excessive pressure in the medial heel and forefoot. Fig. 11.8 illustrates the forces travelling through the feet during a single stance phase in the gait cycle. The diagram is derived from a scan of an individual with a marked pes planus and excessive pressure through the medial longitudinal arch of the foot (the green line) "*GaitScan*" from *The Orthotic Group* was the pressure analysis tool used to generate the images.

These more sophisticated tools can help a practitioner to more precisely identify the nature of the biomechanical faults in patients' feet and assist the manual therapist in prescribing a pair of foot orthoses that will be uniquely suited to meet the needs of the patient. The prescription and

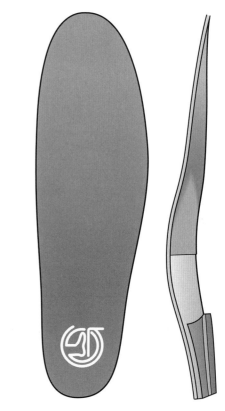

Figure 11.6 • Custom made orthoses.

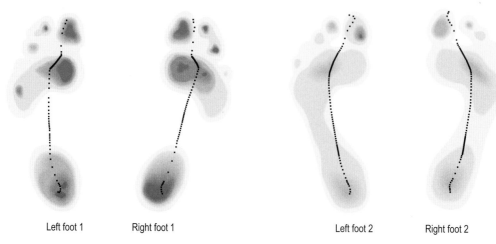

| Left foot 1 | Right foot 1 | | Left foot 2 | Right foot 2 |

Figure 11.7 • Comparison of pressure plate scans of normal and overpronating feet. (a) Left foot 1; (b) right foot 1; (c) left foot 2; (d) right foot 2. Scans (a,b) show **bilateral** overpronation **with** the right foot **more severe than the left**; scans (c,d) are normal.

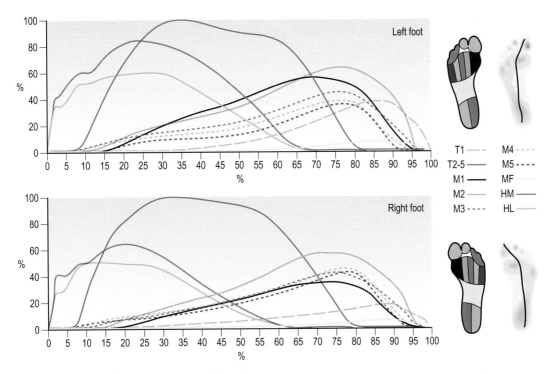

Figure 11.8 • A single stance phase in the gait cycle.
Forces travelling through the feet of an individual with marked pes planus and excessive pressure through the medial longitudinal arch.

implementation of orthotics has been found to facilitate the healing of current complaints and prevent the recurrence of overuse injuries caused by faulty foot biomechanics.

This has been an introduction to some of the alternatives to the standard regime for the management of acute and chronic conditions in the foot and ankle.

11.1　Acupuncture in lower limb dysfunction

Jennie Longbottom

Introduction

The evidence that specifically relates to ankle acupuncture is weak at best; much of the data discussed originate from traditional Chinese medical and military institutions.

Except for one paper (Koo et al 2002), this body of evidence is completely bereft of references to support claims for treatment effects. Much of the older work emanating from China is based on traditional Chinese medicine (TCM) theory, and thus has little in parallel with Western physiological basis.

A study by Erickson & Edwards (1996) found that acupuncture was successful in resolving or reducing persistent foot and ankle pain. However, the strength of this evidence is questionable because there was no control group and a large dropout (27 of 69) at 1-year follow-up.

Eksyma-Sillman et al (1995) hypothesized that muscle spasm interferes with the anterior draw test when assessing ankle instability in stress radiography, and therefore used acupuncture to produce muscle relaxation in the lower limb prior to examination. Joint space widening increased in both groups (67% of the asymptomatic group, 50% of the symptomatic group), although there was a high possibility of errors in measurement and carryover effect.

Koo et al (2002) investigated acupuncture for ankle pain in rats; ankle sprain was 'produced' in Sprague-Dawley rats by manually overextending the lateral ligaments (4 minutes in total) with increasing force, under general anaesthesia. Following this, the pain vocalization threshold was determined by the use of blunt forceps, with a strain gauge attached, applied both before and after acupuncture intervention. Acupuncture was applied at Small Intestine 6 (SI6) and Large Intestine 4 (LI4), which were deemed to be the equivalent of human acupuncture points. Both the threshold of vocalization and stepping force increased following electroacupuncture (EA) administered for 30 minutes. Unfortunately, this paper makes many assumptions, not least that acupuncture points used in humans are equivalent to those in other mammals. Furthermore, there is no rationale for the use of the named points, particularly as they are upper limb points being used for a lower limb problem. Thus, there is a great risk of drawing inconclusive parallels from this study as to the evidence for the efficacy of acupuncture in the management of human ankle sprains.

Hahm (2007) used this same rat ankle sprain model to demonstrate that EA of 2 and 100 Hz is effective for ankle sprain pain, but only 2 Hz was effective in reducing ankle oedema. These findings provide information on the physiological mechanisms, but it is debatable whether the results can be directly extrapolated to the human condition.

Acute sprain

The management and treatment of tendinopathies has been the subject of numerous studies. The literature describes various types of treatment for patients with achilles tendinopathy (AT), including rest, heat, ultrasound, electrical stimulation, anti-inflammatory medications, exercise, and surgery (Alfredson 2003; Kader et al 2002; Paavola et al 2002). Historically, there has been a lack of agreement on management owing to insufficient data (McLauchlan & Handoll 2001).

Very little evidence exists regarding the efficacy of acupuncture as a treatment for tendinopathies and no study has been undertaken that refers its use with AT specifically. Trinh et al (2004) conducted a systematic review of acupuncture for lateral epicondyle pain caused by overuse of the extensor carpi radialis brevis tendon. The study concluded that there was strong evidence suggesting that acupuncture is effective in short-term pain relief for lateral epicondyle pain. This may suggest that the results could be extrapolated for other chronic tendinopathies such as AT. However, Razavi and Jansen (2004) did not find evidence to support the use of acupuncture for rotator cuff tendinitis when compared with placebo transcutaneous electrical nerve stimulation (TENS).

Therefore it must be assumed that acupuncture for pain relief in the case of AT may have the potential to act through a variety of mechanisms, namely the peripheral, spinal, and supraspinal mechanisms of acupuncture analgesia, alterations in sympathetic outflow, and changes in motor output (Lundeberg 1998, cited in Bradnam 2007).

The possibility of myofascial TrPts in the gastrocnemius, soleus, and tibialis posterior muscle must not be overlooked in any tendinopathy. The use of TrPt needling should be incorporated early in any treatment management programme (Mense 2003; Tillu & Gupta 1998), to enhance pain relief and prevent further central nervous alterations. It is hypothesized that the acupuncture needle provides a localized stretch to the contracted cytoskeletal structures, which may disentangle the myosin filaments in the Z-band. Winding up of connective tissue occurs with rotation of the needle and appears to have the effect of straightening the collagen fibres (Langevin et al 2001). Cytoskeleton reorganization and increased interleukins may result from this mechanical stimulation. Additionally, pain may be alleviated as group II fibres register a change in total fibre length, activating the gate control system by blocking nociceptive input from the TrPt (Baldry 2001).

Plantar fasciitis

The available evidence pertaining to acupuncture management of PF is sparse. Tillu and Gupta (1998) showed a statistically significant positive analgesic effect for chronic PF using acupuncture points Kidney 3 (KID3), Bladder 60 (BL60), and Spleen 6 (SP6) for up to 6 weeks. This study also incorporated the use of TrPt acupuncture into the gastrocnemius and plantar fascia at 4 weeks, which statistically improved pain relief. Unfortunately, it must be noted that the reliability of this study is undermined by the lack of blinding or control group and the small sample size.

Medial tibial stress syndrome (shin splints)

Medial tibial stress syndrome (MTSS) is commonly referred to as 'shin splints'. It is usually associated with inflammation of the long toe or ankle flexors at or near their insertion to the posterior medial tibial border (Shultz et al 2000). Predisposing factors include excessive pronation, inflexibility of the calf muscle, AT, or long toe flexors (posterior tibialis and flexor hallucis longus), dorsiflexion weakness or fatigue, and foot conditions such as pes cavus and pes planus, which can change the shock-absorbing or decelerating capabilities of the lower-leg, resulting in transmission of increased stress to the shin and lower leg muscles (Perrin et al 2000).

Research concerning the use of acupuncture with MTSS is limited and much of it is in the form of anecdotal case reports. MTSS is frequently reported to be one of the most common exercise-related overuse injuries (Kortebein et al 2000), producing increased pain along the posteromedial border of the tibia, mostly in the distal two-thirds (Edwards et al 2005; Schulman 2004).

In a study undertaken by Callison (2002), 40 athletes with MTSS were divided into three separate groups receiving acupuncture, sports medicine treatment or a combined approach. Subjects reported their pain level at rest, during and after sport and their non-steroidal, anti-inflammatory drug (NSAID) dose, using a questionnaire. This was done at intake and two further weekly follow-ups over a 3-week period. The study concluded that acupuncture appears to be an effective modality for relieving pain associated with MTSS and for reducing reliance on NSAIDs. Athletes in the acupuncture and combined groups received the most pain relief, were least hindered by pain during sport and/or non-sporting activities, and felt treatments were effective. Perception of pain, pain relief, and effectiveness were unchanged for athletes in the sports medicine group.

Callison's (2002) study was somewhat flawed in that it did not report enough statistical evidence to view the use of acupuncture as a viable treatment source; the study grouping was not randomized, and the group cohorts were small in number. The groups lacked homogeneity, in that the athletes played different sports and, although the frequency of participation may have been equal between groups, the intensity may have differed. The above study did not illustrate how stress reactions or compartment syndromes were ruled out in determining a diagnosis. The self-reported questionnaire adopted was open to bias and inconsistency. This study showed a trend towards acupuncture as a treatment modality for MTSS, but with such a small cohort it is questionable whether these findings can be generalized to the larger population.

In a single case study undertaken by Krenner (2002), acupuncture was utilized with other modalities in the management of MTSS to stimulate endogenous endorphin release into the area. Unfortunately, no definitive conclusions can be made because different treatment disciplines were used, which is a common thread running through the relevant literature.

Mladenoff (1980) successfully treated a group of five patients with MTSS, all five gaining complete recovery of symptoms within a 12-week period, with one patient having 100% resolution in 2 weeks. It was deemed that the addition of acupuncture to the holistic management of patients with MTSS accelerated their rehabilitation, recovery, and return to full training. In this small study, cohort acupuncture was once again used only as an adjunct to treatment, with correction of biomechanical and other pathology, such as TrPt deactivation, rendered concomitantly.

Schulman (2004) illustrated the use of acupuncture as a simple and effective treatment for MTSS only with the identification and management of biomechanical abnormalities that predispose and contribute to injury. Since there are a number of intervention variables, it is speculative to ascribe cause-and-effect entirely to acupuncture.

The aetiology and pathogenesis of MTSS are not definitively known; excessive stress at the facial insertion of the medial soleus or flexor digitorum longus (FDL) muscles appear to be the most likely causes (Kortebein et al 2000). The presence of active or latent TrPts can be observed in soleus, tibialis posterior, and FDL in the setting of athletic injuries (Huguenin 2004) such as MTSS. Therefore it is important to assess for and treat any precipitating or perpetuating factors in the presence of TrPts, in order to maximize the chance of a long-term response to any treatment approaches (Huguenin 2004). Unfortunately, there are few well-designed published studies of TrPt deactivation within the management of MSST.

Case study 1

Anonymous

Introduction

The ankle is one of the most common sites for acute musculoskeletal injuries, and sprains account for 75% of ankle injuries (Barker et al 1997), with more than 40% of ankle sprains having the potential to cause chronic problems (Bennet 1994; Safran et al 1999).

Subjective assessment

A 33-year old female presented with chronic ankle pain, loss of ROM, persistent swelling, and a limping gait pattern caused by pain following a severe inversion injury, suffered whilst wearing high heels. Initial immediate symptoms included gross swelling, bruising, severe pain, and an inability to bear weight. X-rays showed no bony abnormalities noted. No immediate treatment was received until the following month when the subject presented to their general practitioner with no improvement in the ankle. The magnetic resonance imaging (MRI) results showed an os trigonum injury in the posterior aspect of the ankle. Conservative physiotherapy management was chosen prior to consideration of surgical intervention.

On initial presentation, the subject reported an intermittent dull ache extending from the posterior aspect of the knee, throughout the calf and surrounding the anterior, lateral, and posterior aspect of the ankle joint that measured 60/100 on a visual analogue scale (VAS). Aggravating factors included swimming (immediate onset) and walking of more than 10 minutes duration. Persistent swelling was also noted in correlation to the above aggravating factors, a problem that also occurred after flying. Symptoms were reduced with rest, ice, and NSAIDs. The subject was otherwise fit and well, but unable to participate in swimming, walking, or jogging and finding work increasingly difficult. Initial long-term goals for the patient included a reduction in pain levels and a return to activity.

Objective assessment

On assessment, the subject had reduced weight-bearing on the right ankle, with minimal heel strike and push off and marked swelling and thickening at the achilles tendon. ROM testing were as Table 11.1. Functional tests included:

- A squat test limited by reduced ankle dorsiflexion;
- Sitting on heels with ankles in plantar flexion; and
- One-legged heel raise.

These were not possible owing to pain and reduced ROM. Muscle testing revealed atrophy and weakening of the tibialis anterior, gastrocnemius, soleus, and the peroneii with reduced muscle length. On palpation, there was marked tenderness at the posterior aspect of the ankle joint that extended upwards along the achilles tendon to the musculotendinous junction, along the medial gutter, the lateral ligament complex, and anteriorly over the talar dome.

This subject presented with a 9-month history of chronic ankle sprain (CAS), persistent pain, swelling, reduced ROM, and muscular atrophy. These problems had been aggravated by the lack of physical intervention

(Continued)

Case Study 1 (Continued)

Table 11.1 Initial assessment of active ROM

	Pain	ROM
Dorsiflexion (DF)	Posterior & anterior aspect of ankle, VAS 60/100	¾, limited by pain
Plantarflexion (PF)	Posterior & anterior aspect of ankle, VAS 60/100	¾ limited by pain
Inversion (INV)	Lateral ligament complex, VAS 60/100	Full range available, patient apprehensive, lax ligaments
Eversion (EV)	Nil	Full range available

following the initial injury. X-ray and MRI had ruled out possible fractures, talar dome lesions and ligamentous ruptures; however, the os trigonum could be ruled out at this stage as a possible cause of the subject's symptoms.

Clinical reasoning

On deciding an effective treatment regime with which to treat this persistent chronic ankle sprain, acupuncture was considered for its analgesic effects in order to allow the subject's participation in a functional weight-bearing exercise programme. Acupuncture was chosen as an adjunct to the physiotherapy management of CAS in order to alleviate symptoms of pain and facilitate weight-bearing exercises in an attempt to alter pain memory.

Acupuncture point selection

Acupuncture point selection was based on the subject's pain presentation and palpation of the ankle as recommended by Macpherson et al (2003). Various meridians including Bladder (BL), Gall Bladder (GB), Stomach (ST), and Kidney (KID) were used, because of their proximity to all aspects of the ankle. Selected local points along these meridians, including GB40, ST41, and SP5, were used for their spinal analgesic effects; BL60 and KID3 were added in order to target the posterior achilles tendon pain. These latter points were also used to assist circulation and local tissue release pertaining to the thickened persistent swelling at the posterior aspect of this subject's ankle. BL60 was also chosen because of its close proximity to the lateral ligament complex and posterior aspect of the ankle joint, along with KID3, GB40, ST41, and SP5 along the anterior joint line, which was tender on palpation.

Distally, GB34 was used bilaterally in order to achieve stimulation of the ascending and descending spinal pathways for optimum pain modulation (Tillu et al 2001). GB34 is considered by TCM acupuncture theory to be a cardinal point since it is a He-Sea point that promotes the flow of Qi and is identified as a point useful for all joint mobility (Hecker 2005).

Treatment programme

Treatments were biweekly, extending over a period of 4 weeks. A total of 8 treatment sessions were completed after the initial assessment.

Initial assessment and treatment

The mainstay of non-acupuncture treatment consisted of progressive weight-bearing ankle, strengthening, and proprioception exercises. Outcomes measures were reassessed at each contact to evaluate the effectiveness of the treatment. These included VAS (Carlsson 1983; Price et al 1983) and ROM of the ankle, focusing on the most restricted dorsiflexion and plantarflexion. Functional tests including a squat, sitting on heels with ankles plantar flexed, and a one-legged heel raise were also reassessed following the full course of treatment, as outlined in Table 11.2.

Table 11.2 Treatment Programme

Acupoints	Outcome measures	Home exercises
LIV3[B]	VAS 60/100	1-legged calf raises
	MLF pain	
	ROM: dorsiflexion ¾	
	plantarflexion ¾	
GB40	VAS 70/100	As above and gastrocnemius and soleus stretches
ST41	MLF pain	Attempt swimming
SP5	ROM: dorsiflexion ¾	
GB34[DB]	plantarflexion ¾	

(Continued)

Case Study 1 (Continued)

Table 11.2 (Continued)

Acupoints	Outcome measures	Home exercises
BL60	VAS 50/100	As above and
GB34[DB], GB40	MLF pain	Step-ups
KID3	ROM: dorsiflexion ¾	Step-downs
SP5	plantarflexion ¾	
ST41		
BL60	VAS 30/100	As above and
GB34[DB], GB40	MLF pain	1-legged stand on sit fit/wobble board
KID3	ROM: dorsiflexion ¾	
SP5	MLF stiffness	
ST41	ROM plantarflexion ¾	
BL60	VAS 20/100	Progress to step-ups and step-downs with sit fit on step.
GB34[DB], GB40	MLF stiffness	Attempt brisk walking
KID3	ROM: dorsiflexion ¾	Continue stretches
SP5	plantarflexion ¾	
ST41		
BL60	VAS 20/100	As above
GB34[DB], GB40	MLF stiffness	
KID3	ROM: dorsiflexion ¾	
SP5	plantarflexion ¾	
ST41		
BL60	VAS 0/100	As above and
GB34[DB], GB40	MLF stiffness	Attempt a jog, even surface with supportive trainers
KID3	ROM: dorsiflexion ¾	
SP5	plantarflexion ¾	
ST41		
BL60	VAS 0/100	Continue with jogging, stretching, and proprioceptive work
GB34[DB], GB40	ROM full throughout	
KID3		
SP5		
ST41		

Notes: D, distal; B, bilateral; Rx, treatment; MLF, main limiting factor; VAS, visual analogue scale; ROM, range of movement.

Outcome

Following the initial treatment, there appeared to be an increase in the subject's reported VAS scores. The pain scores then dropped progressively until the patient experienced no daily pain. There appeared to be a gradual increase in ankle ROM, as pain levels dropped, allowing more progressive and demanding ankle exercises to be undertaken. During the final course of treatment, the subject was experiencing:

- No pain;
- Minimal swelling;
- A marked reduction in the achilles thickness;

(Continued)

Case Study 1 (Continued)

- Full active ROM;
- Full functional squat with only an occasional twinge;
- A VAS score of 10/100 anteriorly;
  - Sitting on heels; and
  - Achieving 1-legged heel raise.

Conclusion

Rehabilitation of ankle injuries should be structured and individualized. In the acute phase, the focus should be on controlling inflammation, re-establishing full ROM, and gaining strength. Failing this, chronic pain, persistent swelling, muscle weakness, and instability can persist. The outcome of the present case study suggests that analgesic acupuncture is useful in the management of CAS when combined with a functional exercise rehabilitation programme; however, it also highlights the need for future reliable research in this field.

Case study 2

Eghon Murray

Introduction

Medial tibial traction periostitis (MTTP) is one of the most common exercise-induced lower limb overuse injuries. This is a case report detailing an effective acupuncture treatment of a 38-year-old male diagnosed with MTTP. The report also reviews the relevant literature on MTTP management using acupuncture. The case study illustrates the use of acupuncture as an efficacious treatment for MTTP in this instance, though there is limited supporting evidence to justify validity to the larger population.

A male 38-year-old recreational runner presented with a longstanding history of left-sided exercise-induced anteromedial shin pain. He had an acute exacerbation 4 days previously following a sudden increase in his training volume, after a sustained period of inactivity. He was unable to run more than 20 minutes owing to the pain, his symptoms were aggravated by impact and inclines, and he complained of a dull ache into the distal third of the left tibia, with tightness into the posteromedial calf. He did not complain of any paraesthesia.

Subjective and objective assessment

On examination he had fore and rear foot valgus, poor pelvic and hip control during single leg squat, and poor gluteal activation, worse on the left. He was weak into his left inverters, had early fatigue during the calf test, and had a positive hop test for pain on the left. He was also tender on palpation into the medial cortex of the mid-shaft of the tibial deep compartment. He had active TrPts into the soleus and tibialis posterior muscles. Owing to the presentation of bony tenderness, MRI was undertaken in order to rule out any long-term stress reaction; the findings were consistent with MTTP, of which the diagnosis was confirmed.

Acupuncture point rationale

An analysis of the meridian system in relation to the area of pain revealed involvement of the Spleen, Liver, and Kidney meridians (Mladenoff 1980) (Table 11.3). The Liver meridian was selected for its proposed increased blood flow upon soft tissue and the Kidney meridian, because it is hypothesized that they have an effect on osseous inflammation (Mladenoff 1980).

Physiological reasoning for acupuncture selection

There is a substantial body of evidence, albeit not solely based on randomized controlled trials (RCTs), to demonstrate that acupuncture is an effective modulator of pain (Carlsson 2002; Chen 2006) via the stimulation of high threshold, small diameter A-delta (Aδ) nerves that communicate with the dorsal horn of the spinal cord, brainstem, periaqueductal grey (PAG), and hypothalamus via the arcuate nucleus. This stimulation, in turn, triggers descending inhibitory pathways in the shape of endogenous opioid mechanisms (Kaptchuk 2002). Acupuncture thus induces afferent nerve signals that can modulate spinal signal transmission and the brain's perception of pain. Acupuncture stimulation also leads to the release of enkephalins and endorphins, exerting an inhibitory effect on nociceptive reflexes at the segmental level. Central opioid release is thought to produce a global reduction in pain perception by gating spinal cord pain impulse transmission and thereby, inhibiting nociception (Hugeunin 2004). This is known as diffuse noxious inhibitory control (DNIC) (White 1999). In this way ascending Aδ fibres and C fibres, which stimulate the PAG and hypothalamus, can promote the secretion of serotonin and norepinephrine (White 1999).

Another component of this treatment was the use of acupuncture in addressing the myofascial TrPts that

(Continued)

Case Study 2 (Continued)

Table 11.3 Acupuncture point rationale

Acupuncture points	Rationale
LI4 & LIV3 (Bilateral)	'4 gates' was selected in the inflammatory phase because they are distal points and can stimulate the descending inhibitory pathway and thus higher centre opioid release
BL62	A distal point, having an anti-inflammatory effect with cortisol release from the higher centres
LIV8	Used segmentally, in conjunction with BL62 in the proliferation stage, will stimulate local pain relief. It is a local meridian, a He-Sea point, can relax tendons and is used specifically for medial compartment syndrome, for which MTSS can be a determinant
KID9	Can sedate osseous inflammation, induce local pain, is a local meridian, and can aid posterior compartment muscular atrophy (Mladenoff 1980)
Tibialis posterior & Soleus TrPt	Deactivation of dysfunctional motor end-plate, to achieve relief of muscle tension and posteromedial tibial traction and therefore pain. These trigger points were also utilized to good effect by Callison to treat MTSS in another study (Callison 2002)

may produce sensory, motor, and autonomic symptoms. A TrPt point is defined as the presence of exquisite tenderness at a nodule in a palpable taut band of muscle (Travell & Simons 1992). There are two major schools of thought as to the aetiology of TrPts: the energy crisis theory (Travell & Simons 1992) and the motor-end-plate hypothesis (Simons et al 2002). When combined, these schools of thought provide a plausible explanation as to the management of myofascial pain by TrPt needling.

The energy crisis theory postulates that a buildup in ischaemic byproducts is in part responsible for some of the pain produced by sensitization of sensory nerves. An increased demand on the muscle is thought to lead to increased calcium release from the sarcolemma and prolonged shortening of the sarcomeres (Travel & Simons 1992). A compromised circulation and reduced cellular oxidative phosphorylation is thought to equate to insufficient adeno-tri-phosphate (ATP) in order to initiate an active relaxation.

The motor-end-plate hypothesis is thought possibly to coexist with the energy crisis theory in that TrPts have been found to have minute loci that produce characteristic electrical activity; the end-plate activity is insufficient to produce a muscle contraction, but can result in action potentials being propagated within a small distance along the cell membrane. This small amount of propagation may be enough to cause activation of a few contractile elements and be responsible for some degree of shortening (Huguenin 2004; Travell & Simons 1992).

Dry needling involves advancing the needle into the muscle in the region of the TrPt, aiming to reproduce the subject's pain symptoms, producing a local twitch response and, ultimately, achieve relief of muscle tension and pain (Huguenin 2004). As stated there are few well-designed published studies of this technique; the mere action of producing a painful stimulus via the needling technique may be the key to obtaining improvements in pain perception. Dry needling is thought to stimulate type II and III afferents and as a result analgesia and autonomic modulation can occur. The needle is thought to disrupt the dysfunctional end-plate (Baldry 2001), thereby decreasing tension and pain. Mechanical pressure exerted manually or via a needle on the TrPt is thought to reduce the demand for ATP and thus return the muscle to a more homeostatic state (McPartland & Simons 2006).

Outcome measurements and results

The following outcome measurements were used in order to assess the effectiveness of the interventions:
- A verbal rating score (VRS) 0/10;
- A functional performance test (FPT) using the single leg heel raise test (SLHRT) and hop test (HT); and
- The calf stress test (CST) involving the maximum number of single heel raises in 1 minute.

Following the three treatment sessions the patient felt immediate and marked relief, with complete eradication of pain at rest; he was able to perform a SLHRT without pain and reported a significant reduction in pain during the HT. The subject was also able to run, without pain, for 40 minutes (Table 11.4).

Conclusion and limitations

Although underlying biomechanical issues were addressed, this case report suggests that acupuncture may be utilized to good effect in the holistic

(Continued)

Case Study 2 (Continued)

Table 11.4 Treatment summary

Session	Acupuncture point/ trigger point	De Qi/needle grasp	Treatment duration (mins)	Outcome
1	LI4[B] LIV3[B] BL62[L]	Yes	20	Decreased pain at rest
2	LIV3[L] BL62[L] LIV8[L] Tibialis posterior and soleus TrPt	Yes Needle grasp/twitch response	20 1	Decreased functional pain
3	LIV[L] BL62[L] KID9[L] Tibialis posterior and soleus TrPt	Yes Needle grasp/twitch response	20 1	Decreased functional pain

Notes: B, bilateral; L, left.

management of a patient with MTSS. The limitations are such that a case report is largely anecdotal; the validity and generalization are therefore questionable. Medial tibial traction syndrome is a variable condition, with many extrinsic and intrinsic dependents; in this case it was managed with a variant of treatment modalities and it may be speculative to solely ascribe cause and effect entirely to acupuncture intervention. Unfortunately, only three treatment sessions were undertaken due to patient circumstances; it has been documented that at least 5 to 6 treatment sessions are required before efficacy can be determined (Bradnam 2003). Acupuncture treatment sessions were also only 20 minutes in length due to time constraints; for higher centre descending inhibitory pathway opioid release, 30 minutes treatment is indicated (Bradnam 2003).

Discussion

Biomechanical factors and training errors are the likely significant determinants that may predispose to MTSS. The literature is in agreement that these should be addressed concomitantly with any acupuncture treatment modality (Mladenoff 1980; Schulman 2004); hence a conflict arises within this case report, along with many others, in determining the efficacy of acupuncture, as it is not the sole intervention.

Although other issues were addressed concomitantly with the acupuncture, there is evidence that acupuncture intervention produced a result in the management of pain. More specifically, TrPt release appeared to have an immediate and marked effect on the subject's recovery and reported pain scales. It is unlikely that the subject's gluteal and deep flexor muscle strength would have significantly improved within this time factor, as a means of explaining such a dramatic resolution of symptoms and functional progression. Therefore, even as an adjunct in the holistic management, it is important to acknowledge the therapeutic effect acupuncture can have in the treatment of MTSS.

No studies have proclaimed acupuncture as a panacea in the treatment of MTSS, demonstrating that the effectiveness of acupuncture is undoubtedly complex and notoriously complicated by a host of methodological issues. One of these issues is the predicament of sham acupuncture; in the quest for a matching control, one that is inert, identical in appearance and sensation, and without the release of non-specific physiological effects (Kaptchuk 2002). As sham acupuncture has a noxious afferent effect, it must also be considered that absence of evidence should not be equated with evidence of absence of effect.

The case study highlights overuse pathology, MTSS, commonly seen in physiotherapy practice and serves to reinforce the approach that management should be holistic and comprehensive. This case study offers support for the sparse anecdotal evidence in the literature for the successful application of acupuncture in the treatment of MTSS in conjunction with addressing any relevant biomechanical predisposition.

References

Alfredson, H., 2003. Chronic midportion achilles tendinopathy: an update on research and treatment. Clin. Sports Med. 22 (4), 727–741.

Alfredson, H., 2005. The chronic painful achilles and patellar tendon: research on basic biology and treatment. Scand. J. Med. Med. Sports 15 (4), 252–259.

Alfredson, H., Lorentzon, R., 2000. Chronic achilles tendinosis: recommendations. Sports Med. 29 (2), 135–146.

Alfredson, H., Forsgren, S., Thorsen, K., Lorentzon, R., 2001. In vivo microdialysis and immunohistochemical analysis of tendon tissue demonstrated high amounts of free glutamate and glutamate NMDAR1 receptors, but no signs of inflammation, in Jumper's knee. J. Orthop. Res. 19 (5), 881–886.

Andres, B.M., Murrell, G.A., 2008. Treatment of tendinopathy, what works, what does not and what is on the horizon. Clin. Related Orthop. Res. 466, 1539–1554.

Baldry, P.E., 2001. Management of Myofascial Trigger Point Pain. British Medical Acupuncture Society, Spring Scientific Meeting, Bournemouth, UK.

Balduini, F.C., Vegso, J.J., Torg, J.S., et al., 1987. Management and rehabilitation of ligamentous injuries to the ankle. Sports Med. 4, 364–380.

Barker, H.B., Beynnon, B.D., Renstron, P.A., 1997. Ankle injury risk factors in sports. Sports Med. 23, 69–74.

Bartold, S.J., 2004. The plantar fascia as a source of pain biomechanics, presentation and treatment. J. Bodyw. Mov. Ther. 8 (3), 214–226.

Bennett, W.F., 1994. Lateral ankle sprains. Part II: acute and chronic treatment. Orthop. Rev. 23, 504–510.

Bjur, D., Alfredson, H., Forsgren, S., 2005. The innervation pattern of the human achilles tendon: studies of the normal and tendinosis tendon with markers for general and sensory innervation. Cell Tissue Res. 320 (1), 201–206.

Bradnam, L., 2003. A proposed clinical reasoning model for Western acupuncture. New Zealand J. Physiotherapy 31, 40–45.

Bradnam, L., 2007. A proposed clinical reasoning model for western acupuncture. J. Acupun. Assoc. Chart. Physiotherap., 21–39.

Callison, M., 2002. Study: acupuncture and tibial stress syndrome (shin splints). J. Chinese Med. 70, 4–29.

Carlsson, A.M., 1983. Assessment of chronic pain. I. Aspects of the reliability and validity of the visual analogue scale. Pain 16 (1), 87–101.

Carlsson, C., 2002. Acupuncture mechanisms for clinically relevant long-term effects-reconsideration and a hypothesis. Acupun. Med. 20 (2–3), 82–99.

Chen, A., Feng, F-J., Wang, L., et al., 2006. Mode and site of acupuncture modulation in the human brain: 3D (124-ch) EEG power spectrum mapping and source imaging. Neuroimage 29 (4), 1080–1091.

Dimou, E.S., Brantingham, J.W., Wood, T.A., 2004. Randomised, controlled trial (with blinded observer) of chiropractic manipulation and achilles stretching vs.orthotics for the treatment of plantar fasciitis. J. Am. Chiropractic Assoc. 41 (9), 32–34.

Dyck Jr., D.D., Boyajian-O'Neill, L.A., 2004. Plantar faciitis. Clin. J. Sport Med. 14 (5), 305–309.

Edwards Jr., P.H., Wright, M.L., Hartman, J.F., 2005. A practical approach for the differential diagnosis of chronic leg pain in the athlete. Am. J. Sports Med. 33 (8), 1241–1249.

Eisenhart, A.W., Gaeta, T.J., Yens, D. P., 2007. Osteopathic manipulative treatment in emergency department for patients with acute ankle injuries. J. Am. Osteopathic Assoc. 103 (9), 417–421.

Eksyma-Sillman, S., Suramo, I., Junnila, S.Y.T., et al., 1995. Effect of acupuncture as seen in stress radiography of the ankle. Acupun. Med. 13 (1), 2–4.

Erickson, R.J., Edwards, B., 1996. Medically unresponsive foot pain treated successfully with acupuncture. Acupun. Med. 14 (2), 71–74.

Fryer, G., Fryer, J., Mudge, P., et al., 2002. The effect of talocrural joint manipulation on ROM of ankle. Therapeutics 25, 384–390.

Gillman, S.F., 2004. The impact of chiropractic manipulative therapy on chronic recurrent lateral ankle sprain syndrome in two young athletes. J. Chiropractic Med. 4 (3), 153–159.

Glick, J.M., Gordon, R.B., Nishimoto, D., 1976. The prevention and treatment of ankle injuries. Am. J. Sports Med. 4, 136–141.

Hahm, T.S., 2007. The effect of 2 Hz and 100 Hz electrical stimulation of acupoint on ankle sprain in rats. J. Korean Med. Sci. 22, 347–351.

Hampson, K., Forsyth, N.R., El Haj, A., et al., 2008 Tendon tissue engineering. In: Ashammakhi, N., Reis, R., Chiellini, F., (Eds.), Topics in tissue engineering, 4, 1–21.

Hart, P.H., Jones, C.A., Finlay-Jones, J.J., 1995. Monocytes cultured in cytokine-defined environments differ from freshly isolated monocytes in their responses to IL-4 and IL-10. J. Leukocyte Biol. 57 (6), 909–918.

Harvie, P., Ostlere, S.J., The, J., et al., 2004. Genetic influences in the aetiology of tears of the rotator cuff. J. Bone Joint Surg. 86 (5), 696–700.

Hassouna, H.Z., Singh, D., 2005. The variation in the management of Morton's metatarsalgia. The Foot 15 (3), 149–153.

Hecker, H.U., 2005. Color Atlas of Acupuncture: Body Points, Ear Points, Trigger Points Complementary Medicine. Thieme Publishing, Stuttgart.

Hertel, J., 2000. Functional instability following lateral ankle sprain. Sports Med. 29 (5), 361–371.

Huguenin, L.K., 2004. Myofascial trigger points: the current evidence. Phys. Therapy in Sport 5, 2–12.

Justus, J., Fiechtner, M.P.H., Brodeur, R., 2002. Manual manipulation techniques for rheumatic disease. Med. Clin. North Am. 86 (1), 91–103.

Kader, D., Saxena, A., Movin, T., et al., 2002. Achilles tendinopathy: some aspects of basic science and clinical management. Brit. J. Sports Med. 36 (4), 239–249.

Kannus, P., Natri, A., 1997. Aetiology and pathophysiology of tendon ruptures in sports. Scand. J. Med. Sci. Sports 7 (7), 107–112.

Kaptchuk, T.J., 2002. Acupuncture: theory, efficacy and practice. Ann. Internal Med. 136 (5), 374–383.

Kerkhoffs, G.M., Rowe, B.H., Assendelft, W.J., et al., 2002. Immobilization and functional treatment for acute lateral ankle ligament injuries in adults. Cochrane Database Syst. Rev. 3, CD003762.

Koo, S.T., Park, Y.I., Lim, K.S., et al., 2002. Acupuncture analgesia in a new rat model of ankle sprain pain. Pain 99 (3), 423–431.

Kortebein, P.M., Kaufman, H.R., Basford, J.R., 2000. Medial tibial stress syndrome (MTSS). Med. Sci. Sports Exer. 32 (2), 27–33.

Krenner, D.C., 2002. Case report: comprehensive management of medial tibial stress syndrome. J. Chiropractic Med. 1 (3), 38–46.

Langevin, H.M., Churchill, D.L., Fox, J.R., et al., 2001. Biomechanical response to acupuncture needling in humans. J. Applied Physiol. 91 (6), 2471–2478.

Lemont, H., Ammirati, K.M., Usen, N., 2003. Plantar faciitis: a degenerative process (fasciosis) without inflammation. J. Am. Podiatry Med. Assoc. 93 (3), 234–237.

Logan, A.L., Rowe, L.J., 1995. Adjustive techniques. In: The Foot and Ankle: Clinical Applications, 1st edn. Jones & Bartlett, Sudbury, MA.

Macpherson, H., Thorpe, L., Thomas, K., et al., 2003. Acupuncture for low back pain: traditional diagnosis and treatment of 148 patients in a clinical trial. Complementary Ther. Med. 12, 38–44.

Martin, J.E., Hosch, J.C., Goforth, W.P., et al., 2001. Mechanical treatment of plantar fasciitis: a prospective study. J. Am. Med. Assoc. 91 (2), 55–62.

McLauchlan, G.J., Handoll, H.H., 2001. Interventions for treating acute and chronic achilles tendinitis. Cochrane Database Syst. Rev. 1 (2), CD000232.

McPartland, J.M., Simons, D.G., 2006. Myofascial trigger points: translating molecular theory into manual therapy. J. Man. Manip. Ther. 14 (4), 232–239.

Mense, S., 2003. The pathogenesis of muscle pain. Curr. Pain Headache Reports 7, 419–425.

Michaud, T.C., 1997. Orthoses and other forms of conservative foot care, self-published.

Mladenoff, E., 1980. Acupuncture treatment of shin splints. Am. J. Acupun. 8 (3), 245–248.

Nashi, M., Venkatachalam, A.K., Muddu, B.N., 1995. Review of Morton's neuroma. The Foot 5 (4), 165–166.

Paavola, M., Kannus, P., Järvinen, T.A., et al., 2002. Treatment of tendon disorders. Is there a role for corticosteroid injection? Foot Ankle Clinic 7 (3), 501–513.

Peterson, D.H., Bergmann, T.F., 2002. Chiropractic glossary of commonly used terms. In: Chiropractic Technique, 2nd edn. Mosby, St Louis, MO.

Pizzorno, J.E., Murray, M.T., 2007. Clinician's Handbook of Natural Medicine, 2nd edn.. Churchill Livingstone, Philadelphia.

Pizzorno, J.E., Murray, M.T., Joiner-Bey, H., 1997. Encyclopedia of Natural Medicine, rev 2nd edn.. Churchill Livingstone, Philadelphia.

Pizzorno, J.E., Murray, M.T., Joiner-Bey, H., 2005. Textbook of Natural Medicine, 3rd edn.. Churchill Livingstone, Philadelphia.

Price, D.D., McGrath, P.A., Rafii, A., et al., 1983. The validation of visual analogue scales as ratio scale measures for chronic and experimental pain. Pain 17, 45–56.

Razavi, M., Jansen, G.B., 2004. Effects of acupuncture and placebo TENS in addition to exercise in treatment of rotator cuff tendinitis. Clin. Rehabilitat. 18 (8), 872–878.

Rompe, J.D., Nafe, B., Furia, J.P., et al., 2007. Eccentric loading, shock wave therapy, wait-and-see policy for tendinopathy of the main body of tendo-achilles: a randomised controlled trial. Am. J. Sports Med. 35, 374–783.

Rose, A., Lee, R.J., Williams, R.M., et al., 2000. Functional instability in non-contact ankle ligament injuries. Brit. J. Sports Med. 34, 352–358.

Ryan, L., 1994. Mechanical stability, muscle strength and proprioception in the functionally unstable ankle. Aust. J. Physiother. 40 (1), 41–47.

Safran, M.R., Benedetti, R.S., Bartolozzi, A.R., et al., 1999. Lateral ankle sprains: a comprehensive review. Part 1: aetiology, pathoanatomy, histopathogenesis, and diagnosis. Med. Sci. Sports Exer. 31 (S7), S429–S437.

Schulman, R., 2004. Tibial shin splint treated with a single acupuncture session: Case report and review of the literature. Med. Acupun. 13 (1), 7–9.

September, A.N., Schwellnus, M.P., Collins, M., 2007. Tendon and ligament injuries: the genetic component. Brit. J. Sports Med. 41, 241–246.

Shalabi, A., Kristoffersen-Wiberg, M., Aspelin, P., 2004. Immediate achilles tendon response after strength training evaluated by MRI. Med. Sci. Sports Exer. 36, 1841–1846.

Shultz, S., Houglum, P., Perrin, D., 2000. Assessment of Athletic Injuries. Human Kinetics, Champaign, IL.

Simons, D.G., Hong, C-Z., Simons, L.S., 2002. Endplate potentials are common to midfiber myofascial trigger points. Am. J. Phys. Med. Rehabilitat. 81, 212–222.

Souza, T.A., 2001. Differential Diagnosis and Management for the Chiropractor Protocols and Algorithms. Aspen, Gaithersburg, MD.

Steinmetz, M., 1999. Treatment choices for plantar faciitis. Am. Fam. Physician 60 (9), 2504.

Tillu, A., Gupta, S., 1998. Effect of acupuncture treatment on heel pain due to plantar faciitis. Acupun. Med. 16 (2), 66–68.

Tillu, A., Roberts, C., Tillu, S., 2001. Unilateral versus bilateral acupuncture on knee function in advanced osteoarthritis of the knee: a prospective randomised trial. Acupun. Med. 19, 15–18.

Travell, J., Simons, D., 1992. Myofascial Pain and Dysfunction: the Trigger Point Manual, Vol. ii: The Lower Extremities. Lippincott Williams and Wilkins, Baltimore.

Trinh, K.V., Phillips, S.D., Ho, E., et al., 2004. Acupuncture for the alleviation of lateral epicondylar pain: a systematic review. Rheumatology 43 (9), 1085–1090.

Van der Wee, P.J., Lenssen, A.F., Hendriks, E.J., et al., 2006. Effectiveness of exercise therapy and manual mobilisation in ankle sprain and functional instability: a systematic review. Aust. J. Physiother. 52 (1), 27–37.

Wang, J.H., 2006. Mechanobiology of tendon. J. Biomech. 39, 1563–1582.

White, A., 1999. Neurophysiology of acupuncture analgesia. In: Ernst, E., White, A. (Eds.), Acupuncture: A Scientific Appraisal. Butterworth-Heinemann, London.

Whitman, J.M., Childs, J.D., Walker, V., 2005. The use of manipulation in a patient with an ankle sprain injury not responding to conventional management: a case report. Man. Ther. 10 (3), 224–231.

Transcutaneous electrical nerve stimulators for pain management

Professor Mark Johnson

CHAPTER CONTENTS

Introduction

Transcutaneous electrical nerve stimulation (TENS) is a peripheral stimulation technique that is non-invasive, allowing patients the ability to self-administer treatment. The purpose of TENS is to deliver pulsed electrical currents across the intact surface of the skin to activate underlying nerves and reduce pain (Fig. 12.1). Effective treatment is facilitated when administered to produce a strong non-painful electrical paraesthesia. The effects are usually rapid in onset and offset, allowing treatment administration throughout the day. TENS is inexpensive and can be purchased without prescription in the UK. However, a practitioner who has been trained in the principles and practice of TENS should supervise patient's use in the first instance and provide a point of contact to troubleshoot any problems.

Electrotherapy became popular in the eighteenth and nineteenth centuries following the invention of electrostatic generators. However, increasing use of pharmacological treatments in the twentieth century meant that electrotherapy disappeared from mainstream medicine until the mid-1960s. Interest in electrotherapy for pain relief increased with the publication of Melzack and Wall's *Pain Mechanisms: A New Theory* (Melzack & Wall 1965). They suggested that large diameter non-noxious transmitting peripheral afferents could be stimulated using electrical stimuli, reducing onward transmission of noxious information arising from tissue damage. In 1967 Wall & Sweet reported that electrical stimulation of peripheral nerves reduced pain in eight chronic pain patients (Wall & Sweet 1967). Pain relief was also demonstrated in patients during electrical stimulation of dorsal columns (Shealy et al 1967) and the periaqueductal grey of the midbrain, forming part of the descending pain inhibitory pathways (Richardson & Akil 1977). Originally, TENS was used to predict

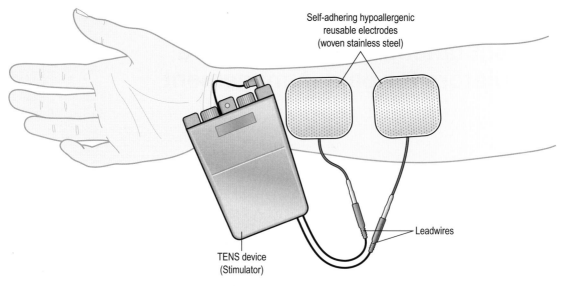

Figure 12.1 • Transcutaneous electrical nerve stimulation (TENS)

the success of dorsal column stimulation implants until it was realized that it could be used as a successful modality on its own (Long 1973; Shealy 1972).

Definition and techniques

Healthcare professionals use the term TENS to refer to currents administered using a 'standard TENS device' (Fig. 12.2). Differences in the design between manufacturers tend to be cosmetic with limited effect on physiological and clinical outcome. Some manufacturers have designed TENS devices that markedly differ from a standard device. These TENS-like devices include interferential therapy, microcurrent therapy, and transcutaneous electrical acupoint stimulation. A critical review of TENS-like devices can be found in Johnson (2001a, b). A standard TENS device should be used for pain in the first instance and will be the focus of this chapter.

The purpose of TENS is to stimulate nerve fibres and to generate nerve impulses that elicit pain modulation. Different techniques are used to stimulate different populations of nerve fibres (Table 12.1). The main techniques are:

• Conventional TENS: low-intensity, high-frequency currents, to elicit segmental analgesia;

• Acupuncture-like TENS: high-intensity, low-frequency currents, to elicit extrasegmental analgesia; and

• Intense TENS: high-intensity high-frequency currents, to elicit peripheral nerve blockade, and segmental and extrasegmental analgesia.

Conventional TENS is used for most patients in the first instance.

Conventional TENS

The International Association for the Study of Pain (IASP) defines conventional TENS as high frequency (50–100 Hz), low intensity (paraesthesia, not painful), small pulse width (50–200 μs) (Charlton 2005). Conventional TENS is used to activate low-threshold, large diameter myelinated afferent fibres (Aβ) normally transmitting information related to non-painful touch and pressure (Fig. 12.3). This inhibits onward transmission of nociceptive information at synapses in the central nervous system (see Mechanism of Action). Patients are instructed to increase TENS pulse amplitude until a strong, comfortable, non-painful paraesthesia is experienced beneath the electrodes, indicating large diameter myelinated afferent fibre activity. A painful TENS paraesthesia beneath the electrodes is not appropriate. Theoretically, high-frequency (~10–200 pulses per second (pps)) currents are optimal because they generate a large afferent barrage leading to greater

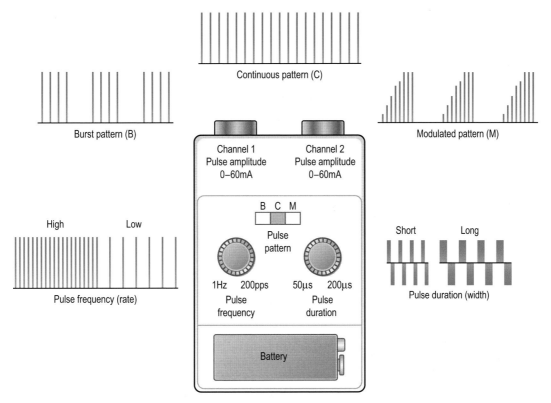

Figure 12.2 • A standard TENS device

Table 12.1 Types of TENS

	Physiological intention	TENS parameters	Patient experience	Electrode location	Analgesic profile	Regimen
Conventional TENS	To stimulate large diameter non-noxious afferents (Aβ) to produce segmental analgesia	Low intensity (amplitude), high frequency (10–200 pps)	Strong, non-painful TENS paraesthesia with minimal muscle activity	Dermatomes Site of pain	Usually rapid onset and offset	Use TENS whenever in pain
AL-TENS	To stimulate small diameter cutaneous and motor afferents (Aδ) to produce extrasegmental analgesia	High intensity (amplitude), low frequency (1–5 bursts of 100 pps)	Strong comfortable muscle twitching	Myotomes Site of pain Muscles Motor nerves Acupuncture points	May be delayed onset and offset	Use TENS for 20–30 minutes at a time
Intense TENS	To stimulate small diameter cutaneous afferents (Aδ) to produce counterirritation	High amplitude (uncomfortable/noxious), high frequency (50–200 pps)	Uncomfortable (painful) electrical paraesthesia	Dermatomes Site of pain Nerves proximal to pain	Rapid onset and delayed offset	Short periods only 5–15 minutes at a time

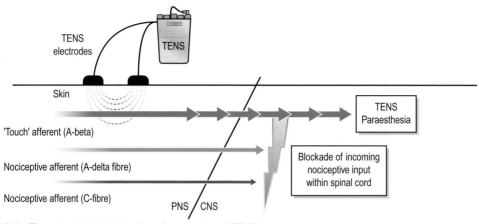

Figure 12.3 • The physiological intention of conventional TENS
Arrows indicate direction of TENS-induced nerve impulses; PNS = peripheral nervous system; CNS = central nervous system.

inhibition of nociceptive transmission. Pulse durations between 50 and 200μs allow optimal precision in achieving the desired intensity when titrating pulse amplitude.

Acupuncture-like TENS (AL-TENS)

AL-TENS was developed to harness the mechanisms of action of TENS and acupuncture by activating segmental and extrasegmental mechanisms (descending pain inhibitory pathways) (Eriksson & Sjölund 1976). IASP define AL-TENS as a form of hyperstimulation achieved using currents that are low frequency (2–4 Hz), higher intensity (to tolerance threshold), and longer pulse width (100–400μs) (Charlton 2005). Intermittent trains or bursts (2–4 Hz) of high-frequency pulses (100–200 pps) are often used in clinical practice to reduce discomfort experienced using high-intensity single pulses. The intention of AL-TENS is to stimulate small diameter, higher threshold afferents (Aδ) using high-intensity, low-frequency TENS. Research suggests that small muscle afferents produce greatest analgesia so some practitioners administer AL-TENS to generate non-painful muscle twitches which indirectly generates impulses in small diameter muscle afferents (Fig. 12.4). Electrodes are positioned at the site of pain, over myotomes, muscles, acupuncture points, and trigger points. AL-TENS is used to treat patients who are resistant to conventional TENS and patients are advised to administer it less frequently than conventional TENS, e.g. 20 minutes, 3 times a day (Eriksson & Sjölund 1976). AL-TENS can also be used for muscle and visceral pain arising from deep-seated structures, radiating neuropathic pain, and in situations where prolonged analgesia is required (Johnson 1998).

Intense TENS

Intense TENS is a counterirritant and is delivered for short periods of time over nerve bundles close to the site of pain. High-frequency (up to 200 pps), high-intensity currents that are painful but tolerable are used. The intention of intense TENS is to stimulate small diameter, higher threshold cutaneous afferents (Aδ) to block transmission of nociceptive information in peripheral nerves (Fig. 12.5). Intense TENS activates diffuse noxious inhibitory controls (Le Bars et al 1979), and can be used for minor procedures such as wound dressing and suture removal.

Contraindications

Manufacturers list cardiac pacemakers, epilepsy, and pregnancy as contraindications because it may be difficult to exclude TENS as a potential cause from a medico-legal perspective. The Chartered Society for Physiotherapy (CSP) suggest that TENS can be used in pregnancy and in epilepsy providing electrodes are placed well away from the abdomen, sacrum, and neck respectively (i.e. local contraindication) (CSP

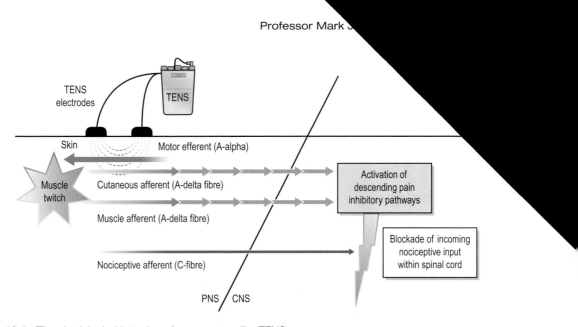

Figure 12.4 • The physiological intention of acupuncture-like TENS.
Arrows indicate direction of TENS-induced nerve impulses; PNS = peripheral nervous system; CNS = central nervous system.

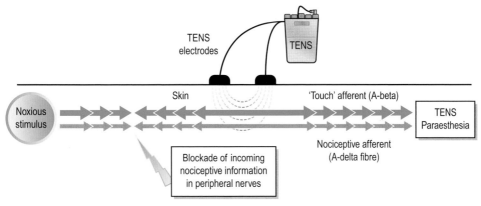

Figure 12.5 • Intense TENS
Arrows indicate direction of TENS-induced nerve impulses and direction of nerve impulses arising from damaged tissue

2006). The CSP also lists bleeding tissue as a contraindication and suggests that TENS should not be delivered over active epiphysis or over an active, treatable tumour.

Precautions

TENS should not be administered over the anterior neck, eyes, and testes or through the chest using anterior and posterior positions. TENS may interfere with foetal and cardiac monitoring equipment and should not be administered close to transdermal drug delivery systems. There is no known evidence that adverse events occur when TENS is used with metal implants, stents, percutaneous central catheters, or drainage systems. It should not be used while driving and should only be given internally using devices designed for that purpose (e.g. incontinence or dental analgesia). TENS devices with timers that automatically switch off are useful to aid sleep and may be used by children with success (Lander & Fowler-Kerry 1993; Merkel et al 1999).

Serious adverse events from TENS occur but are extremely rare (Mann 1996; Rosted 2001). It has

Johnson

CHAPTER 12

ccasionally
retains an
major drug
combined
rug-related
ffeine may
95).

TENS is potentially useful for any type of pain including that of nociceptive, neuropathic, and musculoskeletal origins (Table 12.2). Clinical experience suggests it provides long-term benefit for low back pain (LBP), osteoarthritis (OA), localized muscle pain, and neuropathic pains of peripheral origin such as postherpetic and trigeminal neuralgias, amputee pain, entrapment neuropathies, and radiculopathies (Barlas & Lundeberg 2006). TENS may also benefit metastatic bone disease, nerve compression by a neoplasm, and post-mastectomy and post-thoracotomy pains (Berkovitch & Waller 2005).

Timing and dosage

TENS is ideal when treatment needs to be dynamic as effects are usually rapid in onset and offset, and are maximal during stimulation. Electrodes are left in situ and TENS may be administered intermittently throughout the day on an as-needed basis. Patients can leave TENS switched on for long periods of time and should increase intensity for breakthrough or incident pain. It should be administered before pain becomes moderate or severe but skin hygiene is essential as minor skin irritation under electrodes may occur.

Electrode location

TENS should be delivered over healthy sensate skin; therefore skin sensitivity testing should be undertaken at the site of electrode placement. Electrodes are positioned at dermatomes related to the site of pain for conventional TENS. As TENS activates nerve fibres directly beneath the electrodes the primary site for electrodes is around the

Table 12.2 Clinical Indications

Pain	Chronic pain
Postoperative pain	Osteoarthritis, rheumatoid arthritis, low back pain
Labour pain	Neuropathic pain including amputee pain, postherpetic and trigeminal neuralgias, post-stroke pain, complex regional pain syndrome
Dysmenorrhoea	Localized muscle pain including muscle tension, myofascial pain, post-exercise soreness
Angina pectoris	Nociceptive pain including inflammatory pains and chronic wound pain
Orofacial pain	Cancer-related pain
Physical trauma including fractured ribs and minor medical procedures	Acute pain

site of pain (Fig. 12.6), or positioned paravertebrally at the appropriate spinal segment or on contralateral dermatomes. If it is not possible to site electrodes close to the pain because of hypersensitivity or skin damage (e.g. open wound, eczema), then electrodes should be positioned on nerves proximal to the pain. TENS may aggravate pain if electrodes are placed on skin with tactile allodynia.

TENS on acupuncture points

The use of TENS to supplement acupuncture analgesia over specific points, such as trigger and acupuncture points, is done sparingly within clinical application. A common misconception is that AL-TENS must be delivered at acupuncture points, which is not the case, but it may be effective. A review of research on TENS and acupuncture points concluded that it may be useful when given over acupuncture points but there were few studies that compared TENS at acupuncture points versus TENS at the site of pain (Walsh 1996).

Transcutaneous electrical acupoint stimulators (TEAS) are watch-like devices worn on the underside of the wrist over the Pericardium 6 (P6) acupuncture point (Fig. 12.6). Good quality randomized controlled trials (RCTs) have found that TEAS reduced

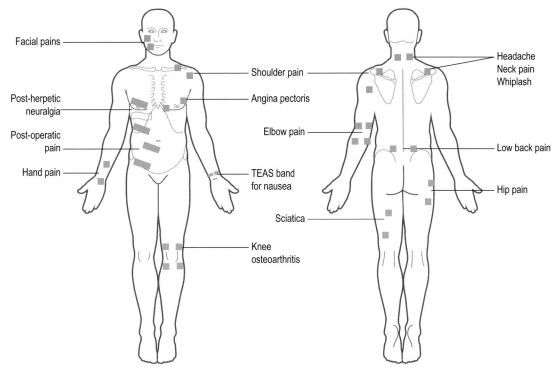

Figure 12.6 • Common sites for positioning electrodes during TENS

postoperative and chemotherapy-induced nausea and vomiting (Coloma et al 2002; Zarate et al 2001).

Electrical characteristics of TENS

The key determinant of TENS outcome is titration of the pulse amplitude to activate different nerve fibres (Table 12.1). For conventional TENS the user should titrate pulse amplitude to produce a strong, comfortable, non-painful paraesthesia beneath the electrodes. Practitioners should be cautious of claims about the best pulse frequencies, durations, and patterns for different pain conditions. A systematic review of studies investigating the effects of different pulse frequencies on experimental pain in healthy humans concluded that research to find optimal TENS settings for different conditions is confusing (Chen et al 2008) suggesting that the parameters may influence subjective comfort of paraesthesia rather than having clinically meaningful effects on TENS outcome (Johnson et al 1991a, b). For this reason, pulse frequency, pattern, and duration are selected by trial and error according to 'personal comfort' for the pain at that time. Patients are encouraged to experiment with settings within and

between treatments whilst maintaining a strong but comfortable intensity.

Research evidence

Mechanism of action

TENS causes antridromic activation of peripheral nerves so that impulses travelling away from the central nervous system will collide and extinguish afferent impulses arising from peripheral receptors. This may lead to peripheral blockade of impulses arising from tissue damage (Fig. 12.5).

Animal studies show that conventional TENS inhibits central transmission of nociceptive information in the spinal cord when applied to somatic receptive fields (Garrison & Foreman 1994, 1996; Leem et al 1995). The inhibitory neurotransmitter gamma-amino butyric acid (GABA) appears to be critical for conventional TENS effects (Duggan & Foong 1985; Maeda et al 2007). It has also been shown to reduce inflammation-induced sensitization of dorsal horn neurons in anaesthetized rats (Ma & Sluka 2001).

Higher intensities, e.g. AL-TENS, act via extrasegmental mechanisms and activate structures on the descending pain inhibitory pathways (e.g. periaqueductal grey and ventromedial medulla) and inhibit structures on descending pain facilitatory pathways (Ainsworth et al 2006; Chung et al 1984a, b). Higher intensities cause long-term depression of central nociceptor cells for up to 2 hours post stimulation (Sandkühler et al 1997, 2000). Activation of deep tissue peripheral afferents appears to produce largest effects (Duranti et al 1988; Radhakrishnan & Sluka 2005). Brief, intense, painful TENS probably elicits counterirritant mechanisms via diffuse noxious inhibitory controls (Le Bars et al 1979).

Recent research has shown low-frequency TENS to involve mu opioid receptors and high-frequency TENS to involve delta opioid receptors (Kalra et al 2001; Sluka et al 1999, 2000). Cholinergic, adrenergic, and serotinergic systems also seem to be involved (King et al 2005; Radhakrishnan et al 2003; Sluka & Chandran 2002).

Clinical effectiveness

There are over 500 RCTs cited in PubMed (10 September 2009) but many have methodological shortcomings due to inappropriate technique and/or under dosing. Systematic reviews of clinical research for acute pain have been inconclusive for a mix of acute pain conditions (Walsh et al 2009), positive for primary dysmenorrhoea (Proctor et al 2003) and negative for labour pain (Carroll et al 1997; Dowswell et al 2009) and postoperative pain (Carroll et al 1996). However, a systematic review of 21 RCTs on TENS for postoperative pain revealed shortcomings in RCTs that may have contributed to negative findings (Bjordal et al 2003). The meta-analysis demonstrated TENS reduced analgesic consumption during postoperative care, provided it was administered using a strong, sub-noxious electrical stimulation at the site of pain.

Systematic reviews for chronic pain are often inconclusive (Nnoaham and Kumbang 2008; Khadilkar et al 2005) although authors are often positive about TENS effects. It may be of benefit for, knee OA (Osiri et al 2000; Bjordal et al 2008), rheumatoid arthritis of the hand (Brosseau et al 2003), post-stroke shoulder pain (Price & Pandyan 2000), whiplash, mechanical neck disorders (Kroeling et al 2005), and chronic recurrent headache (Bronfort et al 2004). A meta-analysis of 38 studies on TENS and peripheral electrical nerve stimulation (PENS) for chronic musculoskeletal pain reported significant decreases in pain at rest and on movement (Johnson & Martinson 2007). There is insufficient evidence to judge the effects of TENS for cancer pain (Robb et al 2009)

   ## Case Study 1

Anonymous

Introduction

Complex regional pain syndrome type 1 (CRPS 1) was previously classified as reflex sympathetic dystrophy (RSD) (Evans 1946) and refers to a functional disorder of the spinal cord that involves the dorsal and ventral horns, and the intermediolateral columns, to varying degrees so as to produce sensory, motor, and autonomic abnormalities (Loeser 2005; Wilson et al 2005a). Type I CRPS is distinguished from type II solely by the presence or absence of a clinically detectable injury or nerve involvement. The condition is a form of neuropathic pain, but not all neuropathic pain are caused by CRPS and not all neuropathies lead to presentations of this type (Loeser 2005). The symptoms of CRPS 1 may be caused by an injury or by spontaneous events, manifesting via pain and sensory changes disproportionate in intensity, distribution, and duration to the underlying pathology (Dunn 2000). Additional dysfunctional features may involve motor changes, autonomic changes, trophic changes, and psychological dysfunction.

CRPS 1 is now regarded as a systemic condition involving the entire neuroaxis with manifestations of inflammatory changes at the central and peripheral nerve levels. It is a syndrome that represents a spectrum of changes involving a myriad of multiple systems including neurogenic both peripheral (PNS) and central nervous systems (CNS); endocrine; vascular; musculoskeletal; and biopsychosocial (Wilson et al 2005b). The condition appears to have a cyclical presentation, with recurrences of symptoms after dormant periods ranging from 6 months to 2 years; recurrent episodes are reported as occurring in 10 to 30% of patients diagnosed with the condition (Dunn 2000).

Current evidence is far from conclusive and a wide variety of causative mechanisms have been described (van Griensven 2005), with generalized sensory and motor changes not explained by the peripheral innervation (Rommel et al 1999) and even altered brain responses (Juottonen et al 2002). There appears to be no evidence of CRPS as a psychogenic condition, merely

(Continued)

Case Study 1 (Continued)

anxiety and stress linked to the physical presentation alongside sympathetic dysfunction (Covington 1996). With this in mind, many treatment approaches have been tried, but there is almost no reliable evidence of genuine efficacy (Bengtson 1997). Early treatment, pain modulation, and functional rehabilitation are essential, together with a respectful approach to a highly sensitized CNS and PNS; each treatment must be judged on individual merits for each patient. The emphasis must lie with the functional restoration or improvement of the affected area. If untreated, CRPS 1 will progress through acute, subacute (dystrophic), and finally, atrophic phases. Each stage results in progressively greater dysfunction and disability, with a diminishing chance of successful resolution (Keller et al 1996).

The IASP renamed both types with their present nomenclature in 1995. The IASP has agreed on four diagnostic criteria for CRPS 1, the last three of which must be present to confirm the diagnosis:

- The presence of an initiating noxious event or a cause for immobilization;
- Continuing pain, allodynia, or hyperalgesia, which is disproportionate to any inciting event;
- Evidence of oedema, changes in skin blood flow, or abnormal sudomotor activity in the region of pain; and
- The exclusion of other pathology that would otherwise account for the degree of pain and dysfunction.

With such a myriad of complex and debilitating symptoms it is not surprising that physiotherapy provides the mainstay of treatment of CRPS 1. If left unrecognized and therefore untreated, atrophy, contracture, and irreversible disablement can lead to despondency, depression, and, in rare cases, amputation. The treatment of CRPS still engenders much controversy because by its very nature no single treatment produces predictable results in every patient. Each treatment programme must be individually tailored to the specific symptoms and the personality of the patient. It is precisely because pain in these patients is so pronounced and intractable that gentle handling is essential.

Subject's history

The subject was a male, aged 49 years, who sustained a complex fracture to his left distal radius after falling downstairs. X-rays detected a fracture of the left wrist, and 2 days later he had an open surgical reduction with internal fixation and bone grafting of the fractured ulna; postoperatively he was placed in a plaster cast in which he remained for 6 weeks. The subject presented 1 week after the plaster was removed, having returned to work as a project manager in the construction industry, but he was experiencing problems with all aspects of daily living and work.

The subject described his pain as sharp, deep, and burning, affecting most of his wrist and hand, particularly over the operation scars and in the interphalangeal (IP) joints of his fingers over the radial aspect. The visual analogue scale (VAS) was reported as 80.5/100 on any activities involving the use of his hand. Changes in temperature aggravated his pain, especially cold weather. The subject reported no sleep disturbance, although his wrist and fingers were stiff and painful in the morning.

Objective examination

The following objectives signs were demonstrated:
- Swelling and oedema of the hand.
- Trophic skin changes which was dry and flaky.
- Active wrist movements were greatly limited by pain and stiffness, particularly extension was only 10°. flexion to 30°; and supination was so minimal it was too difficult to measure accurately.
- Extension at the interphalangeal joint (IPJ) and metacarpophalangeal joints (MPJ) were full, but flexion was severely restricted, measured at 70 mm from the palm.
- There were sensory changes to light touch to which he was hypersensitive, particularly on his fingertips; and
- Passive accessory movements were not examined because of severe pain.

From the subjective history and objective examination it was concluded that the patient's problems were:
- Pain, severe and debilitating in nature;
- Oedema;
- Decreased range of movement (ROM);
- Altered sensation; and
- Decreased function.

Treatment

Initial treatment consisted of:
- An explanation of CRPS 1;
- A full explanation of the need for exercise, desensitization, and pacing; and
- Restoration of full functional independence.

The subject was instructed into the use of contrast baths and self-massage; desensitization of the skin with different textures; and gentle active wrist and finger exercises. During the next four treatments, with increased handling and some gentle accessory glides to the wrist and IPJ, he reported a definite improvement in pain levels and light functional use; the subject felt generally more comfortable, but ROM demonstrated little improvement.

The patient returned to see the consultant who confirmed the diagnosis of CRPS 1 and also brought up the possibility that, having viewed recent X-rays, perhaps

(Continued)

Case Study 1 (Continued)

some of the internal fixating metalwork could be acting to block wrist extension.

A change in treatment was indicated as progress had plateaued and more active pain inhibitory mechanisms were required to facilitate restoration of function. As wrist hypersensitivity remained the overwhelming problem, acupuncture was considered too invasive into an already sensitized sympathetic nervous system (SNS); the skin texture and circulatory quality of the limb were not sufficiently robust to tolerate needling into the area.

TENS using AL-TENS at 4 Hz was administered to Large Intestine 4 (LI4) bilaterally, LI10, and LI11 on the left arm. This treatment was administered in the clinic and the subject asked to use it at home for two periods of 30 minutes, twice daily whilst all the normal physiotherapy rehabilitation activities were continued.

At treatment three further use of conventional TENS current was applied to the extra Baxie acupuncture points between the second and third, third and fourth, and fourth and fifth metacarpal heads found proximal to the folds between the fingers (Hecker et al 2001). Again, the patient was instructed to use this as a daily home treatment whilst passive, active, and accessory joint mobility was undertaken during the physiotherapy intervention.

Outcome

After the first TENS treatment the subject complained of aching and soreness in his hand which was different in nature from his presenting pain and eased the following day; the VAS was now 40/100, increasing to a 70/100 after mobilizations and stretches but settling after treatment. Active ROM had also improved: wrist extension was now 25°; supination was 70°, but difficult to maintain. The hand appearance has been the most dramatic improvement, with resolution of oedema over the dorsum of the hand and wrist; there was no longer a general shiny appearance to the hand or increased sweating, and the hypersensitivity in the fingertips had resolved. There is unfortunately the appearance of fixed flexion contractures in the distal IPJ of the little and ring fingers; these digits remain very stiff and lacked full ROM. Functionally there has been great improvement and the subject has returned to driving, although this involved changing gear, which remained awkward.

Clinical reasoning

It is clear from both the subjective and objective findings of the initial and subsequent examination that this patient demonstrated CRPS 1 according to the recognized signs and symptoms described in the literature (Janig et al 1991; Koman et al 1999; Mitchell et al 1864). The subject demonstrated classic hyperaesthesia, allodynia, and vasomotor and labile sudomotor changes.

Research into the effect of TENS on the nervous system is well recognized (Johnson et al 1991b; King et al 2005) and the analgesic effect produced by the secretion of endorphins, enkephalins, dynorphin, serotonin, and adrenaline as a result of TENS will enhance descending inhibitory control (Johnson 1998).

After the first two treatments, the treatment was extended to include acupuncture points as the hand sensitivity had reduced and the subject was now able to tolerate enhanced exercise and practitioner handling of the affected limb. The non-meridian, extra, Baxie points were used in between the metacarpal heads of the index, middle, and ring fingers in the contralateral limb, chosen for their action of alleviating pain, stiffness, and swelling in the hand (Hecker 2008). The He-Sea points, Pericardium 3 (PC3), Lung 5 (LU5), and LI11 were used on the affected side to increase the circulation and Qi flow to the hand and forearm. The extra point Yintang was added to help with relaxation and induce sleep.

Reflective practice

One limitation of this single case study is the use of other physiotherapy modalities alongside that of TENS; mobilizations, exercises, and gentle massage, along with an extensive home exercise programme were all used concurrently. The improvement in the symptoms and objective measurements cannot be solely attributed to the application of one modality.

The choice of acupuncture points appeared appropriate for the condition but perhaps bilateral application of LI4, into the affected tissue may have added to the sensitization but it appeared to be well tolerated by the subject. It would have been interesting to have the opportunity to continue with a progression of active acupuncture treatments for the stiffness in the ring and little fingers, but unfortunately time constraints prevented this progression from taking place.

Conclusion

CRPS 1 is a multifactorial condition that requires clear diagnosis and an individually tailored treatment plan. No two cases will respond in the same way; this case study demonstrated the successful integration of TENS and acupuncture into a complex management programme, as a means of facilitating greater pain modulation, empowering the subject in a home management programme, and providing a cost-effective means of managing a very complex, long-term condition.

(Continued)

Case Study 2

Matthew Walmsley

Introduction

This case study presents a 78-year-old male with acute on chronic cervical (Cx) and associated right arm pain. After an episode of chronic pain in 1996, he underwent a Cx laminectomy at the levels of C4 to C7 inclusively and following his operation the pain resolved. He subsequently received no physiotherapeutic follow-up. During 2008, he experienced an acute onset of Cx pain following a rotation of his Cx spine whilst sitting. Pain was initially centralized in his Cx spine, then peripheralized, developing clawing and weakness in his right arm and hand following an ulnar nerve distribution. During initial assessment this patient had severe functional difficulties. He presented with a pain-evoked Cx block into right rotation and side flexion, limiting his movement to approximately 50 and 30%, respectively, compared to the opposite side. He had associated ulna nerve pain with affected C7 to T1 myotomes and dermatomes on his right. Manual therapy commenced with exercise and taping and after three sessions of physiotherapy he reported some level of satisfaction in terms of pain resolution; however he still had moderate pain and some functional limitations.

Following initial assessment, the priority was to reduce pain, then unload the nerve and gain increased movement at his Cx spine. Treatment included education, taping, electroacupuncture (EA), and progressive Cx stabilization exercises. After 8 sessions of the above treatment over a period of 2 months, the patient reported an 85% improvement in pain and a 75% improvement in functional capacity. Moreover, clawing of his right hand was completely eradicated and he was able to complete all functional rehabilitation.

During the next five physiotherapy treatments acupuncture was used to reduce pain further and help stimulate nerve growth and effectiveness of C7 to T1 myotomes. Following these sessions the patient's strength in his right hand became similar to his left and functional tasks were now manageable.

Subjective and objective examinations

The locations of symptoms, with frequency and intensity, are summarized on the body chart in Fig. 12.7.

The objective assessment is summarized in Table 12.3.

Clinical reasoning and underlying mechanisms

Considering this patient's previous surgery and the aggravating factors it is likely that he has had a degree of ulnar nerve damage. Therefore, the most likely pain presentation is mechanism with a peripheral neuropathic component, together with some nociceptive pain owing to local tissue trauma. Neuropathic pain (NP) is initiated by nervous system damage or dysfunction. It is often difficult to manage due to a complex history with diverse causes and it is often difficult to identify a specific cause of NP; symptoms can include perceived temperature changes, weakness, radiating pain, pins and needles, numbness, and changes in skin condition (Colvin et al 2000; NICE 2008). Axons within the ulnar nerve may have been damaged; therefore early intervention is imperative in order to create the best environment for axonal healing to help resolve and prevent further problems (Colvin et al 2000).

Since the onset of pain, the subject had become increasingly frustrated and was struggling to sleep. He had commenced on a low dose of Amitriptylin to help decrease pain, improve his low mood, and improve sleep quality (Gilron 2006). Sleep is an important aspect of self-healing, since during sleep hormones are released that boost the immune system and promote self-healing (Moldofsky 1995). However, the physiological functions of sleep are partly unknown (Kryger et al 1994; Parmeggiani 1994). Lack of sleep may lead to lower pain threshold, centrally sensitising this subject to the neural injury (Moldofsky et al 1975). As he had experienced insomnia for the past 4 weeks, his pain threshold would have been significantly reduced, increasing his NP and further reducing his mood and ability to cope. Taking this in to account, reducing this subject's NP and insomnia would help resolve his problems.

Treatment selection

During the first two sessions of physiotherapy attention was paid to offloading the ulnar nerve, together with positions of comfort for the Cx to decrease the subject's acute pain (Wheeless 2009). By the third session, acupuncture was considered for reduction of insomnia and pain and facilitate to improvement in function. In this case, it was hypothesized that damage to the neural tissue had taken place in the ulnar nerve, resulting in a short onset of afferent impulses, termed injury discharge which has been linked to the onset of NP (Kryger et al 1994).

Many studies have been completed using acupuncture for the treatment of NP, with varied results and many conclude that traditional acupuncture, using meridian points, is much more beneficial when treating nociceptive pain rather than neuropathic pain (Bradnam 2003; Budh et al 2006). This is thought to be due to a difference in neuropeptides needed during pain modulation (Han 2003). However, many studies have found EA to be an effective analgesic and a good treatment for NP, without any observed negative side effects (Stener-Victorin et al 1999). EA has been demonstrated to activate inhibitory systems within the spinal cord, which results in segmental inhibition of the sympathetic outflow (Sato et al 1997) and pain pathways, as predicted by the gate control theory (Melzack & Wall 1965). In this instance the C7 to T1 segments could be

(Continued)

Case Study 2 (Continued)

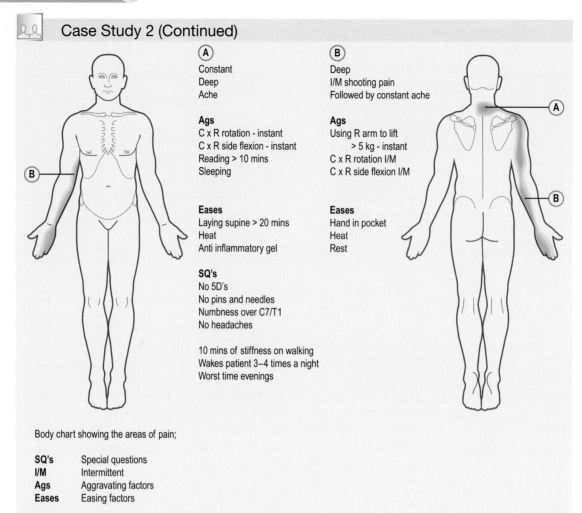

A
Constant
Deep
Ache

Ags
C x R rotation - instant
C x R side flexion - instant
Reading > 10 mins
Sleeping

Eases
Laying supine > 20 mins
Heat
Anti inflammatory gel

SQ's
No 5D's
No pins and needles
Numbness over C7/T1
No headaches

10 mins of stiffness on walking
Wakes patient 3–4 times a night
Worst time evenings

B
Deep
I/M shooting pain
Followed by constant ache

Ags
Using R arm to lift
    > 5 kg - instant
C x R rotation I/M
C x R side flexion I/M

Eases
Hand in pocket
Heat
Rest

Body chart showing the areas of pain;

SQ's	Special questions
I/M	Intermittent
Ags	Aggravating factors
Eases	Easing factors

Figure 12.7 • Symptom location.

utilized by relevant, adjacent acupuncture points in order to decrease localized pain, whilst other points may be utilized to give the patient systemic relief.

Stener-Victorin (2003) used a combination of high- and low-frequency (80 and 2 Hz, respectively) EA, and found it lowered pain experienced by 24%, compared to the control, using acupuncture points Governor Vessel 20 (GV20) and Stomach 29 (ST29) at 80 Hz; Triple Energizer 5 (TE5) and LI4 at 2 Hz; and ST36 with manual stimulation. This identical study design was carried out (Taguchi 2007) with a variation on point selection; however, they found no statistical difference between the two groups. These two studies identified 11 and 8% reductions in anaesthetic requirement when using EA at auricular points, respectively (Taguchi 2007). In contrast, Morioka et al (2002) and Stener-Victorin et al (2003) stimulated three acupoints ST36, GB34, and Bladder 60 (BL60), failing to reduce anaesthetic need.

Nedstrand et al (2005), using acupuncture in an attempt to reduce hormonal symptoms in women, found a decreased generalized pain threshold by using EA. The points used were BL15, BL23, BL32, Heart 7 (H7), Spleen 6 (SP6) and SP9, LIV3, PC6, and GV20. The choice of acupuncture points demonstrated no significant decrease in pain scales that had been found in previous studies during treatment of dysmenorrhoea. Within all studies reviewed, there was no consistency of points used; there was, however, a general consensus about the use and the amount of stimulation to use for NP relief. High frequency (100 Hz) was seen to be better than low frequency (2 Hz) at reducing pain (Han et al 1999; Liang et al 2002; Morioka et al 2002).

Recent studies showed that EA in specific frequencies applied to certain points could facilitate the release of neuropeptides, eliciting profound physiological effects, activating self-healing mechanisms (Han 2004).

(Continued)

Case Study 2 (Continued)

Table 12.3 Objective assessment baseline measurements

Observation	Right trapezius lengthened No muscle bulk loss Protracted Cx and rounded shoulders Kyphotic at Tx spine
Palpation	Tenderness over whole Cx spine, worse over R facets between C3 and C7
AROM	Right side flexion = ⅓ Right shoulder full ROM Right rotation = ½ Pain on all movements ROM blocked by pain No active movement of middle, ring, and small No end-feel gained. fingers on right
Neural function	No absence of triceps reflex No absence of coracobrachialis and or biceps reflex Diminished RC7 to T1 dermatome and myotome sensation
Functional tests	Instant pain on picking up anything heavier than 5 kg with R hand
Muscle tests	Unable to assess Cx spine due to pain All GHJ muscles at R and L full power R hand myotomal weakness in C7 to T1
Special tests	Repeated flexion and extension of Cx spine increased pain Combined movements of Cx spine into R rotation, R side flexion and extension increased both A and B pain Upper limb tension test (ULTT) 3 positive on R
Investigations	Nil since X-ray following laminectomy 1997 No MRI
Medications	Anti-inflammatory gel, atenolol, ramipril, and lansoprazole
Hobbies	Before injury; walking, looking after grandchildren, and reading

Notes: ULTT, upper limb tension test; Tx, thoracic spine; Cx, cervical spine; R, Right; L, Left.

At different frequencies, different neuropeptides are released; these are most commonly dynorphin and enkephalin (Han 2003). Using EA at 2 Hz accelerates the release of enkephalin, whilst that of 100 Hz increases the release of dynorphin (Han 2003). However, a combination of the two frequencies produces a simultaneous release of both, resulting in a maximal therapeutic effect (Han 2004). This result was in direct contrast with the hypothesis summarized by Verge et al (1991) that central neuropeptides can be released only by high-frequency stimulation. It is therefore hypothesized that a combination of 2- and 100-Hz EA, applied in unison, will result in two sites of stimulation, which become merged and are perceived as 102 Hz, almost indistinguishable from 100 Hz. As a result, only dynorphin will be released (Han 2004).

In addition to decreasing pain, EA was found to improve physical activity, sense of well being, and quality of sleep, whilst reducing the need for medication (Hamza 2000). Hamza (2000) found that using frequencies of 15 and 30 Hz, repeated every 3 seconds, and using 0 Hz for the sham treatments, respectively, the EA group reported needing significantly less medication than the sham group, which remained the same. Although this study had some good findings, the acupuncture points used were not disclosed.

There is also some evidence that EA can be beneficial in treating insomnia (Hamza et al 2000; Spence et al 2004). Spence et al (2004) found that 10 sessions of acupuncture could produce significant improvement in sleep quality; however, this study failed to mention the points used. With decreased sleep, an increase in nociceptive substances such as substance P, bradykinin, histamine, and prostaglandins would be released; this would lead to greater central sensitization and reduce the subject's peripheral pain threshold, leading to a further reduction in deep sleep (Ishimaru et al 1995; Kitade et al 1979; Taguchi 2007).

(Continued)

Case Study 2 (Continued)

Outcome measurements and results

Outcome measures were active Cx right rotation and side flexion measured with a cervical goniometer. Subjective information including pain and uninterrupted sleep were measured with the VAS scale and patient records, respectively. Table 12.4 gives an overview of the points used and Table 12.5 summarizes the outcome measures recorded in all physiotherapy sessions that included acupuncture treatment. Following this treatment the patient reported decrease in both pain and improved sleep.

Limitations

Undoubtedly, there are some limitations; the subject is undergoing a natural healing process, and therefore it is difficult to ascertain how much EA had improved

Table 12.4 Acupuncture point rationale

Session	Aim	Points used	De Qi	Rationale	Time/frequency
1	Familiarize patient to acupuncture and gain general well being and improved sleep	LI4 + LIV3^B Extra point Yintang	√ √ √	Four gaits used for general anaesthesia. Ying tang for sleep.	20 mins De Qi gained again @ 10 mins
2	Encourage neural regeneration and decrease pain. Plus improve sleep	LI4 + LIV3^B GB10^B BL10^B BL11^B EA 80 Hz	√ √ √ √ √ √ √ √	Segmental approach for anaesthesia (BL11) HFEA to stimulate opioid release.	30 mins 80 Hz pulsed @ 2-s intervals. De Qi gained 10 mins at manual points
3	Encourage neural regeneration and decrease pain. Plus improve sleep	LI4 + LIV3^B GB10^B BL10^B BL11^B EA 80Hz HJJ 80Hz GV14	√ √ √ √ √ √ √ √ √ √ √	Expand on segmental anaesthesia (HJJ and GV) using HFEA and LFEA to stimulate dorsal horn effect	30 mins 80 Hz and 2 Hz separately pulsed @ 2-s intervals. De Qi gained 10 mins @ manual points
4	Encourage neural regeneration and decrease pain. Plus improve sleep	LI4 + LIV3^B GB10 ^{B} BL10^B BL11^B EA 80Hz HJJ 100Hz GV14 LI11^R LI15^R	√ √ √ √ √ √ √ √ √ √ √ √ √√ √	As above plus adding points on the LI meridian as it passes over the affected myotome.	30 mins 100 and 2 Hz separately pulsed @ 2-s intervals. De Qi gained 10 mins @ manual points
5	Encourage neural regeneration and decrease pain. Plus improve sleep	LI4 + LIV3^B GB10^B BL10^B BL11^B EA 80Hz HJJ 100Hz GV14 LI11^R LI15^R	√ √ √ √ √ √ √ √ √ √ √ √ √ √	As above.	30 mins 100 and 2 Hz separately pulsed @ 2-s intervals. De Qi gained 10 mins @ manual points

Notes: B, Bilateral; R, Right; L, Left; GB, Gall Bladder; BL, Bladder; LIV, Liver; GV, Governor Vessel; LI, Large Intestine; HJJ, Huatuojiaji points; EA, Electroacupuncture; HFEA, high-frequency, electroacupuncture; LFEA, low-frequency, electroacupuncture.

(Continued)

Case Study 2 (Continued)

Table 12.5 Outcome measurements

Day	Power/grip strength	Pain VAS	Cx ROM	C7/T1 myotomal function Oxford Scale	Sleep
1	0.3 kg	80/100	R rotation 50% R side flexion 30%	Full active elbow extension, nil finger abduction and or wrist flexion	5.6
8	0.5 kg	71/100	R rotation 50% R side flexion 50%	Full active elbow extension, 0/5 finger abduction and 2/5 wrist flexion	6.7
22	1 kg	71/100	R rotation 60% R side flexion 65%	Full active elbow extension, 3/5 finger abduction and 3/5 wrist flexion	6.5
29	3 kg	50/100	R rotation 60% R side flexion 70%	Full active elbow extension, 3/5 finger abduction and 3/5 wrist flexion	7
36	5 kg	14/100	R rotation 80% R side flexion 85%	Full active elbow extension, 4/5 finger abduction and 5/5 wrist flexion	7.2

Notes: Power/grip, tested with a grip dynamometer; ROM, compared to L with a Cervical Goniometer; Sleep, average hours per night.

symptoms. Secondly, the measure of the amount of sleep was very subjective and did not address quality of sleep; a more specific questionnaire could have been used to determine well being, tiredness, energy, and mood (Hamza 2000). Finally, the acupuncture protocol used in this study was not previously validated, as no study has fully concluded specific points and or frequencies of EA to use in the treatment of NP.

Discussion

This case study attempted to analyse the use of EA and physiotherapeutic interventions on NP. Although acupuncture is not commonly recognized for treating such conditions, it was considered in this case, as it was coupled with other interventions to help treat the subject's pain, insomnia, and reduced motor function.

During the first 3 sessions of physiotherapy the patient made very limited improvement and EA was considered in conjunction with the exercises regime. Following 5 treatments of EA, outcome measurements all improved significantly. Pain levels reduced from 92/100 to14/100 (VAS), Cx ROM in right side flexion improved from 30 to 80%, and the average amount of sleep improved from 5.6 to 7.2 hours per night.

According to traditional Chinese medicine, the 'four gates', LI4 and LIV3 (Liang et al 2002) combined with a segmental approach at C7 to T1, exhibit a powerful analgesic effect (Han 2003) whilst the extra point Ying Tang and EA in general can improve sleep (Hamza 2000).

Many theories can be considered to explain the positive outcomes regarding pain relief. Manual acupuncture given to healthy volunteers, at acupuncture points LI4 and LIV3 has been shown to deactivate areas in the brain that regulate pain modulation (Yan et al 2005). Acupuncture has been shown to be much more effective when used with low-frequency EA, stimulating the dorsal horn and giving longer lasting relief (Mo et al 1996; Han 2003 Hamza 2000). This effect is further enhanced when alternated with high-frequency EA at segmental levels, in order to offer an overall global analgesia (Hamza 2000; Morioka et al 2002; Han 2003).

Two studies demonstrated the improvement in sleep with the use of EA (Hamza 2000; Nedstrand et al 2005). Although the results of both of these studies appeared conclusive, different acupuncture points were used and no relationships were formed with biochemical changes at cellular level. Many authors consider this effect to be psychological and may even be due to acupuncture intervention facilitating increased time to rest whilst the treatment is taking place (Renckens 2002; Spiller 2007).

Considering the above, it appears that specific molecular and chemical factors account for acupuncture-induced pain modulation. However, it is impossible to discount the power of suggestion associated with expectancy and belief for pain reduction (Pariente et al 2005). In some patient interactions this could play a significant role, as human pain modulating areas have been found to be activated in both conditions, starting a chemical process that enabled the release of neuropeptides crucial for the relief of pain (Han 2003, 2004). Therefore, it is impossible to be definitive concerning the specific and non-specific factors in facilitating decrease in the subject's pain, increase in motor function, and improvement in sleep.

(Continued)

Case Study 2 (Continued)

Conclusion

In conclusion, integration of manual therapy and EA for this subject demonstrated good results. Initially the advice and exercises approach helped to increase and normalize movement, gain increased stability, and desensitize the CNS. Later, EA was effective in producing systemic and segmental analgesia, decreasing right arm pain, and improving neural growth, function, and strength. Furthermore, average hours of sleep increased with the use of EA; however, further studies are needed to determine the exact effect of EA on the neuronal structures.

References

Ainsworth, L., Budelier, K., Clinesmith, M., et al., 2006. Transcutaneous electrical nerve stimulation (TENS) reduces chronic hyperalgesia induced by muscle inflammation. Pain 120, 182–187.

Barlas, P., Lundeberg, T., 2006. Transcutaneous electrical nerve stimulation and acupuncture. In: McMahon, S., Koltzenburg, M. (Eds.), Melzack and Wall's Textbook of Pain. Elsevier Churchill Livingstone, Philadelphia, pp. 583–590.

Bengtson, K., 1997. Physical modalities for complex regional pain syndrome. Hand Clin. 13 (3), 453–454.

Berkovitch, M., Waller, A., et al., 2005. Treating pain with transcutaneous electrical nerve stimulation (TENS). In: Doyle, D., Hanks, G., Cherny, N.I. (Eds.), Oxford Textbook of Palliative Medicine. Oxford University Press, Oxford, pp. 405–410.

Bjordal, J.M., Johnson, M.I., Ljunggreen, A.E., 2003. Transcutaneous electrical nerve stimulation (TENS) can reduce postoperative analgesic consumption A meta-analysis with assessment of optimal treatment parameters for postoperative pain. European Journal of Pain 7, 181–188.

Bjordal, J.M., Johnson, M.I., Lopes-Martins, R.A., Bogen, B., Chow, R., Ljunggren, A.E., 2007. Short-term efficacy of physical interventions in osteoarthritic knee pain. A systematic review and meta-analysis of randomised placebocontrolled trials. BMC Musculoskelet Disord 8, 51.

Bradnam, L., 2003. A proposed clinical reasoning model for Western acupuncture. NZ J. Physiother. 31, 40–45.

Bronfort, G., Nilsson, N., Haas, M., et al., 2004. Non-invasive physical treatments for chronic/recurrent headache. Cochrane Database Syst. Rev., CD001878.

Brosseau, L., Judd, M.G., Marchand, S., et al., 2003. Transcutaneous electrical nerve stimulation (TENS) for the treatment of rheumatoid arthritis in the hand. Cochrane Database Syst. Rev., CD004377.

Budh, C., Kowalski, J., Lundeberg, T., 2006. A comprehensive pain management programme comprising education, cognitive and behavioural interventions for neuropathic pain following spinal cord injury. J. Rehabil. Med. 38 (3), 172–180.

Carroll, D., Tramer, M., McQuay, H., et al., 1996. Randomization is important in studies with pain outcomes: systematic review of transcutaneous electrical nerve stimulation in acute postoperative pain. Br. J. Anaesth. 77, 798–803.

Carroll, D., Moore, A., Tramer, M., et al., 1997. Transcutaneous electrical nerve stimulation does not relieve in labour pain: updated systematic review. Contemp. Rev. Obstet. Gynaecol. (September), 195–205.

Charlton, J., 2005. Core Curriculum for Professional Education in Pain, third ed. IASP Press, Seattle pp 93–96.

Chartered Society of Physiotherapy (CSP), 2006. Guidance for the clinical use of electrophysical agents.

Chen, C.C., Tabasam, G., Johnson, M.I., 2008. Does the pulse frequency of transcutaneous electrical nerve stimulation (TENS) influence hypoalgesia? A systematic review of studies using experimental pain and healthy human participants. Physiotherapy 94 (1), 11–20.

Chung, J.M., Fang, Z.R., Hori, Y., et al., 1984a. Prolonged inhibition of primate spinothalamic tract cells by peripheral nerve stimulation. Pain 19, 259–275.

Chung, J.M., Lee, K.H., Hori, Y., et al., 1984b. Factors influencing peripheral nerve stimulation produced inhibition of primate spinothalamic tract cells. Pain 19, 277–293.

Coloma, M., White, P.F., Ogunnaike, B.O., et al., 2002. Comparison of acustimulation and ondansetron for the treatment of established postoperative nausea and vomiting. Anesthesiology 97, 1387–1392.

Colvin, L.A., 2000. Practical management of pain. Br. J. Anaesth. 101, 119–127.

Covington, E., 1996. Psychological issues in reflex sympathetic dystrophy. In: Stanton-Hicks, M., Janig, W. (Eds.), Reflex Sympathetic Dystrophy. IASP, Seattle.

Dowswell, T., Bedwell, C., Lavender, T., Neilson, J.P., 2009. Transcutaneous electrical nerve stimulation (TENS) for pain relief in labour. Cochrane Database Syst Rev (2) CD007214.

Duggan, A.W., Foong, F.W., 1985. Bicuculline and spinal inhibition produced by dorsal column stimulation in the cat. Pain 22, 249–259.

Dunn, D., 2000. Chronic regional pain syndrome, type 1: part 1. AORN J. 72 (3), 422–449.

Duranti, R., Pantaleo, T., Bellini, F., 1988. Increase in muscular pain threshold following low frequency-high intensity peripheral conditioning stimulation in humans. Brain Res. 452, 66–72.

Eriksson, M., Sjölund, B.H., 1976. Acupuncture-like electroanalgesia in TNS resistant chronic pain. In: Zotterman, Y. (Ed.), Sensory Functions of the Skin. Pergamon Press, Oxford/New York, pp. 575–581.

Evans, J., 1946. Reflex sympathetic dystrophy. Surg. Clin. North Am. 26, 780–790.

Garrison, D.W., Foreman, R.D., 1994. Decreased activity of spontaneous and noxiously evoked dorsal horn cells during transcutaneous electrical nerve stimulation (TENS). Pain 58, 309–315.

Garrison, D.W., Foreman, R.D., 1996. Effects of transcutaneous electrical nerve stimulation (TENS) on spontaneous and noxiously evoked dorsal horn cell activity in cats with transected spinal cords. Neurosci. Lett. 216, 125–128.

Gilron, I., Watson, C.P.N., Cahill, C.M., et al., 2006. Neuropathic pain: a practical guide for the clinician. Can. Med. Assoc. J. 175, 265–275.

Hamza, M., White, P., Craig, W., et al., 2000. Percutaneous electrical nerve stimulation. A novel analgesic therapy for diabetic neuropathic pain. Diabetes Care 23, 365–370.

Han, S.J., 2003. Acupuncture: neuropeptide release produced by electrical stimulation of different frequencies. Trends Neurosci. 26 (1), 145–149.

Han, S.J., 2004. Acupuncture and endorphins. Neurosci. Lett. 361, 258–261.

Han, Z., Jiang, Y.H., Wan, Y., et al., 1999. Endorphin-1 mediates 2 Hz but not 100Hz electroacupuncture analgesia in the rat. Neurosci. Lett. 274, 75–78.

Hecker, H.U., Steveling, A., Peuker, E., et al., 2001. Color Atlas of Acupuncture. Thieme Publishing, Stuttgart.

Hecker, H.U., Steveling, A., Peuker, E., et al., 2008. Color Atlas of Acupuncture Body Parts, Ear Points, Trigger Points. Thieme Publishing, Stuttgart.

Ishimaru, K., Kawakita, K., Sakita, M., 1995. Analgesic effects induced by TENS and electroacupuncture with different types of stimulating electrodes on deep tissues in human subjects. Pain 63, 181–187.

Janig, W., Blumberg, H., Boas, R.A., et al., 1991. Reflex sympathetic dystrophy syndrome. Consensus statement and general recommendations for diagnosis and clinical research. Pain Res. Clin. Manag. 4, 372–375.

Johnson, M.I., 1998. The analgesic effects and clinical use of acupuncture-like TENS (AL-TENS). Phys. Ther. Rev. 3, 73–93.

Johnson, M.I., 2001a. Transcutaneous electrical nerve stimulation (TENS) and TENS-like devices. Do they provide pain relief? Pain Rev. 8, 121–128.

Johnson, M.I., 2001b. A critical review of the analgesic effects of TENS-like devices. Phy. Ther. Rev. 6, 153–173.

Johnson, M., Martinson, M., 2007. Efficacy of electrical nerve stimulation for chronic musculoskeletal pain: a meta-analysis of randomized controlled trials. Pain 130, 157–165.

Johnson, M.I., Ashton, C.H., Thompson, J.W., 1991a. The consistency of pulse frequencies and pulse patterns of transcutaneous electrical nerve stimulation (TENS) used by chronic pain patients. Pain 44, 231–234.

Johnson, M.I., Ashton, C.H., Thompson, J.W., 1991b. An in-depth study of long-term users of transcutaneous electrical nerve stimulation (TENS) Implications for clinical use of TENS. Pain 44, 221–229.

Juottonen, K., Gockel, M., Silén, T., et al., 2002. Altered central sensorimotor processing in patients with complex regional pain syndrome. Pain 98 (3), 315–323.

Kalra, A., Urban, M.O., Sluka, K.A., 2001. Blockade of opioid receptors in rostral ventral medulla prevents antihyperalgesia produced by transcutaneous electrical nerve stimulation (TENS). J. Pharmacol. Exp. Ther. 298, 257–263.

Keller, T., Goldstein, L., Chappell, T., 1996. Gamekeepers thumb variant complicated by reflex sympathetic dystrophy. J. Trauma 40, 660–662.

Khadilkar, A., Milne, S., Brosseau, L., et al., 2005. Transcutaneous electrical nerve stimulation (TENS) for chronic low-back pain. Cochrane Database Syst. Rev., CD003008.

King, E.W., Audette, K., Athman, G.A., et al., 2005. Transcutaneous electrical nerve stimulation activates peripherally located alpha-2A adrenergic receptors. Pain 115, 364–373.

Kitade, T., Hyodo, M., 1979. The effects of stimulation of ear acupuncture points on the body's pain threshold. Am. J. Chin. Med. 7, 241–252.

Koman, L.A., Poehling, G.G., Smith, T.L., 1999. Complex regional pain syndrome: RSD and causalgia. In: Greens Operative Hand Surgery, 4th ed. Churchill Livingstone, Philadelphia.

Kroeling, P., Gross, A.R., Goldsmith, C.H., 2005. A Cochrane review of electrotherapy for mechanical neck disorders. Spine 30, 641–648.

Kryger, M.H., Roth, T., Carskadon, M., 1994. Circadian rhythms in humans: an overview. In: Kryger, M.H., Roth, T., Dement, W.C. (Eds.), Principles and Practice of Sleep Medicine. WB Saunders, Philadelphia, pp. 301–308.

Lander, J., Fowler-Kerry, S., 1993. TENS for children's procedural pain. Pain 52, 209–216.

Le Bars, D., Dickenson, A.H., Besson, J.M., 1979. Diffuse noxious inhibitory controls (DNIC). Effects on dorsal horn convergent neurones in the rat. Pain 6, 283–304.

Leem, J., Park, E., Paik, K., 1995. Electrophysiological evidence for the antinociceptive effect of transcutaneous electrical stimulation on mechanically evoked responsiveness of dorsal horn neurons in neuropathic rats. Neurosci. Lett. 192, 197–200.

Liang, X.B., Liu, X.Y., Li, F.Q., et al., 2002. Long-term high-frequency electro-acupuncture stimulation prevents neuronal degeneration and up-regulates BDNF mRNA in the substantia nigra and ventral tegmental area following medial forebrain bundle axotomy. Mol. Brain Res. 108, 51–59.

Loeser, J., 2005. Introduction to complex regional pain syndrome. In: Wilson, M., Stanton-Hicks, M., Harden, R. (Eds.), CRPS: Current Diagnosis and Therapy. IASP, Seattle, pp. 3A–7A.

Long, D.M., 1973. Electrical stimulation for relief of pain from chronic nerve injury. J. Neurosurg. 39, 718–722.

Ma, Y.T., Sluka, K.A., 2001. Reduction in inflammation-induced sensitization of dorsal horn neurons by transcutaneous electrical nerve stimulation in anesthetized rats. Exp. Brain Res. 137, 94–102.

Maeda, Y., Lisi, T.L., Vance, C.G., et al., 2007. Release of GABA and activation of GABA (A) in the spinal cord mediates the effects of TENS in rats. Brain Res. 1136, 43–50.

Mann, C., 1996. Respiratory compromise: a rare complication of transcutaneous electrical nerve stimulation for angina pectoris. Journal of Accident and Emergency Medicine 13, 68.

Marchand, S., Li, J., Charest, J., 1995. Effects of caffeine on analgesia from transcutaneous electrical nerve stimulation. N. Engl. J. Med. 333, 325–326.

Melzack, R., Wall, P., 1965. Pain mechanisms: a new theory. Science 150, 971–979.

Merkel, S.I., Gutstein, H.B., Malviya, S., 1999. Use of transcutaneous electrical nerve stimulation in a young child with pain from open perineal lesions. J. Pain. Symptom Manage. 18, 376–381.

Mitchell, S.W., Morhouse, G.R., Keen, W.W., 1864. Gunshot Wounds and Other Injuries of Nerves. Lippincott, Philadelphia.

Mo, X., Chen, D., Ji, C., et al., 1996. Effect of electroacupuncture and transcutaneous electric nerve stimulation on experimental diabetes and its neuropathy. Chen Tzu Yen Chiu 3, 55–59.

Moldofsky, H., 1995. Sleep, neuroimmune and neuroendonocrine functions in fibromyalgia and chronic fatigue syndrome. Adv. Neuroimmunol. 5, 39–56.

Moldofsky, H., Scarisbrick, P., England, R., et al., 1975. Musculoskeletal symptoms and non-REM sleep disturbance in patients with 'fibrositis syndrome' and healthy controls. Psychosom. Med. 37, 341–351.

Morioka, N., Akça, O., Doufas, A.G., et al., 2002. Electro-acupuncture at the Zusanli, Kanglingquan, and Kunlun points does not reduce anaesthetic requirement. Anaesthesiol. Analogue 95, 98–102.

National Institute of Clinical Excellence (NICE), 2008. Spinal cord stimulation for chronic pain of neuropathic or ischaemic origin.

Nedstrand, E., Wijma, K., Wyon, Y., et al., 2005. Vasomotor symptoms decrease in women with breast cancer randomised to treatment with applied relaxation or electro-acupuncture: a preliminary study. Climacteric 8 (3), 243–250.

Nnoaham, K.E., Kumbang, J., 2008. Transcutaneous electrical nerve stimulation (TENS) for chronic pain. Cochrane Database Syst Rev (3) CD003222.

Osiri, M., Welch, V., Brosseau, L., et al., 2000. Transcutaneous electrical nerve stimulation for knee osteoarthritis. Cochrane Database Syst. Rev., CD002823.

Pariente, J., White, P., Frackowiak, R.S., et al., 2005. Expectancy and belief modulate the neuronal substrates of pain treated by acupuncture. Neuroimage 25, 1161–1167.

Parmeggiani, P.L., 1994. The autonomic nervous system in sleep. In: Kryger, M.H., Roth, T., Dement, W.C. (Eds.), Principles And Practice of Sleep Medicine. WB Saunders, Philadelphia, pp. 194–203.

Price, C.I., Pandyan, A.D., 2000. Electrical stimulation for preventing and treating post-stroke shoulder pain. Cochrane Database Syst. Rev., CD001698.

Proctor, M.L., Smith, C.A., Farquhar, C.M., et al., 2003. Transcutaneous electrical nerve stimulation and acupuncture for primary dysmenorrhoea (Cochrane Review). Cochrane Database Syst. Rev., CD002123.

Radhakrishnan, R., Sluka, K.A., 2005. Deep tissue afferents but not cutaneous afferents mediate transcutaneous electrical nerve stimulation-Induced antihyperalgesia. J. Pain 6, 673–680.

Radhakrishnan, R., King, E.W., Dickman, J.K., et al., 2003. Spinal 5-HT (2) and 5-HT (3) receptors mediate low but not high frequency TENS-induced antihyperalgesia in rats. Pain 105, 205–213.

Renckens, C.N., 2002. Alternative treatments in reproductive medicine: much ado about nothing: the fact that millions of people do not master arithmetic does not prove that two times two is anything else than four. Hum. Reprod. 17, 528–533.

Richardson, D.E., Akil, H., 1977. Long-term results of periventricular gray self-stimulation. Neurosurgery 1, 199–202.

Robb, K., Oxberry, S.G., Bennett, M. I., Johnson, M.I., Simpson, K.H., Searle, R.D., 2009. A Cochrane systematic review of transcutaneous electrical nerve stimulation for cancer pain. J Pain Sympton Manage 37 (4), 746–753.

Rommel, O., Gehling, M., Dertwinkel, R., et al., 1999. Hemisensory impairment in patients with complex regional pain syndrome. Pain 80 (1–2), 95–101.

Rosted, P., 2001. Repetitive epileptic fits–a possible adverse effect after transcutaneous electrical nerve stimulation (TENS) in a post-stroke patient. Acupunct. Med. 19, 46–49.

Sandkühler, J., 2000. Long-lasting analgesia following TENS and acupuncture: Spinal mechanisms beyond gate control. In: Devor, M., Rowbotham, M.C., Wiesenfeld-Hallin, Z. (Eds.), Progress in Pain Research and Management. IASP Press, Seattle, pp. 359–369.

Sandkühler, J., Chen, J.G., Cheng, G., et al., 1997. Low-frequency stimulation of afferent Adelta-fibers induces long-term depression at primary afferent synapses with substantia gelatinosa neurons in the rat. J. Neurosci. 17, 6483–6491.

Sato, A., Sato, Y., Schmidt, R.F., 1997. The Impact of Somatosensory Input on Autonomic Functions. Springer-Verlag, Heidelberg.

Shealy, C.N., 1972. Transcutaneous electroanalgesia. Surg. Forum 23, 419–421.

Shealy, C.N., Mortimer, J.T., Reswick, J.B., 1967. Electrical inhibition of pain by stimulation of the dorsal columns: preliminary clinical report. Anesth. Analg. 46, 489–491.

Sluka, K.A., Chandran, P., 2002. Enhanced reduction in hyperalgesia by combined administration of clonidine and TENS. Pain 100, 183–190.

Sluka, K.A., Deacon, M., Stibal, A., et al., 1999. Spinal blockade of opioid receptors prevents the analgesia produced by TENS in arthritic rats. J. Pharmacol. Exp. Ther. 289, 840–846.

Sluka, K.A., Judge, M.A., McColley, M.M., et al., 2000. Low frequency TENS is less effective than high frequency TENS at reducing inflammation-induced hyperalgesia in morphine-tolerant rats. Eur. J. Pain 4, 185–193.

Spence, D.W., Kayumov, L., Chen, A., et al., 2004. Acupuncture increases nocturnal melatonin secretion and reduces insomnia and anxiety: a preliminary report. J. Neuropsy-chiatry Clin. Neurosci. 16, 19–28.

Spiller, J., 2007. Acupuncture, Ketamine and Piriformis Syndrome – A case report from palliative care. Acupunct. Med. 25, 109–112.

Stener-Victorin, E., Waldenstrom, U., Nilsson, L., et al., 1999. A prospective randomised study of electro-acupuncture versus alfentanil as anaesthesia during oocyte aspiration in in-vitro fertilization. Hum. Reprod. 14, 2480–2484.

Stener-Victorin, E., Waldenstrom, U., Wikland, M., et al., 2003. Electro-acupuncture as a preoperative analgesic method and its effects on implantation rate and neuropeptide Y concentrations in follicular fluid. Hum. Reprod. 18 (7), 1454–1460.

Taguchi, R., 2007. Acupuncture anaes-thesia and analgesia for acute pain in Japan. Ann. Oncol. 5, 153–158.

van Griensven, H., 2005. Pain in Practice: Theory and Treatment Strategies for Manual Therapists. Butterworth Heinemann, Oxford.

Verge, V.M., Richardson, P.M., Hockfelt, T., 1991. Differential influence of nerve growth factor on neuropeptide expression in vivo: a novel role in peptide suppression in adult sensory neurons. J. Neurosci. 15, 2081–2096.

Wall, P.D., Sweet, W.H., 1967. Temporary abolition of pain in man. Science 155, 108–109.

Walsh, D.M., 1996. Transcutaneous electrical nerve stimulation and acupuncture points. Complement. Ther. Med. 4, 133–137.

Walsh, D., Howe, T., Johnson, M.I., Sluka, K.A., 2009. Transcutaneous electrical nerve stimulation for acute pain. Cochrane Database of Systematic Reviews 138 (2), 1–72.

Wheeless, C., 2009. Textbook of Orthopaedics. Data Trace Internet Publishing.

Wilson, P., Stanton-Hicks, M., Harden, R. (Eds.), 2005a. CRPS: Current Diagnosis and Therapy. IASP Press, Seattle.

Wilson, P., Stanton-Hicks, M., Harden, R., 2005b. Progress in Pain Research and Management. IASP Press, Seattle.

Yan, B., Li, K., Xu, J., et al., 2005. Acupoint-specific fMRI patterns in human brain. Neurosci. Lett. 383, 236–240.

Zarate, E., Mingus, M., White, P.F., et al., 2001. The use of transcutaneous acupoint electrical stimulation for preventing nausea and vomiting after laparoscopic surgery. Anesth. Analg. 92, 629–635.

Index